More Praise for *The Spectrum*

"Dr. Ornish's wonderful new book can make an important difference in the health of the world at a time when it most needs it."

> —GRO BRUNDTLAND, M.D.,
> *former Director General, World Health Organization, United Nations,*
> *former Prime Minister, Norway*

"Dr. Dean Ornish knows more about inspiring people to eat well, live well, do well, and be well than anyone on the planet. *The Spectrum* is a powerful book for living longer and better and it shows how to live a healthful, joyful, and loving life."

> —QUINCY JONES

"Dr. Dean Ornish is one of my best students, and I agree with what he is telling you. I have known him well for many years now. So you should pay good attention to what he tells you in his new book."

> —ALEXANDER LEAF, M.D.,
> *Chairman, Department of Medicine (emeritus),*
> *Chairman, Department of Preventive Medicine and Clinical Epidemiology*
> *(emeritus), Harvard Medical School and Massachusetts General Hospital*

"Dean Ornish has written the definitive guide to caring for your health."

> —RACHEL NAOMI REMEN,
> *author of* Kitchen Table Wisdom

"*The Spectrum* provides unparalleled guidance and ideas from the sage of preventive medicine."

> —LARRY BRILLIANT, M.D., M.P.H.,
> *Executive Director, Google Foundation and Google.org*

"This is a must-read book for those seeking accurate information for how to optimize their personal health."

> —JAMES O. HILL, PH.D.,
> *Director, Center for Human Nutrition, University of Colorado,*
> *Co-founder, America on the Move*

"This country is in the midst of an unprecedented epidemic of obesity and inactivity, which is fueling the spiraling increase in the cost of health care. In *The Spectrum*, Dean Ornish again shows us how to escape this medical quagmire and start a wellness movement in this country. I highly recommend this book."

> —KENNETH COOPER, M.D., M.P.H.,
> *Founder and President, The Cooper Aerobics Center*

ALSO BY DEAN ORNISH, M.D.

Love and Survival

Everyday Cooking with Dr. Dean Ornish

Eat More, Weigh Less

Dr. Dean Ornish's Program for Reversing Heart Disease

Stress, Diet, and Your Heart

THE SPECTRUM

A SCIENTIFICALLY PROVEN

PROGRAM TO FEEL BETTER,

LIVE LONGER, LOSE WEIGHT,

AND GAIN HEALTH

THE
SPECTRUM

DEAN ORNISH, M.D.

WITH RECIPES BY

ART SMITH

BALLANTINE BOOKS | NEW YORK

No book can replace the diagnostic expertise and medical advice of a trusted physician. Please be certain to consult with your doctor before making any decisions that affect your health, particularly if you suffer from any medical condition or have any symptom that may require treatment.

Copyright © 2007 by Dean Ornish, M.D., LLC

Published in the United States by Ballantine Books, an imprint of The Random House Publishing Group, a division of Random House, Inc., New York.

BALLANTINE and colophon are registered trademarks of Random House, Inc.

As of press time, the URLs displayed in this book link or refer to existing websites on the Internet. Random House, Inc., is not responsible for the content available on any such site (including, without limitation, outdated, inaccurate, or incomplete information).

Grateful acknowledgment is made to the following for permission to reprint previously published materials:

The Cartoon Bank: *The New Yorker* Cartoon by Roz Chast, copyright © The New Yorker Collection 2003 Roz Chast from cartoonbank.com. All rights reserved. Reprinted by permission of The Cartoon Bank.

Donald S. Coffey: Human development and the change of diet chart from "Similarities of Prostate and Breast Cancer: Evolution, Diet, and Estrogens" by Donald S. Coffey (*Urology* 57, April 2001), copyright © 2001 Elsevier Science, Inc. Reprinted by permission of Donald S. Coffey.

John L. Hart F.L.P. and Creators Syndicate, Inc.: The Wizard of Id comic strip by Brant Parker and Johnny Hart, copyright © 1992 Creators Syndicate, Inc. Reprinted by permission of John L. Hart F.L.P. and Creators Syndicate, Inc.

Insert photographs by Kipling Swehla; food stylists: Domenica Catelli and Constance Pikulas.

Library of Congress Cataloging-in-Publication Data
Ornish, Dean.
The spectrum: a scientifically proven program to feel better, live longer, lose weight, and gain health / by Dean Ornish; with recipes by Art Smith.
p.   cm.
Includes bibliographical references.
ISBN 978-0-345-49630-0 (hardcover: alk. paper)
1. Health.   2. Nutrition.   3. Weight loss.   4. Physical fitness.   5. Stress management.   I. Smith, Art, 1960–   II. Title.
RA776.O758 2007
613.2—dc22   2007037188

Printed in the United States of America

www.ballantinebooks.com

9 8 7 6 5 4 3 2 1

First Edition

Book design by Jo Anne Metsch

This book is gratefully dedicated to Anne and Lucas,
with all my heart . . .

your happiness is my happiness
yet again, like never before
now and forever

∞

CONTENTS

PART II
WELCOME TO ART'S KITCHEN: AN ABUNDANT
SPECTRUM OF FOODS TO ENJOY

PART I

WELCOME: HOW TO PERSONALIZE A WAY OF EATING AND LIVING JUST RIGHT FOR YOU

1

IT WORKS!

The one thing more difficult than following a regimen is not imposing it on others.

—Marcel Proust

■ ■ ■ ■ ■ ■ ■ ■ ■

I just had a piece of chocolate. Dark chocolate. Really high-fat gourmet dark chocolate. It was delicious. I have a little chocolate almost every day.

Now, you may be wondering if I'm cheating on my very own diet. Well, no, I'm not. I'm *enjoying* my very own diet.

I'm writing this book to help you understand that you have a broad spectrum of choices when it comes to what you eat, how much you exercise, how you manage stress, and how you live. It's not all or nothing. In the process, I hope to dispel some misconceptions about what I recommend.

In short, this book will show you how to personalize a way of eating and living that's just right for you, based on your own needs and preferences. It has been scientifically proven to help you feel better, live longer, lose weight, and gain health.

It works! Why? Because it's based on pleasure, not pain; abundance, not deprivation; science, not myth; freedom and power, not restriction and manipulation. Joy of living is sustainable; fear of dying is not.

There are many myths and false choices that are confusing to many people. These include:

- If I live and eat healthfully, am I going to live longer or is it just going to *seem* longer?
- Is it fun for me or good for me?
- Low-fat or low-carb?
- Fast food or good food?
- Atkins indulgent or Ornish ascetic?

You really don't have to make these choices.

This is a book about how to enjoy life more fully while enhancing your health and well-being. It's based on our latest research showing that you can actually change how your genes are expressed just by changing what you eat and how you live.

In short, this book can empower you to transform your own life.

By now, many people are thoroughly exasperated by the seemingly contradictory information they read about what a sound nutrition and lifestyle program should be. Nowhere are the claims more conflicting than in the area of diet. I often hear, "Those damn doctors! They can't make up their minds. To hell with 'em, I'll eat and do whatever I want and quit worrying about it!"

I understand why many people feel that way. It can be really confusing when even the experts don't seem to agree.

Fortunately, at a time when people are more confused than ever, there is an emerging consensus about what to eat and how to live. The jury is in: a convergence of scientific evidence can help us resolve conflicting claims and distinguish what just sounds good from what is proven to be true.

Now it is possible to cut through the confusion and to customize a diet and lifestyle program just right for you based on your own needs and preferences. You have a spectrum of choices.

People have different needs, goals, and preferences. The medicine of the future is personalized medicine, which this book brings you today.

The recipes and cooking instructions, by the renowned chef Art Smith, are for foods that taste good and also make you look good and feel good. Many of them have several versions, so you can customize them to meet your own needs and preferences.

It seems that many people have misconceptions about what I eat and how I live my own life. For example, a few years ago, the playwright and producer Mike Nichols came up to me at a benefit for a foundation and said, "Hey, Dean, I'm on your diet—if it tastes good, I can't eat it"—echoing Mark Twain, "The only way to keep your health is to eat what you don't want, drink what you don't like, and do what you'd rather not."

This is the most common misunderstanding about my work—that I recommend one really strict diet and lifestyle program for everyone. "Yes, it works, but it's almost impossible to follow."

It's understandable why so many people believe this. Many of the media stories on the work my colleagues and I have conducted have focused on our research showing that heart disease and other chronic diseases can be reversed—and they often can!—just by making comprehensive lifestyle changes. Reversing a disease does require the stricter version of the diet and lifestyle program—the pound of cure—whereas if you're just trying to feel good and stay healthy you need only the ounce of prevention. However, for people who aren't sick, I recommended a spectrum of choices.

In this book, I'm not trying to get you to do—or not do—anything. Food and lifestyle choices are deeply personal decisions. Having seen what a powerful difference changes in diet and lifestyle can make, I want to share these findings with you so that you can make intelligent choices in what you eat and how you live. How much or little you want to change, if at all, is entirely up to you. More on this later.

Whenever I go out to dinner, people often comment on what I'm eating or apologize for what they're eating—"I have to be careful what I eat around you"—as though I'm going to be the sheriff or the vice principal of the high school waving my finger at them, judging them, and shaming them into eating differently.

In reality, nothing could be further from the truth. So I usually make a sign of the cross and say, jokingly, "You are forgiven," and we all have a good laugh about it. I then tell them that it doesn't matter to me what they eat or how they live as long as they're happy. When I order dessert, they often feel both surprised and relieved.

This misperception of who I am and what I believe was best encapsulated in a *New Yorker* cartoon that made me smile:

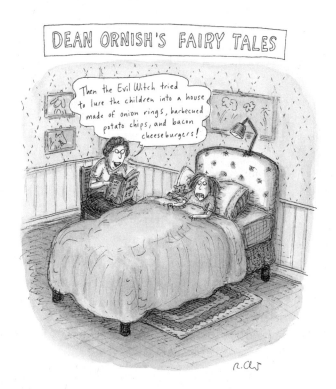

PROVEN PROGRAM

What makes this book unique is that it's based on three decades of research proving what works, what doesn't, for whom, and under what circumstances. Most books are written based on anecdotal testimonials (which are often unreliable), or on the experience of others, or on wishful thinking. They may make promises that often remain unfulfilled.

Instead, this program is grounded in science, and it's been proven to work:

• My colleagues and I at the nonprofit Preventive Medicine Research Institute have proven that this program works to help prevent, and to slow, stop, and even reverse the progression of the most common and most deadly diseases, including coronary heart disease, prostate cancer, diabetes, hypertension, obesity, elevated cholesterol levels, arthritis, and many other chronic diseases.

• We recently conducted the first study in men with prostate cancer showing that our program of comprehensive lifestyle changes may change how your genes are expressed—in general, turning on (upregulating) the good parts of the genes and turning off (downregulating) the harmful ones. More on this in chapter 4.

• We recently conducted the first study showing that comprehensive lifestyle changes may improve how quickly your cells age. Telomeres are the ends of your DNA, and they affect longevity. As they become shorter and their structural integrity is weakened, cells age and die more quickly. In simple terms, as your telomeres get shorter, your life gets shorter. In our new study, we found that the telomerase enzyme (which repairs telomeres) increased significantly in those who went through our diet and lifestyle program after only three months.

• We learned what really works to motivate people to make and maintain comprehensive lifestyle changes in the real world. We've consistently shown that our program can motivate many people to make and maintain bigger changes in diet and lifestyle, and to achieve better clinical outcomes and larger cost savings in diverse groups of people than have ever before been demonstrated.

Let's examine these.

THE PROGRAM WORKS TO PREVENT
AND REVERSE DISEASE

People often think that advances in medicine have to be a new drug, a new laser, or a surgical intervention to be powerful—something really high-tech and expensive. They often have a hard time believing that the simple choices we make in our lives each day—what we eat, how we respond to stress, whether or not we smoke, how much we exercise, and the quality of our relationships—can make such a powerful difference in our health, our well-being, and our survival, but they often do.

Awareness is the first step in healing. When we become more aware of how powerfully our choices in diet and lifestyle affect us—for better and for worse—then we can make different ones. It's like connecting the dots. In my experience, many people are not afraid to make big changes in their lives if they understand the benefits of doing so and how quickly they may occur.

Part of the value of science is to raise our awareness by helping us understand the powerful effects of the diet and lifestyle choices we make each day and how changing these may significantly—sometimes dramatically— improve our health and well-being. In many cases, these improvements may occur much more quickly than people once believed possible.

In our studies, we used the latest in high-tech, expensive, state-of-the-art measures to prove how robust these very simple, low-tech, and low-cost interventions can be.

For more than thirty years, I've directed a series of scientific research studies showing, for the first time, that the progression of even severe coronary heart disease can often be reversed by making comprehensive lifestyle changes. These include a very-low-fat diet including predominantly fruits, vegetables, whole grains, legumes, and soy products in their natural, unrefined forms; moderate exercise such as walking; various stress management techniques, including yoga-based stretching, breathing, meditation, and imagery; and enhanced love and social support, which may include support groups.

In these studies, we also documented that other chronic diseases may be reversible simply by making comprehensive lifestyle changes. Our findings are giving literally millions of people worldwide new hope and new choices, options that are more caring and compassionate as well as more cost-effective and competent.

More recently, we published the results of a randomized controlled trial in collaboration with Peter Carroll, M.D. (Chair, Department of Urology, School of Medicine, University of California, San Francisco) and William

Fair, M.D. (Chief of urologic surgery and Chair of urologic oncology, Memorial Sloan-Kettering Cancer Center, now deceased) showing that the progression of early-stage prostate cancer may be slowed, stopped, or perhaps even reversed by making similar changes in diet and lifestyle. This may be the first randomized controlled trial showing that the progression of *any* type of cancer may be modified just by changing what we eat and how we live. What's true for prostate cancer may be true for breast cancer as well, as I describe in chapter 14.

Our research has been conducted in collaboration with the most credible scientific investigators at major academic medical centers. Our findings have been published in the leading peer-reviewed medical journals, including *The Lancet, The Journal of the American Medical Association, The American Journal of Cardiology, Circulation, Journal of Cardiopulmonary Rehabilitation, Journal of Urology, Yearbook of Medicine, Yearbook of Cardiology, The New England Journal of Medicine, Homeostasis, Urology, Journal of the American Dietetic Association, Hospital Practice, Cardiovascular Risk Factors, World Review of Nutrition and Dietetics, Journal of Cardiovascular Risk, Obesity Research, Journal of the American College of Cardiology,* and others.

Our program has also been featured in the leading standard medical textbooks, including *Harrison's Principles of Internal Medicine, Clinical Trials in Cardiovascular Disease* (companion to *Heart Disease,* the Braunwald standard cardiology textbook), *Harrison's Advances in Cardiology,* and *Clinical Trials in Cardiovascular Disease* (second edition), as well as a number of general-interest books, including Bill Moyers's *Healing and the Mind,* among others.

Research findings documenting the benefits of our program have been presented at numerous scientific meetings, including the annual scientific meetings of the American College of Cardiology, beginning in 1982; the American Heart Association, beginning in 1983; and the Society of Behavioral Medicine, beginning in 1988, as well as many other scientific and medical conferences. On several occasions, our research was highlighted at these meetings and featured at press conferences convened by these organizations.

I say this just to emphasize that the program described in this book has been proven to work in the most rigorous and credible peer-reviewed evaluations. And that matters. A lot.

I have spent so much of my time conducting scientific research because it's important to be able to substantiate and validate whatever health promises are made. In 2000, I was appointed to the White House Commission on Complementary and Alternative Medicine Policy. More than a thousand people testified before our committee.

I learned that more money is spent out of pocket for alternative medicine than for traditional medicine. Why? Many people have become disenchanted with conventional medicine and have embraced a variety of alternative interventions. However, they may find themselves disillusioned with some of these approaches as well because many of them do not have scientific evidence to support their claims.

Seen from this perspective, our program is (as of this writing) one of the most scientifically documented alternative medicine approaches. It integrates the best of traditional and nontraditional approaches to health and healing.

I also understand the limitations of science. As Albert Einstein once said, "Not everything that can be counted counts; and not everything that counts can be counted"—for example, love and joy, as I'll describe later—but many things that are meaningful are also measurable. Also, part of the reason that the public receives so much conflicting information is that there is a lot of bad science out there. In this book, I'll show you how to critically analyze some of these studies.

In our cardiac studies, beginning in 1977, we found that there was a 91 percent reduction in the frequency of angina (chest pain) after only a few weeks, and most of these patients became pain-free. These were patients with very severe coronary heart disease, many of whom literally could not walk across the street without getting severe chest pain and shortness of breath when they began.

After one year, there was a 40 percent average reduction in LDL cholesterol levels. This is comparable to what can be achieved with statin drugs like Lipitor without the costs (more than $15 billion last year) or side effects (both known and unknown).

In the Lifestyle Heart Trial, there was significant reversal in coronary artery blockages in the group that went through our program after only one year, whereas those in the randomized control group, who made more conventional changes, showed a worsening of their coronary artery blockages.

Based on these findings, we received peer-reviewed funding from the National Heart, Lung, and Blood Institute of the National Institutes of Health to extend the study intervention for four additional years. We wanted to find out if patients could continue to maintain these comprehensive lifestyle changes for five years and, if so, what the long-term effects would be. We found that most patients continued to follow this program for five years even though they had initially volunteered only for a one-year study.

There was even more reversal in coronary artery blockages after five years than after one year, whereas patients in the randomized control group showed even more worsening after five years than after one year. These differences were highly statistically significant; see the following graph.

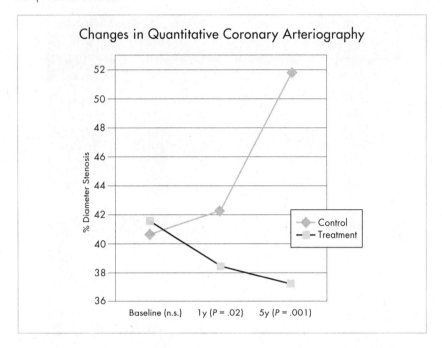

There are two basic ways of measuring the severity of coronary heart disease: anatomical (which measures the severity of coronary artery blockages) and functional (which measures the amount of blood flow to the heart and also how well it pumps). In our research, we used state-of-the-art tests: quantitative coronary arteriography to measure the degree of coronary artery blockages and cardiac PET (*Positron Emission Tomography*) scans to measure blood flow to the heart.

The following figure shows a representative patient in our study. This is what reversing heart disease looks like. He entered our study in 1986 at age 64. At that time, he had severe coronary artery disease involving all of his major coronary arteries and was advised to undergo coronary bypass surgery due to severe angina. When he entered the study, he was unable to walk more than a few steps without severe chest pain.

After six weeks, he was pain-free and was no longer advised to undergo bypass surgery. By the end of the first year, he was able to climb 130 floors per day on a StairMaster with no angina. His PET scan revealed a 300 percent improvement in blood flow to his heart, and his angiogram revealed reversal of coronary atherosclerosis. He also lost 30 pounds.

The picture in the upper-left-hand corner is the "before" picture of his angiogram, showing a significant narrowing in the coronary artery. One year later, in the upper-right-hand photo, that area is significantly wider.

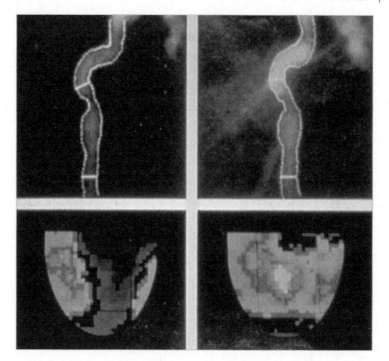

The PET scans of the same patient are shown in the bottom two pictures. Different shadings correspond to how much blood flow each region of the heart received—the darker areas are receiving very little blood flow to the heart, whereas the brighter ones are receiving the most blood flow.

The picture at the lower left revealed that much of this patient's heart was not receiving adequate blood flow, as shown by the large dark areas. One year later, in the lower-right-hand picture, you can see that most of the darker areas are now gone, replaced by brighter ones, showing substantially more blood flow.

These tests were read by scientists who did not know which group the patient was in—in other words, whether or not the patient had changed his or her lifestyle. This helped prevent any possible bias from affecting how the studies were read and interpreted.

Amazingly, 99 percent of patients on our program were able to stop or reverse the progression of their heart disease. There were also 2½ times fewer cardiac events such as heart attacks, bypass surgery operations, angioplasties, and hospital admissions.

We found a direct correlation between the amount of change in diet and lifestyle and the amount of change in these patients' coronary artery disease after one year and also after five years.

In other words, *the more people changed, the better they got.* This is a

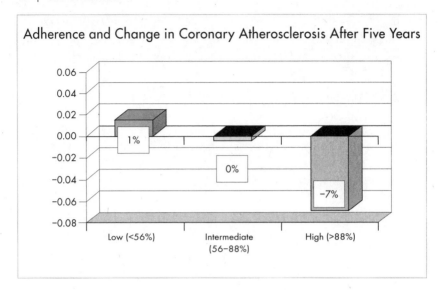

Adherence and Change in Coronary Atherosclerosis After Five Years

theme that I will be repeating throughout the book, and it is one of the foundations of *The Spectrum*.

Similar findings were published five years later by Dr. Caldwell Esselstyn and his colleagues at The Cleveland Clinic. In a follow-up medical journal article, he reported that none of the patients who remained adherent to the nutrition and lifestyle program showed progression of their coronary heart disease.

THE PROGRAM WORKS IN THE REAL WORLD

When I first began conducting research as a second-year medical student in 1977, the idea that the progression of heart disease could be reversed was thought to be impossible by most doctors. They thought that, at best, diet and lifestyle changes might slow down the rate at which the disease progressed, but it could only get worse over time. Equally improbable was the belief that most people would be able to change their diet and lifestyle.

After we and others proved that the progression of coronary heart disease and other chronic diseases could often be reversed by making comprehensive lifestyle changes, these misconceptions slowly began to change. Now most doctors believe that heart disease *is* reversible.

Then the skepticism shifted. Although most physicians believe that the diet and lifestyle program I recommend works, they often think that the majority of people can't follow it because it's too strict, too hard, and too boring. So why bother? "Okay, your patients changed, but you live in California. It's an altered state. They'll do anything there. And you're some kind of guru; you can somehow brainwash people to change."

All About the Benjamins

When we published our research findings, I thought these would significantly change medical practice, but I was a little naive. With all the talk about evidence-based medicine, we really live in an era of what I call "reimbursement-based medicine."

I realized that it wasn't enough to have good science; we also needed to change reimbursement. We doctors do what we are paid to do, and we are trained to do what we are paid to do. Therefore, if we could change reimbursement, then we would improve both medical practice and medical education. As Sean Combs sings, "It's all about the Benjamins" (Benjamin Franklin on hundred-dollar bills).

Beginning in 1993, my colleagues and I began training personnel in more than fifty hospitals and clinics around the country in our diet and lifestyle program via our nonprofit research institute. We conducted three demonstration projects—one with Mutual of Omaha, a second with Highmark Blue Cross Blue Shield, and most recently with Medicare.

We began in 1993 with a demonstration project sponsored by Mutual of Omaha. The questions we wanted to answer were: (a) Could people in Omaha, Des Moines, and South Carolina (where they told me "gravy is a beverage") follow this program as well as those in San Francisco, Boston, or New York? (b) Could we train other health professionals to intervene with their patients as effectively as we could? (c) Was this medically effective as well as cost-effective?

In this first demonstration project, we trained personnel in eight hospitals: Beth Israel Medical Center in New York; Beth Israel Medical Center at Harvard Medical School in Boston; the University of California, San Francisco; Scripps Institute in La Jolla; Alegent Medical Center in Omaha; Richland Memorial Hospital in Columbia, South Carolina; Broward General Hospital in Fort Lauderdale, Florida; and Mercy Hospital in Des Moines, Iowa. Our data-coordinating center was at Harvard Medical School, directed by Alexander Leaf, M.D., who was chair of the Department of Medicine at Harvard Medical School.

Reimbursing comprehensive lifestyle changes is not only medically effective, it's also cost-effective.

In brief, we found that almost 80 percent of patients who were eligible for bypass surgery or angioplasty were able to safely avoid it for at least

THE WIZARD OF ID   Brant parker and Johnny hart

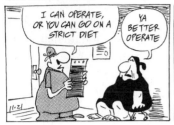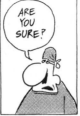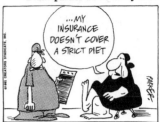

three years. Mutual of Omaha found that it saved almost $30,000 per patient in the first year! We published these findings in the peer-reviewed *The American Journal of Cardiology.*

By then, more than forty insurance companies besides Mutual of Omaha were covering our program, on either a defined-benefit or case-by-case basis. One of these was Highmark Blue Cross Blue Shield, which had such great results that it decided to provide the program in three sites as well as to reimburse it.

Highmark Blue Cross Blue Shield conducted its own demonstration project. As in the Mutual of Omaha demonstration project, it compared people who went through our program with similar patients who did not (called a "matched control group study").

Highmark found that its overall health care costs were reduced by 50 percent in the first year and by an additional 20 to 30 percent in subsequent years. At a time when health care costs (really, disease care costs) are reaching a tipping point, these findings are even more important today.

After the success of these two demonstration projects plus the earlier randomized controlled trials, we approached Medicare to see if it would provide coverage. It initially said no.

In 1995, Chip Kahn (who was then the staff director of the House Ways and Means Health Subcommittee) introduced me to Bruce Vladeck, Ph.D., who was the administrator (Director) of Medicare at the time. In that meeting, Dr. Vladeck said, "Dean, before I'll consider doing a Medicare demonstration project, you first need to get a letter from the director of the National Heart, Lung, and Blood Institute of the National Institutes of Health stating that your program is safe."

"You mean that it's safe as an alternative to bypass surgery or angioplasty?"

"No, just that it's safe."

I was incredulous. "You want me to get a letter saying that it's safe for older Americans to walk, meditate, quit smoking, and eat fruits and vegetables?"

"That's right."

So I met with Dr. Claude Lenfant, who was Director of the National Heart, Lung, and Blood Institute at the time, and his colleagues, and we reviewed the medical literature. Not surprisingly, we found that these are not high-risk activities—especially when compared with having your chest sawed open for a bypass operation. In our earlier research, we had found that older patients improved as much as younger ones, whereas the risks of bypass surgery and angioplasty increased in older patients. So these lifestyle changes are especially beneficial for older patients in the Medicare population.

Dr. Lenfant then sent a letter to Dr. Vladeck saying that the nutritional program I recommend is safe, whatever the age of the patients following it.

A month went by. Dr. Vladeck then wrote a letter back to Dr. Lenfant saying that although he had said that the nutritional program is safe, is it okay for people over sixty-five to do moderate exercise and stress-management techniques?

Not surprisingly, Dr. Lenfant replied that these were of "minimal risk" provided that patients are offered all proven treatments.

Four years later, in 1999, with strong bipartisan support from then President Clinton, then Speaker of the House Newt Gingrich, Representatives Nancy Pelosi, Charles Rangel, Alcee Hastings, Lynn Woolsey, and Dan Burton, Senators Barbara Boxer, Arlen Specter, Dianne Feinstein, Ted Stevens, Hillary Clinton, Bill Frist, Maria Cantwell, Chuck Robb, Jay Rockefeller, and Barbara Mikulski, and others across the political spectrum, Medicare agreed to conduct a demonstration project.

We've gotten to a point in medicine where it's considered "conservative medicine" to cut open someone's chest or to inflate balloons and put stents inside his or her coronary arteries even in the absence of data showing that these approaches prevent heart attacks or extend life in stable patients with heart disease, yet it's considered high risk or even radical to ask people to walk, meditate, quit smoking, and eat fruits and vegetables.

In January 2005, after we completed our Medicare demonstration project, a Medicare Coverage Advisory Commission hearing was convened at the Centers for Medicare and Medicaid Services headquarters in Baltimore to peer-review our findings. I presented data from more than 2,000 patients who had participated in our three demonstration projects (with Mutual of Omaha, Highmark Blue Cross Blue Shield, and Medicare). At this daylong hearing, seventeen experts who were on the Medicare Coverage Advisory Commission reviewed data from our program and others similar to it.

At the end of that day, these experts voted that there was sufficient scientific evidence for Medicare to cover our program for reversing heart disease.

Based on these findings, the Centers for Medicare and Medicaid Services recently agreed to provide Medicare coverage for our program for reversing heart disease and other programs like it. This was a major breakthrough, as it was the first time that Medicare covered an integrative-medicine program of comprehensive lifestyle changes. Since reimbursement is a major determinant of medical practice and medical education, Medicare coverage may help make programs of comprehensive lifestyle changes much more sustainable and widely available to those who most need them.

Now my colleagues and I at the nonprofit Preventive Medicine Research Institute are training health professionals worldwide and providing free licenses to them in an open-source model. These include physicians, nurses, registered dietitians, yoga and meditation teachers, clinical psychologists, chefs, exercise physiologists, and so on. Those we train are making our program available in hospitals, clinics, and other venues and sharing their data with us so we can collect data on large numbers of people at low cost.

This allows us to learn from the experience and best practices of many other people on an ongoing basis, thereby enabling us to continue to refine and improve our program in an organic process. Over time, we can collect data on large numbers of patients and gain greater insight about the effects of comprehensive lifestyle changes in large numbers of people around the world.

HEALING YOURSELF

Our research has shown that your body often has a remarkable capacity to begin healing itself—and much more quickly than people once realized—when we address the underlying causes of illness. For many people, the choices we make each day in what we eat and in how we live are among the most important underlying causes.

When most people are prescribed medications to lower their blood pressure, cholesterol, or blood sugar, they are usually told, "You will have to take this for the rest of your life," often in ever-increasing dosages. Why? Because the underlying causes are not being addressed. When I lecture, I often show a slide of doctors busily mopping up the floor around an overflowing sink without also turning off the faucet.

It's important to treat not only the problem but also its underlying causes. Otherwise, the same problem often recurs (for example, bypass grafts or angioplastied arteries clogging up again), a new set of problems may happen (such as side effects from medications), or there may be painful choices (such as keeping 47 million Americans from having health insurance because it's too expensive to treat everyone with the drugs or surgery that they may need).

We found that many people with coronary heart disease, diabetes, high blood pressure, elevated cholesterol levels, and other chronic conditions are able to reduce or even discontinue these medications (under their doctor's supervision) when they make the diet and lifestyle changes that are outlined in this book.

With the legitimate concerns about pandemics of AIDS and avian flu, it's easy to forget that cardiovascular disease kills more people each year worldwide than any other disease. It's the biggest pandemic of all time. Heart disease is so common that we've become accustomed to it, thinking of it as a natural cause of death. Yet there's nothing natural about it.

Diabetes and obesity are also becoming pandemic. In just the past ten years, the incidence of diabetes in the United States has increased 70 percent among people in their thirties, in large part because of the obesity pandemic. In India, a recent study conducted by the Delhi Diabetes Research Centre among schoolchildren ages 10 to 16 found nearly one in five to be either overweight or clinically obese. A major complication of diabetes is heart disease, along with nerve, eye, and kidney damage.

However, coronary heart disease, type 2 diabetes (once known as adult-onset, though an increasing number of younger people are now getting it), and obesity can be prevented in almost everyone simply by making sufficient changes in diet and lifestyle. We don't have to wait for a breakthrough in technology or a new drug; we just need to put into practice what we already know. If we did, these pandemics could be as rare as malaria is in the United States.

In addition to our research, the landmark INTERHEART study, led by Canadian scientists, followed 30,000 men and women in fifty-two countries on six continents. It found that nine factors related to nutrition and lifestyle accounted for almost 95 percent of the risk of a heart attack in men and women in almost every geographic region and in every racial and ethnic group worldwide. These factors were: smoking, cholesterol level, hypertension, diabetes, obesity, diet, physical activity, alcohol consumption, and psychosocial issues such as emotional stress and depression.

In other words, *the disease that kills the most people each year worldwide and accounts for the single largest expenditure of health care dollars is almost completely preventable just by changing diet and lifestyle in ways described in this book.*

Despite this, relatively little of the money spent by most insurance companies has gone toward teaching people how to prevent or treat cardiovascular disease and other chronic diseases by changing their diet and lifestyle. Much of it goes to pay for surgical procedures such as angioplasty and bypass surgery.

You may be surprised to learn that angioplasty does not reduce the risk of a heart attack and does not prolong life in patients with stable coronary heart disease. This was the remarkable conclusion of a study published in June 2005 in *Circulation,* the American Heart Association's lead scientific journal, in which researchers reviewed all eleven randomized controlled trials of angioplasty. The same conclusion was found in a recent large-scale randomized controlled trial published in *The New England Journal of Medicine.*

It's hard for many people to believe that comprehensive lifestyle changes work even better than drugs and surgery in treating heart disease, but they often do. For example, a major study, also published in *Circulation,* found that regular physical exercise worked even better than angioplasty for preventing heart attacks, strokes, and premature deaths. Another study, published in *The New England Journal of Medicine,* found that those taking the cholesterol-lowering statin Lipitor had 36 percent fewer cardiac events after eighteen months than those undergoing angioplasty.

Several randomized controlled trials have shown that coronary bypass surgery prolongs life only in those with the most severe disease, which is only a small percentage of those who receive it. Angioplasty and bypass surgery may reduce the frequency of angina (chest pain), but most people can reduce angina at least as much in only a few weeks just by changing their diet and lifestyle, if these changes go far enough in the healthy direction on the Spectrum.

In short, most insurance companies have been paying billions of dollars for surgical procedures that are invasive, dangerous, expensive, and largely ineffective, whereas they pay little or nothing for the diet and lifestyle interventions described in this book, which are noninvasive, safe, inexpensive, and powerfully effective in treating coronary heart disease as well as many other chronic diseases. And the only side effects are good ones.

The managed care approach of shortening hospital stays, limiting reimbursement, capitation, and forcing doctors to see more patients in less time leaves everyone frustrated and unhappy because this approach does not address the more fundamental causes of why people get sick. It's a different type of bypass.

Last year, more than one million coronary angioplasties and more than 400,000 coronary bypass operations were performed in the United States at a cost of more than $100 billion. Among Medicare beneficiaries, the number of these operations increased 543 percent between 1984 and 1996 despite the absence of clear outcome benefits. This challenges the sustainability of Medicare.

These health care costs (as mentioned earlier, these are really disease care costs) are also challenging the viability of many businesses and corporations. General Motors spends more on medical care for its employees than it does to buy steel. Howard Schultz, the founder and chairman of Starbucks, said that he spends more on health care for his employees than for coffee beans. As the population ages and health care costs continue to outpace inflation, many corporations project that they will reach a tipping point in only a few years in which health care costs exceed their entire profits. Clearly, this is not sustainable.

At Safeway, this has already happened. Profit margins are lower in the grocery business than in many others, so grocery stores are like the "canary in the coal mine" that sees trends before they affect other businesses.

According to Steven Burd, the chief executive officer of Safeway, "In 2005, our health-care costs for our employees reached $1 billion and were exceeding our net income by about 20 percent." Clearly, this was not sustainable. I consulted with him and his colleagues there (including Kenneth Shachmut and Michael Minasi) to help develop incentives for wellness and prevention services in their health plan. The following year, Safeway's health care costs declined by 11 percent and remained flat in 2007.

What I especially like about this approach is that it is bringing together Democrats and Republicans and labor and management toward a common goal of lowering health care costs, providing universal coverage, and improving the quality of care.

Unfortunately, most insurance companies pay only for drugs and surgery, not for diet and lifestyle. They will pay $30,000 to amputate a diabetic foot, for example, but not a few hundred dollars for foot care and nutrition counseling that can prevent the need for amputation in most people. Most diabetes-related amputations are preventable with scrupulous care, but foot care is not usually covered. Similarly, they'll pay $40,000 for an angioplasty and stents or for coronary bypass surgery but won't cover comprehensive lifestyle changes that can prevent the need for these. I see perverse incentives and disincentives that reward surgical procedures and drugs over preventive approaches throughout medicine.

All of the doctors I know are genuinely interested in helping their patients. However, since we're trained to use drugs and surgery but not lifestyle interventions and preventive approaches, and we're reimbursed to use drugs and surgery but not lifestyle interventions and preventive approaches, it's not surprising that most physicians rely primarily on drugs and surgery. As the pressures of managed care cause doctors to spend less and less time with more and more patients, there is not enough time to talk about diet and lifestyle issues. This is profoundly unsatisfying for both doctors and patients.

Thus, at a time when the limitations and unaffordable costs of high-tech interventions such as angioplasty and stents are becoming better-documented, the power of and cost savings from low-tech interventions such as the diet and lifestyle changes described in this book are also becoming clearer—when they are most needed.

In one of the more extreme examples of how powerful changes in diet and lifestyle can be, my colleagues and I worked with a few men and women who had such severe coronary heart disease that they were waiting for a heart transplant.

Patients with especially severe coronary heart disease sometimes require cardiac transplantation because the heart is pumping blood so inadequately. Unfortunately, there is a shortage of organ donors, so the average waiting time for a donor to become available in most parts of the country is one to two years. (Unlike giving blood, most people are not willing to donate their hearts.) Approximately half of the patients waiting for a heart transplant die before a donor becomes available. And heart transplantation is quite expensive, costing from $250,000 to $500,000 per patient.

Also, in perhaps the ultimate example of what happens when you don't address the underlying cause of a problem, patients who undergo heart transplants often need another one just a few years later. It's a little like changing your oil filter without also changing the oil—it just clogs up again fairly quickly.

Since these patients were just waiting around for a new heart anyway, we offered a few of them the opportunity to go through our program of comprehensive lifestyle changes while waiting for a donor. After one year, some improved so much that they no longer needed a heart transplant! It's amazing to me that these low-tech interventions of comprehensive lifestyle changes may be, at times, even more powerful than the most high-tech interventions such as a heart transplant. Unlike our other research, this is anecdotal data but it is still intriguing.

We published findings on a larger number of patients with impaired ability of their hearts to pump and found that they improved as much as those with hearts that were not as impaired when they entered our program.

Art Smith (no relation to Chef Art Smith) is a seventy-one-year-old man with heart disease so severe that he was told that he was a candidate for a heart transplant in 1992. "I had trouble walking even twenty feet then, I was so short of breath."

In 1994, he entered the program for reversing heart disease based on my work at the Alegent Immanuel Medical Center in Omaha (in other words, the healthiest end of the Spectrum). "I followed it to a 'T,' " he said. "I had so much more energy and was feeling so much better that I was able to go on a heart walk for four miles around the lake. My wife and son were with me, and they couldn't believe how well I was doing."

According to his wife, Shirley, "He had more pep. He was a new man. It gave us new hope. I couldn't believe how much our lives changed for the better. I didn't think he'd ever go back to work again."

As Art explained, "I went back to work driving a bus and wheeling wheelchairs for handicapped people for five years, twelve-hour days, four to five days a week. It was a really big change from when I couldn't walk more than twenty feet. Now, even fifteen years after I started your program, I never get short of breath."

Art not only *felt* better, he *was* better. A state-of-the-art test called a PET scan revealed that his heart was receiving significantly more blood flow after one year of being on the program for reversing heart disease.

Also, the PET scan showed that a lot of his heart muscle that had looked as if it were dead, or scar tissue, was actually "hibernating"—some dead tissue interlaced with heart muscle that was alive but not functioning. After a year of making comprehensive lifestyle changes at the healthy end of the Spectrum, much of his heart muscle that was hibernating began to "wake up" and function again. Another test called an echocardiogram confirmed that his heart muscle was pumping blood so much more effectively that he no longer needed a heart transplant!

Unlike our earlier studies, which were randomized controlled trials, these heart-transplant patients are only anecdotal case reports. Nevertheless, they indicate just how powerful these simple, low-tech, low-cost changes in diet and lifestyle can be.

In other words, when you go all the way to the healthy end of the Spectrum, your body often has a remarkable capacity to begin healing itself.

In a related investigation, we studied forty patients whose hearts were pumping blood poorly, many of whom were on the way to needing a heart transplant. All of these patients were eligible for surgery (bypass surgery or angioplasty). We compared twenty-seven patients who chose our program as an alternative to surgery with thirteen patients who underwent surgery. The two groups were comparable in age, disease severity, and heart function.

After three months, there were six cardiac events (cardiac death, congestive heart failure, stroke, heart attack) in the thirteen patients who had surgery compared with only one cardiac event in the twenty-seven patients who chose our program of comprehensive lifestyle changes. Put another way, there were six events in thirteen patients (46 percent) in the surgical group but only one event in twenty-seven patients (4 percent) in the lifestyle-change group—in other words, ten times fewer cardiac events in the lifestyle-change group than in the surgical group. Not surprisingly, these differences were statistically significant.

After three years, 96 percent of the patients in the lifestyle-change group were still alive, and only three had undergone surgery. In the surgical group, only 77 percent of the patients were still alive, and these differences were also statistically significant.

Thus, even really sick heart-disease patients were able to safely avoid bypass surgery and angioplasty and, if anything, did even better than those who were operated on. Although this is a small sample of patients without a randomized control group, the differences are striking and encouraging.

In the next chapter, I'll describe why these patients were able to make and maintain comprehensive lifestyle changes in the real world—and how you can do so as well.

2

WHY IT WORKS

Listen, here's what I think. I think we can't go around measuring our goodness by what we *don't* do. By what we deny ourselves. What we resist, and who we exclude. I think we've got to measure goodness by what we embrace, what we create, and who we include.

—From the movie *Chocolat*

■ ■ ■ ■ ■ ■ ■ ■ ■

Like most things in life, the longer you do something and the more experience and practice you have, the more successful and skillful you become at doing it.

During the past three decades of conducting research on the powerful effects of making comprehensive lifestyle changes, my colleagues and I at the Preventive Medicine Research Institute have learned a lot about what really works to motivate people to make and maintain lasting changes in diet and lifestyle. A lot of what we once thought was true turned out to be wrong. We have made many mistakes and learned from them, so you don't have to make the same mistakes—you can make new ones!

Here's a summary of what we have learned so far.

HOW TO TRANSFORM YOUR LIFESTYLE AND YOUR LIFE

When people make the diet and lifestyle changes I recommend in this book, most of them find that they feel so much better so quickly that it reframes the reason for changing from fear of dying to joy of living. Joy and love are powerful, sustainable motivators, but fear and deprivation are not.

1. You have a full spectrum of nutrition and lifestyle choices.

As I mentioned in chapter 1, it's not all or nothing. To the degree that you move in a healthful direction along this spectrum, you're likely to look better, feel better, lose weight, and gain health. You're likely also to smell better and taste better, because your body excretes wastes via your breath and perspiration.

People have different needs, goals, and preferences. What matters most is your *overall* way of eating and living. If you indulge yourself one day, you can eat more healthfully the next. If you're a couch potato one day, you can exercise a little more the next. If you don't have time to meditate for twenty minutes, you can do it for one minute—consistency is more important than duration. Then you're less likely to feel restricted. Studies have shown that the people who eat the most healthfully overall are those who allow themselves some indulgences.

If you're trying to reverse heart disease or prevent the recurrence of cancer, you may need the "pound of cure"—that is, bigger changes in diet and lifestyle than someone who just wants to lower his or her cholesterol level a few points or lose a few pounds. If you have a strong family history, or if genetic testing shows you to be at higher risk, this information can be a powerful motivator to make bigger changes in diet and lifestyle than you might otherwise have made. Also, it may be possible to tailor pharmacologic interventions more effectively and efficiently.

If you're like me, basically healthy, you can thrive on the "ounce of prevention." And if you're somewhere in between—if you have some worrisome risk factors for heart disease (high cholesterol, high blood pressure)—you can begin by making moderate changes in diet and lifestyle, progressively more intensive as needed. If that's enough to achieve your goals, great; if not, you may want to consider making bigger changes.

For example, most people in this country have elevated cholesterol levels. They are initially advised to follow a diet based on the National Cholesterol Education Program or American Heart Association guidelines—less red meat, more skinless chicken, and so on. For some people, that's sufficient to lower their cholesterol levels enough, but not for most. Many are then told, "Sorry, it looks like diet didn't work for you" or "You failed diet." Then they are usually prescribed cholesterol-lowering drugs, which they are told they will need to take for the rest of their lives.

In reality, most people can make progressively bigger changes in nutrition and lifestyle to achieve their goals—often without medication. If moderate changes in diet and lifestyle aren't sufficient to lower your cholesterol sufficiently, bigger changes in diet and lifestyle usually are.

How much you want to change is up to you; I just want to make sure you know what your options are so you can choose intelligently and wisely. In this book, I'll show you how.

If you don't have a serious illness such as coronary heart disease, it usually doesn't matter if you indulge yourself on occasion. However, if you do have heart disease, even a single meal that's high in saturated fat may cause acute changes in how stickily your blood clots and how constricted your arteries may become, both of which may increase the risk of chest pain or even a heart attack.

2. Even more than feeling healthy, most people want to feel free and in control.

The food police are counterproductive. "Doctor's orders" don't work, at least not for long.

If I tell people, "Eat this and don't eat that" or "Don't smoke," they immediately want to do the opposite. It's just human nature, and it goes back to the very first dietary intervention that failed—"Don't eat the apple"—and that was God talking, so we're not likely to do better than that! And if that person's wife or husband says, "Honey, you *know* you're not supposed to be eating that," people sometimes start to feel a little violent.

Nobody wants to feel controlled or treated like a child. Even my child, Lucas, doesn't like to be treated like a child. I said to him, "No one can tell you what to eat, not even me. You don't ever have to eat anything you don't want. However, you can't have dessert unless you've first eaten your dinner; part of my job is to make sure that you grow up to be big and strong, and if you fill up with dessert first, there won't be room for the nutritious foods."

One day, Lucas drank a box of sweetened lemonade on an empty stomach. He started bouncing around the room in a sugar rush, then found himself lying lethargically on our kitchen floor. So I used this as a teaching moment.

"This is what too much sugar does. It makes your blood sugar zoom up, and you get a little crazy and overexcited; then your blood sugar goes way down and you crash, and you don't have much energy, like in the movie *Over the Hedge*."

"How much sugar is too much?"

"Well, it depends. Whenever you buy a package of food, you can read the label and it will tell you how much sugar it contains." And I showed him the label on the carton of lemonade. "This one has thirty grams of sugar per serving, which is a lot. Better to find something that has no more than six to eight grams of sugar per serving, unless it's a treat."

So, at the age of six, he loves to read labels. Whenever we buy food, he checks out the label—"Oh, Daddy, that has too much sugar. Let's get something different."

The point is that he feels empowered and in control, and he also feels regarded and respected, so he feels free to make healthful choices that are sustainable. He understands the reasons for eating this way, which is better than me telling him "Because I said so!"

Kids develop their taste preferences for foods when they're young. The noted pediatrician Dr. William Sears refers to this as "shaping young kids' tastes." They also tend to copy what their parents eat.

So in our home, we serve mostly healthful foods. As a result, Lucas enjoys eating mostly fruits, vegetables, whole grains, legumes, soy products, some cheese, eggs, and a little fish. And, like his dad, he likes to eat a little chocolate most days.

If he wants a treat or some dessert and he's eaten his meal, then he gets it. But since there isn't a charge around it, it's not a "forbidden fruit," so he doesn't feel compelled to pig out. For example:

"Can I have some dessert?"

"Sure, what would you like?"

"Some M&Ms."

"Okay, how many?"

"Five."

So he has five M&Ms and feels very happy. He doesn't feel the need to eat the whole package because there's nothing forbidden.

Whether you're six or sixty, if you go on a diet and lifestyle program and feel constrained, you're likely to go off it sooner or later. Offering a spectrum of choices is much more effective; then, you feel free. If you see your food and lifestyle choices each day as part of a spectrum, as a way of living, you are more likely to feel empowered and to be successful.

Just to digress—I was with Lucas and my wife, Anne, in our kitchen recently. It was one of those beautiful spring days when I felt lucky to be alive and enjoying the day together with them.

I said, "I just feel so happy, maybe I should pinch myself to make sure I'm not dreaming."

Lucas replied, "Daddy, never pinch yourself when you're happy."

3. Eating bad food does not make you a bad person.

The language of behavioral modification often has a moralistic quality to it that turns off a lot of people (like "cheating" on a diet). It's a small step from thinking of foods as "good" or "bad" to seeing yourself as a "good person" or a "bad person" if you eat them, and this creates downward spirals in a vicious cycle. You flog yourself, saying that gluttony is one of the seven deadly sins.

For example, once you feel as if you're a bad person for eating some ice cream, it's all too easy to say, "Well, I blew it, so I might as well finish the entire pint." In reality, although we often project moral qualities onto it, food is just food.

Also, the term "patient compliance" has a fascist, creepy quality to it, sounding like one person manipulating or bending a patient's will to his or her own. In the short run, I may be able to pressure you into changing your diet, but sooner or later (usually sooner), some part of you will rebel. That's why I said earlier that I'm not trying to get you to do anything; in this book, I'm just sharing information that you can use to make informed and intelligent choices.

4. *How* you eat is as important as *what* you eat.

When I eat mindlessly, I have more calories and less pleasure. When I eat mindfully, I have more pleasure with fewer calories.

If I eat mindlessly while watching television, reading, or talking with someone else, I can go through an entire meal without tasting the food, without even noticing that I've been eating. The plate is empty, but I didn't enjoy the food—I've had all of the calories and none of the pleasure. Instead, if I eat mindfully, paying attention to what I'm eating, smaller portions of food can be exquisitely satisfying.

Also, when you pay attention to what you're eating, you notice how different foods affect you, for better and for worse. More-healthful foods make you feel good—light, clear, energetic. Less-healthful foods make you feel bad—heavy, dull, sluggish. Then it comes out of your own experience, not because some doctor or book or friend told you.

To paraphrase Gertrude Stein, a calorie is a calorie is a calorie in terms of its effect on your weight but not in terms of how much pleasure it provides. Later in this book, I'll show you how to meditate on your favorite foods. Then you will have all the pleasure and a lot fewer calories.

5. Joy of living is a much better motivator than fear of dying.

Trying to scare people into changing doesn't work very well. Telling someone that he's likely to have a heart attack if he eats too many unhealthful foods or that she may get lung cancer if she doesn't quit smoking doesn't work very well, at least not for long. Efforts to motivate people to change based on fear of getting sick or dying prematurely are generally unsuccessful.

Why? It's too scary. We all know we're going to die one day—the mortality rate is still 100 percent, one per person—but who wants to think about it? Even someone who has had a heart attack usually changes for only a few weeks before he goes back to his old patterns of living and eating.

For the same reasons, talking about "prevention" or "risk factor reduction" is boring to most people. Telling people that they're going to live to be eighty-six instead of eighty-five is not very motivating—even when they're eighty-five—for who wants to live longer if they're not enjoying life?

Sometimes, people say, "I don't care if I die early—I want to *enjoy* my life." Well, so do I. That's a false choice—is it fun for me, or is it good for me? Why not both? It's fun for you *and* good for you to look good, feel good, have more energy, think more clearly, need less sleep, taste better, smell better, and perform better athletically—and sexually.

Ironically, some of the behaviors that many people think are fun and sexy—like smoking cigarettes, overeating, abusing alcohol and other substances, and being superbusy and stressed out—are the same ones that leave them feeling lethargic, depressed, and impotent. How fun is that?

The latest studies show how much more dynamic our bodies are than had previously been believed. For example, there are minute-to-minute changes in how much blood flow different parts of your body receive. What you eat and what you do can increase or decrease this blood flow very quickly, with powerful effects—for better and for worse.

A meal high in fat, sugar, and calories causes your arteries to constrict, so blood flow is reduced. So does chronic stress. So does nicotine in cigarettes. So do stimulants such as caffeine, cocaine, and amphetamines. So does a lack of exercise.

How do you feel after you've just finished a holiday feast? Sleepy, as if you want to take a nap. Why? Because your brain is receiving less blood flow and oxygen. So is your skin, so you look older. So is your heart, so you may have less stamina. So are your sexual organs, and this interferes with your sexual potency.

When you eat a healthier diet, quit smoking, exercise, meditate, and have more love in your life, your brain receives more blood and oxygen, so you think more clearly, have more energy, and need less sleep. Your face gets more blood flow, so your skin glows more and wrinkles less. Your heart gets more blood flow, so you have more stamina and can even begin to reverse heart disease. Your sexual organs receive more blood flow, so you may become more potent—the same way that drugs like Viagra work (without troubling side effects such as going blind). For many people, these are choices worth making—not just to live longer but also to live better.

Life is to be fully enjoyed. One of the most effective antismoking campaigns was conducted in California by the Department of Health Services. It dressed up an actor like the Marlboro Man in full cowboy regalia, and put his photograph on billboards and in magazines everywhere with a limp cigarette hanging out of his mouth. The large headline was IMPOTENCE, not a warning about lung cancer, heart disease, or emphysema.

This approach was brilliant because it went to the heart (no pun intended) of how smoking is marketed: smoking is sexy. But studies show that half of men who smoke are impotent—how sexy is that?

Nicotine makes your arteries constrict—which reduces blood flow to your sexual organs, causing impotence. Nicotine also diminishes blood flow to your brain (which may cause a stroke) and reduces blood flow to your heart (which may cause a heart attack). In fact, studies have shown that men who are impotent have a higher risk of having a heart attack, because if your penis is not receiving enough blood flow, chances are that your heart isn't, either.

Another effective antismoking campaign was, "Smoking Is Ugly" (www.smokingisugly.com). It featured supermodel Christy Turlington, whose father died of lung cancer. She talked about how smoking accelerates aging because it decreases blood flow to your face and makes it wrinkle prematurely (which is why smokers look about ten years older than they really are and often have that gray pallor). Another campaign asked, "Do you want to taste like an ashtray when your lover kisses you?" That brings it into the here and now: joy of living, not fear of dying.

So, to the degree that you move in a healthy direction on the Spectrum, you're likely to look better, feel better, lose weight, and gain health, as well as smell better, taste better, and love better.

6. It's important to address the deeper issues that underlie our behaviors.

Information is important but not usually sufficient to motivate lasting changes in diet and lifestyle. If it were, no one would smoke. Everyone who smokes knows it's not good for them—the surgeon general's warning is on every package of cigarettes, at least in this country. Yet lots of smart people still smoke—30 percent of Americans still smoke and, in some parts of Asia, more than 80 percent of people still do so. We need to work at a deeper level.

In our studies, I spent a lot of time with the participants over a period of several years. We got to know each other very well, and a powerful trust emerged.

I asked them, "Teach me something. Why do you smoke? Overeat? Drink too much? Work too hard? Abuse substances? Watch too much television? Spend too much time on the Internet? These behaviors seem so maladaptive to me."

They replied, "Dean, you just don't get it. These behaviors aren't maladaptive, they're *very* adaptive—because they help us get through the day."

Loneliness, anxiety, and depression are epidemic in our culture. If we address these deeper issues, it becomes easier for people to make lasting changes in their behaviors.

Hey, I don't want to be the first to break the news to you, but you're going to die. One day. So will I. So will everyone.

Of course, we already know this, but do we really know this? Once we really internalize this, once we accept fully that we're going to die one day, 100 percent certain, we can start to ask, "How can I live more fully?" As Frank Sinatra once said, "Live every day like it's your last, and one day you'll be right."

For some people, it's easy to get into a place of nihilism: It's all in my genes. Who cares? So what? Big deal. Nothing matters. Why bother? I'll eat and do whatever I want; what difference does it make?

I understand nihilism and depression, and I wrote about my experiences with these in two of my earlier books, *Dr. Dean Ornish's Program for Reversing Heart Disease* and *Love and Survival.* They were my catalyst and doorway for transforming my life.

On the other hand, if I focus on what brings real joy and meaning into my life, it makes it much easier to make more of my choices each day on the healthier end of the Spectrum.

Medicine today focuses primarily on drugs and surgery, genes and germs, microbes and molecules. Yet love and intimacy are at the root of what makes us sick and what makes us well. If a new medication had the same impact, failure to prescribe it would be malpractice.

Connections with other people affect not only the *quality* of our lives but also the *quantity* of our lives—that is, our survival. Many well-conducted studies throughout the world have shown that people who feel lonely, depressed, and isolated are many times more likely to die prematurely from virtually all causes than those who have a strong sense of love and intimacy, connection, and community. I'm not aware of any other factor in medicine—not diet, not smoking, not exercise, not genetics, not drugs, not surgery—that has a greater impact on our quality of life, incidence of illness, and premature death.

In part, this is because people who are lonely are more likely to engage in self-destructive behaviors. Telling someone who's lonely and depressed that he's going to live longer if he changes his diet and lifestyle is not very motivating—I mean, who wants to live longer when he's unhappy?

A patient once said to me, "I watch TV and see all the people whose lives seem so much happier than mine, and I say to myself, 'I don't think this is much fun.' I don't want to kill myself, but I'd rather put more energy into numbing the pain than trying to find joy. Because I don't think joy's out there. So I'm just going to keep distracting myself as quickly and as often as I can and fill in the gaps with ways to deaden myself and my pain."

Getting through the day becomes more important than living a long life when you have nothing to live for. As one patient told me, "You know, I've got twenty friends in this pack of cigarettes. They're always there for me, and no one else is. You want to take away my twenty friends? What are you going to give me instead?"

Other patients take refuge in food. As one said to me, "When I feel lonely, I eat a lot of fat—it coats my nerves and numbs the pain. I can fill the void with food." There's a reason why fatty foods are often referred to as "comfort foods." Or people may numb their pain with too much alcohol or other drugs, too much television, too much time on the Internet, or working too hard. We have many ways of numbing, bypassing, and distracting ourselves from pain.

Our experience was confirmed by a recent study published in the *Journal of Marketing* about the connection between people's moods and the type and quantity of food they eat. Researchers found that people who are feeling unhappy eat larger amounts of foods they consider tasty but unhealthy than do happy people.

In this study, test subjects were asked to watch the movie *Love Story,* the maudlin 1970 romance in which the heroine dies at the end (I hope I didn't spoil it for you). They ate, on average, almost 125 grams of buttered, salty popcorn (the amount found in a medium-size bag at the movies)—about 28 percent more than did those watching *Sweet Home Alabama,* the 2002 romantic comedy about a fashion designer going home to the rural South, even though the movies are about the same length.

In another study described in the same journal, college students reading about the deaths of seven children in a fire ate more than four times as many M&Ms as raisins from nearby bowls of snacks. In contrast, students reading about four old friends having an evening together after a chance reunion ate more raisins than M&Ms.

Change isn't easy. But if you're in enough pain, the idea of making changes may start to seem more attractive. I often hear, "Boy, I'm in so much pain, I'm ready to try just about anything."

Awareness is the first step in healing. Part of the benefit of pain is to get our attention, to help us make the connection between when we suffer and why so we can make choices that are a lot more fun and healthful.

The experience of emotional pain and unhappiness can be a powerful catalyst for transforming not only behaviors such as diet and exercise but also for dealing with the deeper issues that really motivate us. We are most successful when we also address the emotional and spiritual dimensions that most influence what we choose to do or not do.

It's very hard to motivate most people to make even simple changes in their behavior such as altering their diet or exercising when they feel depressed, lonely, or fearful, which are epidemic in our culture these days. It is only when the deeper issues of pain, self-esteem, apathy, and purposelessness are addressed that people become willing to make lifestyle choices that are life-enhancing rather than ones that are self-destructive.

7. Make small, gradual changes or big, rapid changes to create sustainable transformations in your diet and lifestyle.

In my experience, there are two basic strategies that work to make and maintain changes in diet and lifestyle.

The first approach is to make small, gradual changes. The barriers to change are low, so they don't seem too intimidating or overwhelming. This approach is seen in organizations like America on the Move (www.americanonthemove.org), whose approach is "Keep it simple." They ask people to get a pedometer, walk 2,000 extra steps per day, and eat 100 calories (about one cookie) fewer per day. Over time, small changes add up and are often sustainable.

The second approach is to make comprehensive lifestyle changes all at once. This seems a little strange to many people, especially physicians, who often say, "I can't even get my patients to take their pills. How do you expect them to change their diet, start exercising and meditating, and spend more time with their friends and family? No way!"

In my experience, paradoxically, it's sometimes easier to make big changes than small ones. Why? When you make big changes, you experience big improvements—and quickly. Most people find that they feel so much better so quickly that it reframes the experience from fear of dying (which is too scary) or risk-factor modification (which is too boring) to joy of living. And it comes out of their own experience, not because some doctor or book or authority told them to do so.

Another reason that making big changes can be easier than making small ones is that when you make big transformations in your diet, your taste preferences often change. Have you ever switched from drinking whole milk to low-fat or skim milk? At first, the milk often tastes like water, not very satisfying. After awhile, it begins to taste fine; then, if you go out to dinner and have whole milk, it tastes like cream—too fatty, too greasy, too rich. Of course, the cow didn't change, but your palate adjusted. However, if you were always drinking both whole milk and some skim milk, then your palate would never have a chance to adapt.

This book is all about freedom of choice. Depending where you want and need to be on your spectrum, you can make small or big changes. The more you move to the healthy end of the Spectrum, and the faster, the greater the benefits and the more quickly they occur. The choice is yours, and yours alone.

8. There's no point in giving up something you enjoy unless you get something back that's even better—and quickly.

We're always making choices. In my experience, most people are not afraid to make even big changes in their lives if they understand the benefits and how quickly they may occur.

When I lecture, I'll sometimes ask the audience, "How many of you have at least one child?" Many people raise their hands.

"Was that a big change in your lifestyle?"

"Oh, yes."

"Was it harder than you thought?"

"Definitely. All those sleepless nights, putting money away for college instead of going to Hawaii . . ."

"How many of you have more than one kid?"

Again, many people raise their hands.

"Did you forget? Or were you just careless? Or because it was worth it?"

"It was *so* worth it."

And that's the point—many people aren't afraid to make big changes in their lifestyle—even monumental ones like having and raising a child. It's not as though you can return your kid to the store if it's too hard or it doesn't turn out the way you planned. But lots of people every day do it—and often more than once.

The most important factor in motivating you to make and maintain big changes in your diet and lifestyle is understanding how powerful the benefits are and how quickly they may occur.

The foods I now eat are very different from what I ate growing up in Texas, eating lots of chili con carne, cheeseburgers, and chalupas (deep-fried burritos). So it was a big change in my diet and lifestyle when I began eating and living more healthfully at age nineteen.

I've been eating and living that way for most of my life since then. It wasn't easy to make those diet changes. But I felt motivated when I experienced immediate benefits. My childhood allergies and asthma disappeared. My cholesterol has remained below 150 mg/dl. And I take no medications. I'm six feet tall and weigh 175 pounds, my blood pressure is 110/70, and I have no chronic diseases. I had a heart scan to determine if I had any calcification in my coronary arteries, and my calcium score was zero, meaning I have no significant calcified coronary artery disease.

9. If it's fun, it's sustainable.

If we view changing our diet and lifestyle as deprivation and sacrifice, well, forget about it. You might be able to force yourself to make some changes for a limited period of time. However, in my experience, trying to motivate yourself to maintain these changes from the intention of deprivation and sacrifice is not sustainable.

Instead, if we understand that *what we gain is so much more than what we give up,* it doesn't feel like a sacrifice. We can see lifestyle choices as opportunities to transform our lives in ways that make us feel more joyful.

For example, I'm sitting at my desk writing this book instead of spending the day in the park because it brings meaning and joy into my life knowing that this book may be helpful to many people. This attitude transforms work into joy, deprivation into abundance.

As I wrote earlier in this chapter, having a child can be viewed as a sacrifice or as a joy. I choose to eat foods mostly from the healthy end of the Spectrum because they make me feel so much better, not because someone told me to do so.

How we approach food is how we approach life. Why have any limitations if you don't have to? Why not eat and do everything you want if you can afford it and no one is watching?

Choosing *not* to do something that we otherwise could do helps define who we are, reminds us that we have free will, freedom of choice. Only when we can say "no" are we free to say "yes."

For example, almost all religions have dietary restrictions, but they differ from one another. Whatever the intrinsic benefit in eating or avoiding certain foods, just the act of choosing not to eat or not to do something that we otherwise might choose helps to make our lives more sacred, more special, more disciplined, more meaningful. More fun.

In this context, what we choose to eat—and not eat—can nourish our soul as well as our body. Each meal reminds us that our lives can be much more than they are. We may choose to follow the restrictions of our own religion or tradition not simply to *please* God but rather to *experience* God.

We can begin to heal our separation from God and from one another at a time when our world is becoming increasingly fragmented and cynical.

It doesn't have to be spiritual. Any time we can make what we do more special and meaningful, it becomes more fun. Otherwise, life can get pretty boring and meaningless.

When we consciously choose to limit what we're doing, it liberates us. Discipline can be liberating if it's freely chosen rather than imposed, because it enables us to do things and to express ourselves in ways that we otherwise might not be able to do. For example, musicians practicing scales may feel that it's a little tedious at times, but it enables them to express themselves more freely by being able to play beautiful music.

Many people think that we have to choose between living a moral, spiritual life that's dry and boring or an immoral, secular life that's exciting and interesting. Fortunately, that isn't the choice.

Living a moral life can be fun, although it's not usually taught that way. A lot of repression occurs in the name of morality, and it's been politicized by the "Moral Majority."

When we consciously choose not to do things that we otherwise could do, it makes them sacred. When I was a teenager, I thought "sacred" meant "boring"—something dry and old, gathering mold and dust. Definitely *not* fun.

Now I understand that "sacred" is just another way of describing what is the most special and therefore the *most* fun, the *most* meaningful, the *most* intimate, the *most* erotic, the *most* exciting, the *most* powerful, the *most* ecstatic, the *most* joyful, the *most* playful, the *most* friendly.

That's what the most enlightened spiritual teachers have taught through the millennia: how to live a joyful life, right here and now.

Ultimately, spiritual leaders teach about ways of living in the world that make it a lot more fun and happy. Not just for some external rewards—going to heaven, getting a gold star or an award, or good karma—rather, these are approaches to living that bring happiness and help us avoid suffering. "My religion is happiness," said the Dalai Lama.

We can go through the world any way we want to; there is free will. Some approaches lead to health and joy; others lead to illness and suffering. We have a spectrum of choices in all aspects of our lives.

People are always making choices, sacrifices. The word "sacrifice" has an austere, depriving connotation. But people don't usually think about that when they put their money aside for their kids' college or wedding, and so they don't buy a new car when they could. These choices—what *not* to do as well as what *to* do—bring meaning into our lives.

In this context, choosing to eat and live differently can be a joyful spiritual practice rather than one leaving you feeling deprived or depressed. You can enjoy life more fully by making these conscious choices. Instead of resolving to make changes in diet and lifestyle out of a sense of austerity, deprivation, and asceticism, I find it much more effective—and fun—to be motivated by feelings of love, joy, and ecstasy.

Growing up in the sixties, the common belief then was that morality is booooooooooorinnnnnggg. The "Playboy Philosophy" and others preached that it's liberating to have many sexual partners and boring to be monoga-mous, but, in my experience, the opposite has been true. From my per-spective, it's not that having sex with many people is wrong, just as eating unhealthy foods all the time isn't wrong; it's just not as much fun as making other choices.

If what you gain is more than what you give up, it's sustainable. Abun-dance is sustainable; deprivation is not. Joy is sustainable; repression is not. "It's good for me" is not sustainable; "it's fun for me" is.

A fully committed relationship allows both people to feel complete trust in each other. Trust allows us to feel safe. When we feel safe, we can open our heart to the other person and be completely naked and vulnerable to them—physically, emotionally, and spiritually. When our hearts are fully open and vulnerable, we can experience profound levels of intimacy that are healing, joyful, powerful, creative, and intensely ecstatic. We can sur-render to each other out of strength and wisdom, not out of fear, weakness, and submission.

When Anne and I are having a romantic date, we have complete trust in each other, so we can be open to all possibilities. We never know what's going to happen, so all degrees of freedom are preserved. We're not trying to get to a preconceived place or to replicate a prior experience, so we can more fully enjoy the infinite possibilities contained in each present moment.

Instead of having similar superficial experiences with different people, we continue to have romantic experiences only with each other that are unlike anything either of us has ever had or even imagined. And if we *had* imagined it, that preconception might have limited our ability to experi-ence something totally new and surprising.

Our experiences are ever-changing, yet always the same. Yet again, like never before. Now and forever.

Preconceptions limit perceptions. Seeing is believing, but we often see only what we believe.

Studies show that we are continually filtering our perceptions of how we believe the world is. While this helps provide a sense of order, it also lim-its our experiences. Preconceptions can lead to boredom because they limit our experiences so significantly.

Great artists and scientists are able to see the world without filtering it through the veil of their preconceptions and paradigms. They literally see and experience the world in a new way, and then they can share their vision with others, helping transform the world we experience.

In summary, when we understand that what we gain is so much more than what we give up, our choices become joyful and meaningful. If it's fun, it's sustainable.

10. The most powerful motivating force in the universe is love.

One evening recently, I was putting my son, Lucas, to bed. I was talking with him about the importance of trust and honesty, and how important these are in any meaningful relationship. He thought about it for a few minutes, and then he said, "Daddy, even if you lied to me a thousand times, I would still believe you."

That degree of unconditional love and trust becomes self-fulfilling. We create what we most love, as well as what we most fear. Knowing how much Lucas trusts me motivates me to be completely worthy of that trust. And when I act in impeccable ways, it allows me to respect and love myself more, which, in turn, gives me that much more love to give others. We can't give what we don't have.

I'd throw myself in front of a train if I thought it would help my son. Almost any parent would. Love is even more powerful than survival.

Whatever their political beliefs, all parents want their kids to be happy and healthy. These are profoundly human issues, ones that defy categorization. At a time when our country is more divided than ever—red states, blue states, Democrats, Republicans, liberals, conservatives—it's heartening (in every sense of the word) when people come together around a common goal.

So it was a double dose of good news when Democrat Bill Clinton and Republican Mike Huckabee, the governor of Arkansas, along with the American Heart Association, announced that they had brokered an agreement with the country's three top soft drink companies (PepsiCo, Coca-Cola, and Cadbury Schweppes and their bottlers) to provide healthier beverages in school vending machines and cafeterias. In addition to the nutritional benefits, they showed that our love for our children can help us overcome our barriers. Republicans, Democrats, companies, and NGOs can choose to transcend their significant differences for the love of our kids. In this case, they did.

Under these new guidelines, elementary schools will sell only bottled water, 100 percent juice, and low-fat and nonfat milk in servings no larger than 8 ounces. Middle schools will do the same but with portion sizes increased to 10 ounces. High schools will also allow diet and unsweetened teas, diet sodas, fitness water, low-calorie sports drinks, flavored water, light juices, and sports drinks in servings up to 12 ounces. At least half of available beverages in high schools will be water and no-calorie and low-calorie selections.

A few months later, PepsiCo and four other companies joined with the American Heart Association and Clinton Foundation to establish voluntary guidelines for healthier foods, including snacks, desserts, and treats sold in schools.

"Ensuring that children have healthier food choices at school is another critical step in the fight against childhood obesity," said President Clinton. "I'm proud of these five companies for making an important statement about this health challenge and an even more important commitment to doing something about it. What we are setting in motion with these guidelines will dramatically change the kind of food that children have access to at school. It will take time, but through coalitions like this of industry and the nonprofit sector, we are going to make a real difference in the lives of millions of children by helping them eat healthier and live healthier."

Now, I think this is one of the best things that's happened in public health in a while. As chair of PepsiCo's health and wellness advisory board (which advises the company on making healthful foods and beverages), we collaborated with company executives in meetings with the American Heart Association and the Clinton Foundation.

Beyond the potential health benefits, this collaboration among Democrats and Republicans, nonprofit and for-profit organizations, and private and public corporations is a model for what others can accomplish when they have a shared vision and determination to make a meaningful difference in the world for the sake of our children. Many people will do things for their children that they won't do for themselves, and these shared goals allow us to transcend our differences.

The epidemics of obesity and diabetes affect children throughout the country, in red states and blue states alike. Awareness is the first step in healing, both individually and nationally. When enough people began to realize that these epidemics may cause our children's generation to be the first to have a shorter life span than their parents, a tipping point was reached.

Concern for our children helps overcome significant differences to achieve a desirable outcome. Appealing to fear and greed can, at least temporarily, be seductive, but I truly believe that love is more powerful than fear, at least in the long run, and enables us to make sustainable changes in our lives.

This primal need to help our children can be harnessed to achieve other goals that affect our kids, such as motivating people to change their diet and lifestyle. If I say to parents, "Consider quitting smoking because it will reduce your risk of getting a stroke, a heart attack, or lung cancer," they often reply, "It's not going to happen to me."

But if I say, "You might consider quitting smoking in order to set a good example for your children so they won't start" or ". . . so they won't have their growth stunted" or ". . . so they won't get asthma from breathing your smoke," they're much more likely to give up cigarettes. One of the most effective antismoking strategies has been for schools to educate children about the harmful health consequences of smoking, causing many of them to go home and say, "Mommy, Daddy, please don't smoke. I love you so much, and I don't want you to die."

We can view our choices in diet and lifestyle as austere sacrifice and deprivation—I can't eat this food or enjoy this indulgence—but it is much more effective and sustainable to reframe our choices as acts of love.

Love made manifest.

For example, I'm not one of those people who loves to exercise. It takes effort for me to motivate myself to work out on a regular basis. What motivates me to do so is love:

- I want to live a long, healthy, and happy life with Anne, and look attractive to her.
- I want to be around to watch my son (and future children) grow up.
- I want to see them graduate and fall in love and dance at their weddings.
- I want to remain healthy enough to play vigorously with them.

Sacrifice is not sustainable. Love is.

As I mentioned earlier, the word "sacrifice" conjures up austerity, deprivation, abnegation, self-immolation, and other awful terms. Sustainable choices come from joy and openness, ones that nourish and delight our hearts, rather than from a place of fear and restriction. Maybe it's time we reframe the concept for what it really is: an act of love, the most powerful force in the universe.

3

HOW IT WORKS

Make everything as simple as possible, but not simpler.

—Albert Einstein

■ ■ ■ ■ ■ ■ ■ ■

Here's some good news: it's not that complicated or difficult to eat and live in a healthy way. This book can be your scientifically proven, trusted field guide to help you distinguish fact from fiction, hype from hope.

And it's not very hard.

In my experience, people who don't know very much about a subject often sound a lot like those who have a deep understanding of it. Both can make it sound simple—one from a lack of awareness, the other from extensive experience that allows the person to distill a complex subject to its most important essence. As Albert Einstein once wrote, "You do not really understand something unless you can explain it to your grandmother."

In this chapter, and in the next, I hope to make *The Spectrum* simple without being simplistic. I'll show you how to cut through the confusion and personalize a way of eating and living that's just right for you, based on your own needs and preferences. You have a spectrum of choices.

FOOD FIGHT

I never intended to become a veteran of the diet wars. Here's how it began.

On New Year's Eve at the change of the millennium, as dinner began, one of the people at our table introduced himself, saying, "Hi, I'm Dan Glickman."

"Hi, I'm Dean Ornish, glad to meet you."

"I'm the U.S. Secretary of Agriculture," he continued. I was about to ask him to stop providing substantial subsidies to farmers growing unhealthy foods when he asked, "So what do you think of the Atkins diet?"

I told him my concerns about it. He reflected for a moment and then said, "You know, I'd like to arrange a debate between you and Dr. Atkins."

"Sure," I replied, not thinking that anything was likely to come of it.

Six weeks later, I found myself at the U.S. Department of Agriculture, debating the late Dr. Atkins for the first time in a public forum. Since then I have debated him, as well as several other authors, on numerous occasions in most of the national mainstream media as well as in plenary sessions at the annual scientific meetings of the American Heart Association, the American College of Cardiology, and the American Dietetic Association, among others.

Whenever I debated Dr. Atkins, he was usually described as the "low-carb" doctor and I was the "low-fat" doctor. But that was never accurate. I have always advocated that an optimal diet is low in total fat, very low in "bad fats" (saturated fat, hydrogenated fats, and trans–fatty acids), high in "good carbs" (fruits, vegetables, whole grains, legumes, and soy products), and low in "bad carbs" (sugar, white flour), and has enough of the "good fats" (omega-3 fatty acids) and high-quality proteins.

It's time to call a truce. Rather than hearing experts bicker, most people want practical, clear, scientifically based information they can use.

Although it's understandable that many people feel more bewildered than ever when they hear seemingly contradictory advice about different diets, in fact a convergence of recommendations is evolving. While some significant differences remain, a greater consensus is emerging among nutrition experts than most people realize.

I first presented these ideas at the Robert Wood Johnson Foundation's "Summit on Obesity." This approach was well received, and I was asked to write an essay for a magazine about this, which the editors called, "The Atkins Ornish South Beach Zone Diet," describing the convergence of recommendations.

Here are the basic principles of a healthy diet, on which most experts agree.

1. Consume some omega-3 fatty acids ("good fats") every day.

Like many people, I take omega-3 fatty acids every day. I began doing so more than twenty years ago when I was completing my residency in internal medicine. Dr. Alexander Leaf, who was then Chief of Medicine at the Harvard Medical School and an inspiring mentor, had conducted pioneering research documenting the extraordinary health benefits of these fatty acids.

Omega-3 fatty acids are found in cold-water fatty fish (salmon, mackerel, herring, trout, sardines, and albacore tuna), as well as canola, soybean, flaxseed, and walnut oils. (In contrast, olive oil does not contain much of the omega-3 fatty acids.) In smaller concentrations, they are also present in dark green leafy vegetables such as kale and collard greens.

Omega-3 fatty acids may reduce triglycerides (a form of fat), lower blood pressure, and decrease inflammation (thereby reducing the symptoms of arthritis and other inflammatory illnesses as well as autoimmune diseases such as lupus). The omega-3 fatty acids can help prevent excessive blood clots from forming, which in turn may decrease the risk of heart attack and stroke. They may also help prevent irregular heartbeats such as atrial fibrillation.

Dr. Leaf's studies, confirmed by those of others, revealed that consuming omega-3 fatty acids on a regular basis may reduce the risk of sudden cardiac death (which is as bad as it sounds) by 42 percent to as much as 90 percent by stabilizing your heart rhythm. Because of this, the American Heart Association recommends at least two servings of fish such as salmon per week.

Since sudden cardiac death is the leading cause of premature death in the United States and most of the industrialized world, a 42 to 90 percent reduction in sudden cardiac death is a very big deal.

If that's not enough, there are even more benefits. When given to pregnant women and lactating mothers, omega-3 fatty acids (which are an important part of the brain) may actually increase their babies' IQs and reduce the incidence of allergic disease in the offspring. They may also reduce depression, and may help reduce the risk of Alzheimer's disease and other causes of dementia. Also, some studies suggest that the omega-3 fatty acids may improve immune function and reduce the risk of prostate cancer, breast cancer, and colon cancer.

Omega-3 fatty acids comprise approximately 8 percent of the average human brain, so it's not surprising that they really are "brain food." If you're pregnant or breast-feeding, the omega-3 fatty acids you consume go to your baby as well, making your baby smarter. If you're not breast-feeding, make sure the formula you're using contains omega-3 fatty acids—researchers in Dallas found that babies who were given formula enriched with omega-3 fatty acids scored seven points higher on intelligence tests.

A major article was published in the international medical journal *The Lancet,* stating that the children of mothers who consumed more than 340 grams (12 ounces) per week of seafood high in omega-3 fatty acids had higher IQs, better behavior, fewer problems with their peers, less hyperactivity, fewer emotional disorders, and better communication skills than those whose mothers consumed less seafood.

The Dark Side of Good Fats

Given these amazing benefits, I've been taking fish oil for many years and have been advising just about everyone else to do the same. I take fish oil capsules (3 grams per day) from which pollutants such as mercury, dioxin, and PCBs that are often found in fish have been removed. This gives all the benefits of the omega-3 fatty acids without the extra fat, calories, and pollutants that come from eating fatty fish. Only three 1-gram capsules per day provide all that most people need. Grass-fed animals provide more omega-3 fatty acids, whereas grain-fed animals provide more omega-6 fatty acids (see page 46).

For vegetarians, some companies such as Martek manufacture omega-3 fatty acid capsules derived from algae. Flaxseed oil and canola oil also contain some precursors of omega-3 fatty acids, but they are in a form that is more difficult for your body to convert to the active omega-3 fatty acids, DHA and EPA.

However, like many wonderful things in life, there is also a dark side to the omega-3 fatty acids. A recent *British Medical Journal* analysis of nearly 100 studies of omega-3 fatty acids found mixed benefits. In most people they were beneficial, but not in everyone. Some people actually got worse.

When Dr. Leaf first learned of these puzzling findings, he thought they were a little, well, fishy. But after reviewing the data from his studies and others and communicating with other investigators, he identified a subgroup of people who actually got worse when they consumed omega-3 fatty acids: those with congestive heart failure or chronic recurrent angina (chest pain) due to insufficient blood flow to their heart. Dr. Leaf wrote in the scientific journal *Fundamental & Clinical Pharmacology*, "Any patient with an advanced state of impaired cardiac function should not be prescribed fish oil fatty acids or be urged to eat fish." As he told me in a telephone conversation, "For these people, it may kill them."

Why? When part of a person's heart receives insufficient blood flow due to coronary artery disease, that part of his or her heart becomes starved for blood and the oxygen it carries. If the deprivation is temporary, he may get angina (chest pain). If it is for more than a few hours, that part of the heart muscle begins to die and turn to scar tissue—in other words, a heart attack. If it's a small part of the heart, the person may live; if not, he may die.

If a moderate to large part of the heart muscle turns to scar tissue, that person may suffer from what's called congestive heart failure. This means that the heart is barely able to pump enough blood to keep the person alive. Also, cells that are only barely receiving enough blood flow become hyperexcitable. This, in turn, can lead to an increased risk of irregular heartbeats, which, in turn, can cause sudden cardiac death.

Omega-3 fatty acids stabilize the rhythm of your heart by effectively removing these hyperexcitable cells from functioning, thereby reducing the likelihood of irregular heartbeats and sudden cardiac death. For most people, this is a very good thing, and it accounts for most of the large reduction in the likelihood of sudden cardiac death.

However, if you have congestive heart failure, your heart may be pumping blood barely well enough to keep you alive. Omega-3 fatty acids may eliminate from function so many of these pumping cells that your heart is no longer able to pump sufficient blood to live, causing an increased risk of cardiac death.

For most people, omega-3 fatty acids are highly beneficial, which is why I still take them every day. But if you have congestive heart failure, chronic recurrent angina (chest pain), or other evidence that your heart is receiving insufficient blood flow, talk to your doctor. If so, it may be prudent to avoid taking omega-3 fatty acids or eating foods that contain them.

How different people react to the same intervention—in this case, omega-3 fatty acids—is an example of how important it is to personalize recommendations. For most people, omega-3 fatty acids are highly beneficial, but for a few others, they can be deadly.

Can You Consume Too Many Good Fats?

One of the few remaining differences in the consensus of what constitutes an optimal diet has to do with how much "good fat" to include in your diet. In chapter 5, I'll show you how to determine the right amount for you.

Is olive oil the healthiest fat? In a word, no. It's a better fat but not the best one.

At the Harvard School of Public Health, Dr. Walter Willett and his colleagues and some authors of popular books have been promoting the idea that it really doesn't matter how much fat you consume in your diet as long as it's "good fats" such as olive oil. While good fats are better for you than bad fats, the total amount of fat in your diet also plays an important role.

All oils are 100 percent fat; since fat has 9 calories per gram versus only 4 calories per gram for protein and carbohydrates, it's very easy to eat a lot of extra calories if you consume a lot of fat. I sometimes see people dipping their bread in olive oil and pouring it on their salads, saying, "Wow, this is so *good* for me!" not realizing that they're consuming a lot more calories than they think.

Also, olive oil contains about 14 percent saturated fat. So if you eat a lot of olive oil, you're consuming a significant amount of saturated fat as well as a lot of calories. One tablespoon of any oil has 14 grams of fat, which means 126 calories per tablespoon. So when you pour any oil on your food, you're drizzling on a lot of liquid calories.

For most people, it's a good idea to reduce total fat consumption. You need only about 5 percent of calories from fat, or about 10 grams per day, to provide the essential fatty acids. The average American gets almost 40 percent of calories from fat. Even the healthiest end of the Spectrum has only about 10 percent of calories from fat, or about 20 grams per day.

What about the studies showing that olive oil lowers your cholesterol level? That's only when you *substitute* olive oil in equivalent amounts for butter or oils such as palm oil that are higher in saturated fat. In other words, it's not that the olive oil *lowers* your cholesterol; it just doesn't *raise* it as much.

A study by Dr. Robert Vogel in the *Journal of the American College of Cardiology* found that olive oil significantly reduces your blood flow to various parts of your body, whereas canola oil and salmon do not. Of course, you want to *increase* blood flow to different parts of your body, not decrease it, especially your brain and your sexual organs.

Similar results were found in another study in which olive oil impaired blood flow, whereas walnuts (which contain omega-3 fatty acids) improved blood flow.

The landmark Lyon Study found that a Mediterranean diet significantly reduced the incidence of heart attacks and premature deaths. Many people attribute these beneficial outcomes to an increased consumption of olive oil. However, in this study it was found that increased consumption of canola oil, not olive oil, accounted for these improvements. Also, people in this study consumed more whole-grain bread, more root vegetables and green vegetables, more fish, less red meat (beef, lamb, and pork were replaced by poultry), and more fruit every day. Butter and cream were replaced by margarine made from canola oil.

Why? Because canola oil has significant amounts of omega-3 fatty acids, whereas olive oil does not. The omega-3 fatty acids are truly good fats for most people. They have extraordinary health benefits, as I described earlier.

The omega-6 fatty acids are also essential to your diet. The problem is that most Americans consume too much of the omega-6 fatty acids and not enough of the omega-3 fatty acids. While the omega-3 fatty acids *reduce* inflammation, the omega-6 fatty acids *increase* it if you consume too much of them. Inflammation increases the risk of coronary heart disease and other chronic illnesses (described in more detail later in this chapter).

Ideally, the ratio of omega-6 fatty acids to omega-3 fatty acids should be about 1 to 1, or no more than 2 to 1. Unfortunately, the ratio in the average American diet (and now that of much of the rest of the world) is between 10 to 1 and 30 to 1, which means most people are consuming way more of the omega-6 fatty acids than the omega-3 fatty acids. The best way to improve this ratio is to consume more omega-3 fatty acids and fewer omega-6 fatty acids.

Much of the excessive omega-6 fatty acids come from eating the wrong kinds of oils. Although olive oil has the reputation of being "good for you," it has thirteen times the amount of harmful omega-6 fatty acids as beneficial omega-3 fatty acids. Corn oil is even worse, with a 46 to 1 ratio of omega-6s to omega-3s.

On the other hand, canola oil has a much more balanced ratio of 2 to 1 omega-6s to omega-3s. Flaxseed oil is rich in omega-3 fatty acids, with a ratio of 1 to 3 omega-6s to omega-3s.

So, to improve your ratio, consume more canola oil or fish oil (which contain omega-3 fatty acids) and less olive oil. This doesn't mean you should never have olive oil—I like the taste of olive oil, and I enjoy it sometimes. It's a healthier fat than many others, but it's not nearly as healthy as fish oil, canola oil, or flaxseed oil.

2. Eat more "good carbs" and fewer "bad carbs."

There is a world of difference in how your body metabolizes "good carbs" and "bad carbs."

Although Dr. Atkins and I agreed on the diagnosis—that many Americans eat too many simple carbohydrates—we disagreed about the prescription. Dr. Atkins advocated replacing simple carbohydrates with high-fat, high–animal protein foods such as bacon, sausage, butter, steak, pork rinds, and Brie.

Telling people what they want to believe is part of the reason that the Atkins diet was once so popular. I would love to be able to tell you that these are health foods, but they are not. This doesn't mean you should never eat these foods—remember, I love chocolate—but these are treats, not health foods. In the next chapter, I'll describe how much you may be able to indulge yourself without jeopardizing your health.

Dr. Atkins was partially right in saying that too many "bad carbs" such as sugar, high-fructose corn syrup, white flour, and white rice may promote weight gain and chronic diseases for reasons described below. There are clear benefits to reducing the intake of refined carbohydrates, especially by people who are sensitive to them.

So his diagnosis was partially correct: too many refined carbohydrates can be unhealthful. But his prescription was wrong. The solution is not to go from refined carbohydrates like pasta to pork rinds and from sugar to sausage but to substitute unrefined good carbs for refined bad carbs.

Good carbs include fruits, vegetables, whole grains, legumes, nuts, and soy products in their natural, unrefined forms. Because these good carbs are unrefined, they are naturally high in fiber as well. The fiber fills you up before you eat too much. For example, it's hard to get too many calories from eating apples or whole grains, because these foods are naturally high in fiber, which causes you to feel full before you consume too many calories.

Also, the fiber in good carbs causes your food to be digested and absorbed into your bloodstream more slowly. This helps keep your blood sugar in a normal range.

The glycemic index is a measure of how much a given food will raise your blood sugar—in other words, how rapidly a carbohydrate in food turns into sugar. Good carbs have a low glycemic index, whereas bad carbs have a high glycemic index.

Another way of expressing this is called "glycemic load," which also takes into account a typical serving size as well as how quickly the food is absorbed. Some people believe that glycemic load is a better indicator of how foods will affect your blood sugar than glycemic index is.

For example, a carrot has a high glycemic index but a low glycemic load. Why? Because the carbohydrates in carrots are absorbed very quickly, but there aren't many of them.

Glycemic load is the amount of carbohydrate in a serving of food multiplied by that food's glycemic index. So even though the glycemic index of a carrot is about the same as that of a baked potato, the glycemic load of a potato is much higher because a potato is very dense in carbohydrates, whereas a serving of carrots doesn't contain many carbohydrates. As a result, eating a baked potato causes a sharp rise in some people's blood sugar whereas a carrot does not.

Here's a table that illustrates this.

Carbohydrate Content, Glycemic Index, and Glycemic Load of Various Carbohydrate Foods

FOOD (serving size)	CARBOHYDRATE CONTENT (in grams)	GLYCEMIC INDEX (percent expressed as decimal)	GLYCEMIC LOAD (rounded to nearest tenth)
Potato (1 baked)	37	1.21	45
Carrots (½ cup cooked)	8	1.31	10
Lentils (½ cup cooked)	20	0.41	8
Dry beans (½ cup cooked)	27	0.60	16
White rice (½ cup cooked)	35	0.81	28
Wild rice (½ cup cooked)	18	0.78	14
White bread (2 slices)	24	1.00	22
Whole-grain bread (2 slices)	24	0.64	15
Pasta (1 cup cooked)	40	0.71	28
Cheerios (1 cup)	22	1.06	23
All-Bran (1 cup)	24	0.60	14
Grape-Nuts (½ cup)	47	0.96	45
Cornflakes (1 cup)	26	1.19	31
Corn chips (1 oz.)	15	1.05	16
Popcorn (air-popped, 1 cup)	5	0.79	4

The standard reference for this table is white bread.

Source: Carbohydrate content and GI values are derived from various sources, including the Division of Preventive Medicine, Brigham and Women's Hospital, Harvard Medical School; "International Tables of Glycemic Index," *American Journal of Clinical Nutrition* 62 (1995): 871S–893S; and Corinne T. Netzer, *The Complete Book of Food Counts,* 5th ed. (New York: Dell, 2000).

When whole wheat flour is processed into white flour, or brown rice into white rice, the fiber and bran are removed. This turns a "good carb" into a "bad carb."

Why? Because when the fiber and bran are removed, you get a quadruple whammy:

1. *You can eat large amounts of "bad carbs" without feeling full.* Fiber fills you up before you consume too many calories. Removing fiber allows you to consume virtually unlimited amounts of calories without causing you to feel full.

2. *When you eat a lot of "bad carbs," they are absorbed quickly, causing your blood sugar to rise too rapidly.* When your blood sugar gets too high, your pancreas secretes insulin to bring it back down. However, it may go down below where it started, causing low blood sugar (hypoglycemia). By analogy, when you pull a pendulum to one side and let it go, it doesn't stop at the midpoint; it continues an equal distance to the other side.

   When your blood sugar gets too low, you feel lethargic and a little crabby. There's a good temporary fix for those bad feelings—more bad carbs! This creates a craving for more "bad carbs" to raise your blood sugar, and a vicious cycle is created.

3. *When your body secretes too much insulin, it accelerates the conversion of calories into triglycerides, which is how your body stores fat.* Thus, when you eat a lot of "bad carbs," you consume an excessive number of calories that don't fill you up, and you're more likely to convert these extra calories to body fat. Insulin may also cause your body to produce more of an enzyme called lipoprotein lipase, which increases the uptake of fat into cells, leading to weight gain.

4. *When your body secretes too much insulin, it may lead to insulin resistance and even diabetes.* Insulin binds to what are called insulin receptors on your cells. When your body makes repeated surges of insulin in response to too many "bad carbs," the receptors become less sensitive—a little like Aesop's fable of the boy who cried wolf—as if the insulin receptors were saying, "Oh, not more insulin again, just ignore it." Like a heroin addict who requires more and more of the drug to get the same feeling, insulin resistance causes your body to make more and more insulin just to maintain the same effect on your blood sugar. Over time, this may lead to type 2 diabetes. Too much insulin also enhances the growth and proliferation of arterial smooth muscle cells, promoting atherosclerosis and clogging your arteries.

This doesn't mean you should never eat bad carbs. I do, in moderation. When I eat bad carbs, I try to consume them along with good carbs and other high-fiber foods. That way, the fiber in the good carbs will slow the absorption of the bad carbs. What matters is the glycemic index or glycemic load of the entire meal, not just of individual food items.

As I'll discuss more fully in the next chapters, some people may need to limit their intake of bad carbs more than others, depending where they are on the Spectrum.

Biology versus Willpower

Have you ever tried to lose weight and blamed yourself for not having enough motivation or discipline? Maybe it's not entirely your fault. Individual variations in biology, not just willpower, may play an important role in weight loss.

Dr. David Ludwig is one of the most respected researchers in childhood obesity. He is Director of the Optimal Weight for Life (OWL) Program, based at Harvard's Children's Hospital in Boston, which is among the oldest and largest clinics in the country for overweight children and their families.

Dr. Ludwig asked, "Why can some people do well on weight-loss diets whereas others do poorly on the very same diets?" He recently published a study in *The Journal of the American Medical Association* showing that individual variations in biology may cause some people to have a harder time losing weight and keeping it off than others—and that tailoring their diet accordingly can make a big difference.

In his study, he assigned seventy-three obese young adults to either a conventional low-fat, high-glycemic-load diet (high in bad carbs such as sugar and refined carbohydrates such as white flour) or a low-glycemic-load diet, which is one that stabilizes blood sugar after meals, as described above.

He found that people who secrete insulin slowly lost the same amount of weight on both diets. In contrast, people who secrete insulin rapidly and were on the low-glycemic-load diet lost five times more weight, and they kept all the weight off throughout the eighteen months of the study.

According to Dr. Ludwig, "When it comes to healthy eating, one size may not fit all. It may be unwise to recommend decreasing dietary fat without adequate attention to the carbohydrates that replace them and vice versa. It's not low-fat versus low-carb—both are important. An optimal approach may be a diet that pays equal attention to the quality of the fats as well as the carbohydrates: high-quality, unprocessed low-glycemic carbs and plant-based proteins and fats."

How can you find out if you secrete insulin quickly or slowly? You can ask your doctor for what's called a glucose tolerance test, in which you drink some sugar water, and a blood sample is taken thirty minutes later. The sugar water makes your blood sugar (glucose) increase, and your pancreas secretes insulin to lower your blood sugar back to normal, which is good.

However, some people secrete too much insulin too quickly. These people tend to gain weight for the reasons described above. So it's not surprising that Dr. Ludwig's study found that people who secrete insulin too quickly lose more weight when they eat low-glycemic-index foods (good carbs) that don't provoke an excessive insulin response.

Should you have a glucose tolerance test? Not necessarily. If you eat a diet of predominantly foods with a low glycemic index, it doesn't matter very much if you tend to secrete insulin quickly or slowly, as these foods won't provoke a rapid insulin response even if you're genetically predisposed to secrete insulin quickly. One reason for having the test is that it may motivate you to eat fewer high-glycemic-index foods if you find that you're a rapid insulin secretor.

In summary, to the degree that you substitute whole foods and good carbs for refined bad carbs, there is a corresponding benefit. Again, it's not all or nothing. In the next chapters, I'll show you how you can take this information and customize a spectrum of eating that's just right for you based on your own needs and preferences.

3. Avoid trans fats, saturated fats, and partially hydrogenated fats ("bad fats").

Why do many food manufacturers continue to use these disease-promoting fats? Because they increase the shelf life of their food products, even though they may decrease the "shelf life" of the people who eat them.

Saturated fats are found primarily in animal fats—in meat (including chicken and other poultry), whole-milk dairy products (cheese, milk, and ice cream), egg yolks, and (to a lesser degree) seafood. Some plant foods, including coconut oil and palm oil, are also high in saturated fats.

When liquid vegetable oils are heated in the presence of hydrogen, this produces both partially hydrogenated fats and trans fats. Partially hydrogenated fats act like and are as disease-promoting as saturated fats.

Most nutrition experts agree that trans–fatty acids are especially bad for your health. Trans fats in the American diet are found predominantly in commercially prepared baked goods, margarines, snack foods, and processed foods, as well as many fried foods. Some experts believe that trans fats are even worse for cholesterol levels than saturated fats because they raise bad LDL and lower good HDL, whereas others believe that saturated fats are just as harmful. It's better to avoid both.

Saturated fats, trans fats, and partially hydrogenated fats promote inflammation and raise total blood cholesterol levels and LDL cholesterol levels. They are strongly linked with an increased risk of coronary heart disease, stroke, diabetes, many types of cancer, and other chronic diseases.

Scientists at Wake Forest University recently reported that diets rich in trans fats may cause a redistribution of fat tissue to the abdomen (the worst place to store fat for both health and appearance) and lead to a higher body weight, even when total calorie intake is the same.

To the degree that you reduce your intake of saturated fat and trans–fatty acids, you reduce your risk of a heart attack and other illnesses. In its new dietary guidelines, the American Heart Association now recommends cutting saturated fat to less than 7 percent of total calories and trans fats to less than 1 percent of total calories in your diet.

Realistically, though, most people are not going to calculate the saturated fat and trans fats in their diet each day. So what can you do to protect yourself and your family?

- Reduce your intake of foods high in trans fats. These include most fried foods and many commercially prepared cookies, cakes, crackers, and snack foods. If the label says "hydrogenated" or "partially hydrogenated," avoid the food. In general, steer clear of foods that contain more than 3 grams of trans fats or saturated fats per serving; lower is better.

- Cut your consumption of foods high in saturated fats. These are found in meat and dairy products as well as some tropical oils, such as palm oil and coconut oil. Most people eat four times as much saturated fat as trans fats, so there is even more room for improvement here.

Processed foods now list both saturated fat and trans fats on the labels. Another way to tell is that the more hydrogenated an oil is, the harder it will be at room temperature. For example, soft tub margarine is usually less hydrogenated and has fewer trans fats than margarine that comes in a stick.

When I first began consulting with McDonald's in 1999 and with PepsiCo in 2001 to help them develop more healthful foods, my first recommendation was to remove the trans fats from their products. In the first year, PepsiCo removed the trans–fatty acids from all of its Frito-Lay (a company owned by PepsiCo) products. It showed that it was possible to do so without compromising the flavor and texture of its foods. It was more of a challenge for McDonald's to do so to preserve the flavor and texture of its french fries, but it found a way to accomplish this goal.

McDonald's has more than 50 million customers every day worldwide, and PepsiCo has almost as many. When I began consulting with these companies, I reasoned that even an incremental change on that scale could make an important difference in the health of many people. Also, they could use their extensive advertising and marketing resources to help change the way people view healthy eating and living, as I described in chapter 1—to make it fun, sexy, hip, cool, crunchy, and convenient to eat and live more healthfully.

I helped McDonald's team develop a Fruit & Walnut Salad, which contains apple slices, grapes, walnuts, and low-fat yogurt. Because of that one salad, McDonald's is now the largest purchaser of apples in the world. I also worked with their team on their Asian Salad, which contains sixteen types of greens, edamame (soybeans), almonds, mandarin oranges, snow peas, and red bell peppers.

In addition to my work with McDonald's and PepsiCo, I also chair the Safeway Advisory Council on Health and Nutrition and the Google Health Advisory Council. I am grateful for these opportunities to make a meaningful difference in the lives of so many people.

When making more healthful foods becomes good business—which it is—it becomes sustainable. At PepsiCo, for example, more than two thirds of revenue growth came from its good-for-you and better-for-you products in 2006.

It takes time for companies of this size to migrate their product offerings to include an increasingly greater proportion of healthier foods—a little like turning an aircraft carrier. But it's happening more quickly than I expected. I'm proud of the impact it's having worldwide in making it more convenient and fun to eat more healthfully.

4. Energy balance is important, and calories count.

There's no mystery in how to lose weight: burn more calories and/or eat fewer calories. It's all about energy balance. You lose weight when you burn more calories than you consume.

You can burn more calories by exercising. Simple changes like taking the stairs, parking a little farther from your destination, and walking thirty minutes a day can make a significant difference. Small changes can lead to big improvements over time.

Of course, you can consume fewer calories by eating less food. That's why you can lose weight on any diet that restricts portion sizes or eliminates entire categories of foods, but it's hard to keep it off because people don't like feeling hungry and deprived for very long. So they often lose weight and then gain it back, blaming themselves for not having enough discipline or willpower, when they were just going about it in the wrong way.

When I hear the phrase "portion control," it makes me want to go out and pig out on something. Anything. It makes me feel, well, controlled, and I don't like feeling that way. As I described earlier, "eating mindfully" sounds so much better, and it's much more sustainable.

An easier way than portion control to consume fewer calories is to eat less fat, because fat (whether saturated, monounsaturated, or unsaturated) has 9 calories per gram, whereas protein and carbohydrates have less than half, only 4 calories per gram. Thus, when you eat less fat, you consume fewer calories without having to eat less food, thereby increasing satiety without adding calories.

In other words, as I described in my book *Eat More, Weigh Less,* when you change the *type* of food, you don't have to be as concerned about the *amount* of food because the foods are less dense in calories. You can eat whenever you're hungry and consume an equal or even larger volume of food, yet still lose weight without feeling hungry or deprived.

It's primarily the volume of food that determines how full you feel, not the number of calories. Most good carbs like fruits and vegetables are naturally low in fat (and thus low in caloric density) and high in fiber, so you feel full before you consume too many calories. Fiber enhances satiety without adding significant calories.

At Pennsylvania State University, researchers found that healthy women instinctively ate about three pounds of food per day, whether the foods were high or low in calories. Thus, the primary drive for when people felt as though they had had enough to eat was the volume of food, not the number of calories. They also found that those on a low-fat diet plus a diet high in fruits and vegetables lost more weight than those on a low-fat diet alone.

In a survey of food consumption data from the U.S. Department of Agriculture's National Food Consumption Surveys (NFCS) and the Continuing Survey of Food Intakes by Individuals (CSFII), "Individuals of all ages who consume a diet with fewer than 30 percent of calories from fat consistently have lower energy intakes. The data suggest that reducing fat intake is one effective strategy for also reducing total energy consumption. . . . Given the increasing rates of obesity in the United States at an earlier age, dietary-fat reduction may be an effective part of an overall strategy to balance energy consumption with energy needs."

Another reason that many people may get too many calories is by consuming too many bad carbs, as described above. Because these foods are low in fiber, large quantities of calories can be consumed without the person feeling full. The processing and lack of fiber may cause these foods to have a high glycemic index and often a high glycemic load; they are absorbed quickly, causing blood glucose levels to spike, which causes insulin surges. These surges may cause a reactive hypoglycemia, increasing hunger and a desire to eat more simple carbohydrates in a vicious cycle, sometimes called "carbohydrate cravings."

Thus, an optimal diet is low in both fat and bad carbs. In the next chapter, I'll help you determine how much fat and bad carbs are right for you.

Protein also helps increase satiety. Plant-based proteins achieve this as well as protein derived from animal sources. The spectrum of choices described in the next chapter reflects the fact that, in general, plant-based proteins are more healthful than those derived from animal sources, and seafood-based proteins are generally more healthful than those derived from red meat. Body weight is inversely associated with dietary fiber and carbohydrates and is positively associated with protein intake. Meat has virtually no dietary fiber.

5. What you *include* in your diet is as important as what you *exclude*.

The Spectrum is about abundance, not deprivation; feeling better, not just living longer. I want to emphasize eating more foods that are beneficial rather than just eating fewer foods that are unhealthful.

There are at least 100,000 substances in foods that have powerful anti-cancer, anti–heart disease, and antiaging properties. These include phyto-chemicals, bioflavonoids, carotenoids, retinols, isoflavones, genistein, lycopene, polyphenols, sulforaphanes, and others.

Where do you find these potent substances? With few exceptions, these protective factors are found in fruits, vegetables, whole grains, legumes, and soy products and some fish. These are rich in good carbs, good fats, good proteins, and other protective substances. The recipes in this book are high in these protective substances.

For example, my colleagues and I at the nonprofit Preventive Medicine Research Institute conducted a double-blind, placebo-controlled, randomized controlled trial looking at the effects of pomegranate juice in people with coronary heart disease. After only three months, we found that blood flow to the heart was improved in those who drank one eight-ounce glass of pomegranate juice each day for only three months, whereas patients who were given a placebo got a little worse.

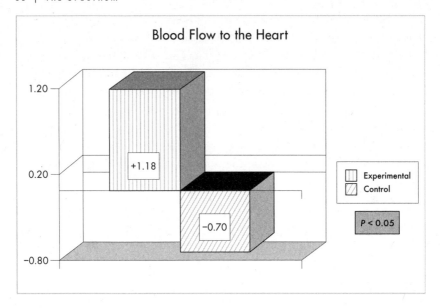

Blood Flow to the Heart

Other studies are showing that pomegranate juice may help prevent and even slow the growth of prostate cancer and other tumors. For example, a study at UCLA showed that a daily eight-ounce glass of pomegranate juice may reduce the recurrence of prostate cancer. Researchers say the effect may be so large that it may help older men outlive the disease.

Several well-designed studies have shown that drinking cranberry juice may significantly reduce the risk of developing urinary tract infections in sexually active women. Whether or not cranberry juice can help treat as well as prevent these infections is not as well established. Another study found that regular consumption of cranberry juice may suppress *Helicobacter pylori* infection, which may reduce the risk of ulcers and gastric cancer.

I'm sure you've heard that red wine may be good for your heart. This may be true, but you can receive essentially the same benefits from drinking unfermented wine, i.e., grape juice. Substances such as flavonoids in grapes help dilate your arteries and keep them flexible, improve blood flow, and reduce the likelihood of blood clots. These substances also help keep cholesterol in your bloodstream from ending up in your arteries.

Antioxidants in grape juice appear to linger in your body longer than those in wine. At the University of California, Davis, researchers took a 1996 cabernet sauvignon, removed all the alcohol, and asked volunteers to alternate between drinking the nonalcoholic wine one day and one with alcohol on the next day. They found that antioxidants remained in the blood 25 percent longer after volunteers drank the nonalcoholic wine than the cabernet with alcohol. Alcohol may hasten the breakdown of antioxidants in your blood.

Recently, researchers at Harvard Medical School and the National Institute on Aging reported that resveratrol, a natural substance found in grapes and red wine, helped reduce the harmful effects of a high-calorie diet in mice and significantly extended their life span. However, the amounts of resveratrol that they gave to these mice were equivalent to drinking 750 to 1,500 bottles of red wine a day.

Here is a table outlining some of the health benefits of various foods. It's not comprehensive, just a few examples of the powerful health benefits they bring.

Health Benefits of Various Foods

ITEM NAME	BENEFITS
FRUITS:	
Apples	An apple a day really may keep the doctor away. The pectin in apples may lower your cholesterol levels and help stabilize your blood sugar. They help prevent lung disease, especially in smokers.
Bananas	Bananas are one of the best sources of potassium, an essential mineral for maintaining normal blood pressure and heart function. Since the average banana contains a whopping 467 milligrams of potassium and only 1 milligram of sodium, a banana a day may help prevent high blood pressure and protect against atherosclerosis. The effectiveness of potassium-rich foods such as bananas in lowering blood pressure has been demonstrated by a number of studies. For example, researchers tracked more than 40,000 American male health professionals over four years to determine the effects of diet on blood pressure. Men who ate diets higher in potassium-rich foods, as well as foods high in magnesium and cereal fiber, had a substantially reduced risk of stroke.
Blueberries	Blueberries contain phytochemicals called anthocyanins that may make you smarter and may improve your memory. And like cranberries, they may reduce the risk of urinary tract infections by keeping *Escherichia coli* bacteria from sticking to your bladder wall.
Cranberries and cranberry juice	Cranberries may reduce the risk of urinary tract infections by keeping *E. coli* bacteria from sticking to your bladder wall.

ITEM NAME	BENEFITS
Grapes (as well as raisins and wine)	Grapes (whether fresh, dried as raisins, or fermented in wine, consumed in moderation) contain antioxidants called polyphenols that help prevent coronary heart disease.
Mangoes	Mangoes are among the best sources of cancer-fighting carotenoids. They are also rich in the antioxidant vitamins C and E. One mango contains 7 grams of digestion-helping fiber, and much of this is soluble fiber, which helps lower your cholesterol level.
Oranges	You may already know that oranges are an excellent source of vitamin C—just one orange supplies 116.2 percent of the daily value for vitamin C—but do you know just how important vitamin C and oranges are for good health? Vitamin C is the primary water-soluble antioxidant in the body, disarming free radicals and preventing damage in the aqueous environment both inside and outside cells. Inside cells, a potential result of free-radical damage to DNA is cancer. In areas of the body where cellular turnover is especially rapid, such as the digestive system, preventing DNA mutations translates into preventing cancer. This is why a good intake of vitamin C is associated with a reduced risk of colon cancer.
Pomegranates and pomegranate juice	Pomegranates and pomegranate juice are loaded with phytochemicals that may help prevent and even reverse the progression of coronary heart disease. They may also help prevent prostate cancer by reducing DNA damage.
Strawberries	Strawberries are filled with phytochemicals that reduce the risk of diabetes and circulatory problems. They may also contain phenols that may lower your risk of cancer and heart disease.
Tomatoes (including tomato sauce and tomato paste)	Tomatoes are rich in lycopene, a powerful antioxidant, which may help reduce your risk of coronary heart disease, breast cancer, lung cancer, and prostate cancer. Cooking tomatoes helps activate lycopene. They also contain vitamins A, C, and E, and potassium.
Watermelon	Watermelon contains even more lycopene than tomatoes do. Lycopene is a powerful antioxidant, which may help reduce your risk of coronary heart disease, breast cancer, lung cancer, and prostate cancer.
VEGETABLES: Artichokes	Artichokes contain silymarin, an antioxidant that helps prevent skin cancer, plus fiber to help control cholesterol.
Bell peppers	Bell peppers, especially red bell peppers, may help boost your immune system. They are excellent sources of vitamin C (they provide three times as much as oranges) and beta-carotene.

ITEM NAME	BENEFITS
Bok choy	Bok choy (Chinese cabbage) contains brassinin (which may help prevent breast tumors), plus indoles and isothiocyanates (which lower levels of estrogen, which helps reduce the risk of breast cancer).
Broccoli	Broccoli is high in beta-carotene, fiber, and phytochemicals that may detoxify cancer-causing substances before they have a chance to cause harm, reducing the risk of breast, colon, and stomach cancers. One cup of broccoli contains more vitamin C than an orange.
Carrots	Carrots are an excellent source of antioxidant compounds and the richest vegetable source of the pro–vitamin A carotenes. Carrots' antioxidant compounds help protect against cardiovascular disease and cancer, and also promote good vision, especially night vision.
Chili peppers	Chili peppers are rich in capsaicin, which is what makes them taste hot. They may help you lose weight by suppressing appetite so you eat less and also by increasing your metabolism, so you burn more calories. They contain antioxidants such as vitamins A and C.
Kale	Kale contains lutein, an antioxidant that protects against macular degeneration, a leading cause of blindness. Kale is also rich in beta-carotene, vitamin C, and vitamin E, as well as folate (which helps prevent heart disease and birth defects) and calcium and magnesium, two minerals important for strong bones. Kale also contains some omega-3 fatty acids.
Onions	Onions are rich in quercetin, which is one of the most powerful flavonoids (natural plant antioxidants) and may help protect against cancer.
Spinach	Spinach is loaded with iron, folate, and two phytochemicals that help prevent macular degeneration. One cup of spinach contains just 41 calories and no fat.
Swiss chard	Swiss chard contains the phytochemical lutein, which lowers the risk of age-related vision loss from macular degeneration and cataracts. A one-cup serving of cooked Swiss chard supplies 47 percent of your RDA (150 milligrams) of magnesium, which helps keep nerve and muscle cells healthy.
LEGUMES: Kidney beans, black beans, peas, and lentils	Beans and lentils—including kidney beans, peas, and black beans—are high in both soluble fiber and folic acid, which help lower cholesterol and decrease homocysteine levels, reducing the risk of heart disease.

ITEM NAME	BENEFITS
NUTS: Walnuts, almonds, and hazelnuts	Nuts are a good source of vitamin E, antioxidants, and protein. The fat supplied in nuts is monounsaturated, which carries a lower risk of cardiovascular disease. Nuts are also an excellent source of magnesium, fiber, B vitamins, and vitamin E. They are high in fat and calories (150 calories per ounce), so watch the portion size.
FOODS RICH IN OMEGA-3 FATTY ACIDS: Cold-water seafood such as salmon, mackerel, herring, bluefish, trout, sardines, albacore tuna; dark green leafy vegetables such as kale and collard greens; and canola, soybean, flaxseed, and walnut oils	Studies have shown that daily consumption of omega-3 fatty acids may dramatically reduce the incidence of sudden cardiac death, reduce triglycerides, lower blood pressure, and decrease inflammation, helping arthritis and lupus. When given to pregnant women and lactating mothers, omega-3 fatty acids may increase a baby's IQ by six points or more and may also reduce the incidence of allergic disease in the offspring. They may also reduce depression and help prevent dementia. Some studies suggest that omega-3 fatty acids may reduce the risk of prostate cancer and breast cancer. Avoid omega-3 fatty acids if you have congestive heart failure.
DAIRY PRODUCTS: Eggs	Eggs are a good source of protein. The egg white provides all of the protein, whereas egg yolks have all the cholesterol. If you have heart disease or high cholesterol, focus on consuming egg whites. Two egg whites can substitute for one egg in most recipes. Some eggs are fortified with omega-3 fatty acids.
Nonfat milk	Nonfat milk provides a significant source of calcium, vitamin B_{12}, and protein. The protein helps keep you feeling full and satisfied until your next meal.
Yogurt	Some yogurt contains live active cultures, which help prevent common gastrointestinal tract problems such as constipation and diarrhea. The calcium present in yogurt also helps maintain weight and bone health.
SOY PRODUCTS: Including tofu, tempeh, soy milk, and edamame	Soy foods are rich in phytoestrogens, which help prevent breast cancer and prostate cancer. They also reduce the risk of coronary heart disease. They are rich in protein, niacin, folate, calcium, copper, iron, magnesium, manganese, potassium, and zinc, and low in saturated fat.

ITEM NAME	BENEFITS
GRAINS: Oatmeal	Oatmeal contains soluble fiber that may help lower your cholesterol level as well as your blood pressure. It fills you up before you consume too many calories, helping you lose weight. Buy old-fashioned steel-cut oatmeal rather than instant, if possible.
Whole-grain breads, cereals, and crackers	Whole-grain breads, cereals, and crackers are "good carbs" because the fiber slows their absorption and keeps your blood sugar level more even. Also, the fiber fills you up before you consume too many calories. The soluble fiber in cereal may reduce your cholesterol level, and the insoluble fiber keeps you regular and may decrease your risk of colon cancer.
OTHER FOODS: Chocolate	Chocolate (my favorite) is rich in flavonols and catechins, which may reduce the risk of heart disease, improve blood flow, and lower blood pressure. Chocolate can be loaded with fat and sugar, but dark chocolate is better than milk chocolate because it's lower in sugar and higher in flavonols. Even a single piece of high-quality dark chocolate can be exquisitely satisfying if you close your eyes and savor it.
Ginger	Ginger contains a compound called gingerol that may lower blood pressure and increase circulation. Ginger also may help relieve motion sickness, morning sickness, and the nausea caused by anesthesia. Other compounds in ginger may help ward off migraines and arthritis pain by blocking inflammation-causing prostaglandins.
Tea: black and green	Tea contains polyphenols, which are powerful antioxidants; they are found even more in green tea than in black tea. The catechins in tea may help prevent cancer throughout your GI tract by helping prevent DNA damage from carcinogens and inhibiting the growth of new blood vessels that would feed tumors. Tea may also help prevent tooth decay. Both green tea and black tea are high in flavonoids, which have many health benefits. Green tea has more than black tea. Drinking tea has been shown to reduce the incidence of coronary heart disease and many gastrointestinal cancers and to enhance immune function.

These foods also may help prevent many forms of cancer by inhibiting the growth of new blood vessels, called angiogenesis. When tumors grow, they send signals for new blood vessels to grow in order to feed the tumor's growth. Many fruits, vegetables, and whole grains have anti-angiogenesis factors that may help prevent the growth of tumors. For more information on this, please go to www.angio.org.

A Spicy Story

Some of your favorite spices also have extraordinary health benefits. When you spice up your meals, you may spice up your life as well. Spices not only help your foods taste better, they can also help you feel better. They have been used since biblical times; what's new is research showing that some of these spices enhance your health as well as your palate.

The average American consumes more than 3½ pounds of spices annually, but nearly half of that is pepper and mustard seed (in prepared mustard). Mustard seeds are mentioned in ancient Sanskrit writings dating back about five thousand years, as well as in the New Testament. They contain lots of protective substances called phytonutrients, which may inhibit the growth of existing cancer cells as well as helping prevent normal cells from turning into cancer cells.

Other spices have some amazing attributes. One of the most exciting is turmeric, an Indian spice that provides the yellow color in curries. Turmeric has powerful anti-inflammatory and antioxidant properties, and has been used in Indian and Chinese medicine for centuries. It reduces the actions of several genes that promote inflammation, which is linked to heart disease, colon cancer, and Alzheimer's disease.

Researchers have found that turmeric may help prevent or even treat Alzheimer's disease. They had some clues about turmeric because the rate of Alzheimer's disease is much lower in India than in the United States— it affects just 1 percent of people over the age of 65 living in some Indian villages. New research is shedding some light on why this may be true.

In Alzheimer's disease, plaques called amyloid are deposited in the brain, which causes the brain to work poorly—almost like a short circuit in the brain's wiring. Researchers at UCLA found that curcumin, one of the most active substances found in turmeric, reduced the number of these plaques by 50 percent. Rats given turmeric also performed better on maze-based memory tests.

Turmeric also enhances immune function, may reduce your risk of a heart attack, and improves digestion. Because of its anti-inflammatory properties, a recent article in *The New England Journal of Medicine* reported that scientists are studying curcumin as a possible treatment for cystic fibrosis and to help prevent Alzheimer's disease. Its anti-inflammatory effects have been shown to be comparable to those of potent steroids such as hydrocortisone without the significant toxic side effects.

Ginger is another spice whose health benefits have been recognized for centuries, especially for reducing gastrointestinal distress. Recent studies have documented that ginger contains compounds that have potent antioxidant and anti-inflammatory effects. Double-blind studies have demonstrated that ginger is very effective in preventing the symptoms of motion sickness, especially seasickness. Ginger has also been shown to be very useful in reducing the nausea and vomiting of pregnancy—just steep an ounce or two of fresh ginger in a cup of hot water. Ginger contains potent anti-inflammatory substances called gingerols, which may be why they help reduce pain and improve function in many people with osteoarthritis or rheumatoid arthritis.

The National Cancer Institute has identified sage, oregano, thyme, rosemary, fennel, turmeric, caraway, anise, coriander, cumin, and tarragon as having some cancer-preventing activity. Cumin, fennel, tarragon, and caraway contain substances called terpenoids that may help slow or even prevent tumor growth, as well as help reduce blood cholesterol levels. Coriander may be particularly useful in combating carcinogens.

Spices such as cinnamon, garlic, sage, and clove may inhibit bacterial growth and help keep cooked food from spoiling. Paprika and saffron may boost your immune system. Nutmeg and cloves, at least in test-tube studies, have been shown to have antibacterial effects. Chili peppers may help block tumor formation.

Rosemary contains substances that are useful for stimulating the immune system, increasing circulation, and improving digestion. Rosemary also contains anti-inflammatory compounds that may make it useful for reducing the severity of asthma attacks. In addition, rosemary has been shown to increase the blood flow to the head and brain, improving concentration.

In my experience, coriander is a little like rap or hip-hop music—people either love it or they hate it. Coriander is especially rich in protective phytonutrients, as well as a good source of iron, magnesium, manganese, and fiber. It contains nine different antibiotics that help prevent the spread of food-borne illnesses such as salmonella.

What's the best way to consume spices? One way, of course, is to add spices to your cooking. Dried spices are available in most supermarkets, but you may find that the ones in your local ethnic market or spice store are more potent and fresher, and it may have a wider selection. Fresh herbs, especially organic ones, are usually more flavorful and better for you than dried herbs.

You can also buy extracts of many spices in capsules or tablets. These have the advantage of being easy to take, even when you eat out, and they are often in higher concentrations than are usually found in foods.

Variety is the spice of life, and enjoying a variety of spices may help you live a healthier life as well as a more flavorful one.

Love Your Guts

Bacteria are bad, right? Well, not always.

Bacteria do have a bad reputation. Many people believe that all they do is cause infections and illness. But some bacteria are actually good for you. These health-enhancing bacteria are called "probiotics"—literally "for life"—in contrast to antibiotics, which kill bacteria.

In short, while harmful bacteria hate your guts, probiotic bacteria love your guts.

There are literally trillions of bacteria in your body that are good for you, especially in the mouth, gut, and vagina. These are sometimes called your "gut flora." These live in a complex ecological equilibrium with other bacteria and help keep the harmful ones from growing. Some are known to produce vitamin K and B vitamins. They may also aid your digestion, improve the absorption of nutrients, help reduce the formation of carcinogens, and enhance your immune function.

But many forces can throw off this delicate balance, among them aging, alcohol, poor diet, stress, chronic illness, and particularly antibiotics, which kill many of the beneficial intestinal bacteria on the way to killing the pathogenic bacteria they're prescribed to treat. When the bacterial balance in the digestive tract is disrupted, some of the harmful intestinal bacteria may grow too numerous, like weeds taking over a lawn, and cause intestinal distress, diarrhea, or worse. Adding probiotic bacteria to your diet (or taking supplements) may help restore the normal balance of intestinal bacteria.

For example, you may have had diarrhea after taking a course of antibiotics. Two randomized controlled trials showed that probiotics such as *Lactobacillus* may shorten the course of infectious diarrhea by 60 percent by restoring the balance of good bacteria to your gut. In another study, 180 people who were hospitalized and suffering antibiotic-related diarrhea were given a placebo or a probiotic supplement. In the placebo group, 22 percent continued to experience significant diarrhea, but in the probiotic group the figure was just 9 percent. Other studies confirm that probiotic supplements reduce the risk of diarrhea while taking antibiotics.

Probiotics are found in foods and dietary supplements that contain good bacteria such as *Lactobacillus acidophilus, Enterococcus,* and *Bifidobacterium.* Dairy products are a common source of probiotics. The Bible and the sacred books of Hinduism mention cultured dairy products such as yogurt, kefir, koumiss, and leben. These foods were often used medically, particularly for intestinal distress and diarrhea, even though ancient peoples had no idea that these foods worked because of the probiotic bacteria they contained.

The vagina, like the gut, contains bacteria in a dynamic equilibrium, which is one of the reasons why women often develop vaginal infections after taking antibiotics that kill good bacteria as well as harmful ones. Spermicides and birth control pills may also disrupt this internal ecology. Several studies show that friendly microorganisms may help prevent vaginal infections in women. For example, *Lactobacillus acidophilus* makes the vagina too acidic for most of the harmful bacteria to survive. In one study, Israeli researchers recruited forty-six women who had suffered at least four vaginal infections caused by yeast or bacteria during the previous year. The researchers gave them yogurt either with or without live probiotic *Lactobacillus* (about 1 cup a day). After two months, the women who ate the yogurt with the probiotic bacteria experienced significantly fewer vaginal infections.

Other research has shown that probiotics may help the large number of people who suffer from irritable bowel syndrome as well as those with Crohn's disease or ulcerative colitis. Several studies have shown that probiotics may help prevent recurrences of these illnesses.

Probiotic bacteria in the intestine also have other benefits. They have two types of antibiotic action: they secrete some antibiotic compounds, and they form a living barrier that helps prevent bad bacteria from attaching to the intestinal wall and entering the bloodstream.

Probiotics also help prevent allergic reactions. Preliminary research suggests that in children, probiotics reduce the risk of eczema. Animal studies suggest cholesterol-lowering and tumor-preventive action. And probiotics have some antioxidant action, which may help prevent the cell damage at the root of heart disease and many cancers.

At birth, infants' digestive tracts contain only small populations of *Bifidobacterium*. But breast milk contains these bacteria, and breast-feeding raises newborns' population of good bacteria in their gut substantially within a few days. That's one reason why breast-fed infants are less likely to contract infectious diarrhea, a major killer in the developing world.

The easiest way to incorporate probiotic bacteria into your life is to eat a few servings a week of live-culture yogurt. Supplements are another option, although they vary in quality and potency. Since the supplements are not regulated by the FDA, there is likely to be more variability in the number and type of probiotic bacteria in them than in foods.

Probiotics cause no serious side effects, but some people notice increased flatulence and constipation. Pregnant women, nursing mothers, and immunosuppressed patients should check with their physicians before taking probiotics.

6. Anti-inflammatory lifestyle changes are very beneficial.

There is a growing awareness that chronic inflammation may be an underlying factor in a number of chronic diseases, including cardiovascular disease, diabetes, arthritis, dementia, autoimmune diseases, and many others.

In the short run, inflammation, like stress, may be beneficial and is a normal part of your body's defense system. Inflammation is one of your immune system's natural responses to invasive agents it perceives as a threat to your body.

For example, when you have a cut and get a bit of dirt in it, the area becomes inflamed. The external signs of this are swelling, heat, and sensitivity. However, inside your body a specific set of chemical events takes place in which your white blood cells and special chemical messengers called cytokines are mobilized to remove the perceived threat to your body. These chemicals "wall off" that bit of dirt and go about destroying it or getting it out of your body.

Sprained ankles, sore throats, and other conditions of this nature are normal, appropriate responses of our defense system to infection or trauma. This kind of acute inflammation is not only natural, it is critical. We need it to survive. It helps us distinguish friendly molecules from unfriendly ones. Without it, that bit of dirt in your cut might rot and become infected, the tissues in the area might die, and, if you had no immune response to the problem, you might end up being killed by a piece of dirt.

The trouble occurs when this defense system runs out of control and is chronically activated. When inflammation becomes chronic and systemic, your body identifies your own tissues as enemy invaders and begins attacking your organs and tissues. As a result, you may end up in an endless cycle where one part of your chemistry is trying to rebuild your body while another part of your chemistry is tearing it down.

What's worse, as the body begins rebuilding and tearing itself apart this way, it tends to become ever more inflamed. Your immune system is desperately using the only means it knows to protect you against a foreign invader that isn't really foreign. Your tissues become progressively more and more inflamed, and the cycle starts spinning out of control.

Usually chronic inflammation of this nature doesn't have the same outward signs that acute inflammation does. You don't experience it as swelling and heat in a particular area. As a result, you may not even realize that inflammation is a problem for you.

A study of an apparently healthy elderly population found that those with the highest levels of C-reactive protein and interleukin-6 (two markers of systemic inflammation) were 260 percent more likely to die during the next four years than were those with lower levels of these markers. The increase in deaths was due to both cardiovascular and other causes. We may feel healthy, but if inflammation is smoldering inside us, we may be in significant trouble.

One of the ways chronic inflammation can be set off is when the part of your genetic code that controls inflammation is upregulated. The genes that tell your immune system to send out the army of inflammation can be "turned on" by a number of environmental factors. It isn't until these genes are "turned off" that the inflammatory response slows down.

Common treatments for inflammation such as anti-inflammatory drugs (such as ibuprofen or aspirin) or steroids (such as prednisone), though often useful for acute problems, interfere with the body's own immune response and may lead to serious side effects. The benefits of statin cholesterol-lowering drugs such as Lipitor may be due as much to their anti-inflammatory effects as to their cholesterol-lowering ones. Low-dose aspirin may help reduce the risk of heart attacks and colon cancer for the same reason.

What causes chronic inflammation? A number of factors in our diet and lifestyle may play a significant role. These include unhealthful dietary choices, lack of exercise, obesity, metabolic syndrome, chronic stress, smoking, environmental toxins and pollution, and chronic infections.

In the Harvard Nurses' Health Study, for example, higher intakes of red and processed meats, sweets, desserts, and refined grains increased blood markers of inflammation, whereas higher intakes of fruit, vegetables, legumes, fish, poultry, and whole grains decreased blood markers of inflammation. Foods low in calories and saturated fats and high in plant sterols, viscous fiber, soy protein, and nuts also decrease inflammation, as do omega-3 fatty acids.

As you move toward the healthy end of the Spectrum, your risk of chronic inflammation decreases. In addition to nutrition, moderate exercise reduces inflammation. So do stress-management techniques. This is one of the rationales for the Nutrition Spectrum, Exercise Spectrum, and Stress-Management Spectrum throughout this book.

By changing the way you eat, how much you exercise, and how well you manage stress, and by increasing the love and intimacy in your life, you may have a significant impact on the amount of inflammation in your body.

Again, it's not all or nothing. The more you move toward the healthy end of the Spectrum, the more likely you are to reduce the environmental influences that cause inflammation. This is a powerful step toward healing your body, losing weight, and feeling healthy. Inflammation is at the root of so many different diseases that reducing its impact on your health may have a profound influence on your life.

The effects of inflammation are not specific to any one organ or system in your body. If you read a journal from virtually any of the medical specialties, you will find many articles about how inflammation is connected to health concerns in that field. It is one of several common pathways that lead to disease. By modulating the inflammatory response, you can allow your body to begin healing and help protect it from future disease.

7. Choose foods that are nutrient-dense.

Foods that are dense in nutrients are packed with beneficial substances that are essential for your optimal health and well-being, and have the highest nutritional value. Nutrient density is simply the amount of nutrients a food contains divided by the number of calories. In other words, foods are dense in nutrients when they have a lot of nutrients and not very many calories.

The foods that are on the most healthful end of the food spectrum described in chapter 5 are dense in nutrients. In simple terms, they are high in the good stuff and low in the bad stuff. They are dense in nutrients but not in calories.

8. Choose quality over quantity.

Many people try to make up in quantity what they don't have in quality. When you eat high-quality, delicious foods, you don't need as much to feel satisfied as when you wolf down food as you leave a drive-through window.

Ideally, high-quality foods are organic, less processed, and locally grown in ways that utilize sustainable agriculture. Now, I know that this might not be possible or affordable for many people, but it's a goal worth striving for.

Alice Waters, Annie Somerville, Michael Pollan, and others have been pioneers in championing the fact that these foods taste better as well as generally being more healthful. Again, you don't have to choose between foods that taste good and ones that are good for you—you can have both.

Smaller portions of good foods are usually more satisfying than larger portions of junk foods, especially if you pay attention to what you're eating. For example, the "French paradox" (why the French have a lower rate of heart disease than one would expect from their diet) is often attributed to red wine, but other factors may play an even more important role. A meal in France may often include some high-fat items, but generally in small portions, and is usually freshly produced and savored with a group of friends in a dinner that may take several hours to consume. (In my book *Love and Survival*, I described why the social support and community of these meals also have a protective effect.) When food is that good, you can have much more pleasure and a lot fewer calories.

As I wrote in the beginning of this book, I enjoy eating chocolate. Rather than eating a package of high-sugar, low-fat cookies (full of bad carbs), I enjoy dark, high-fat, gourmet chocolate. When I walk inside my favorite store on Union Street in San Francisco, which sells high-quality chocolates from around the world, I feel like, well, a kid in a candy store.

I meditate on chocolate. Meditation is the practice of giving something your full attention and awareness. When I eat a chocolate truffle, for example, I focus fully on it and involve as many of my senses as possible. I notice the color and shape with my eyes, I smell it with my nose, and I feel the texture with my fingers. Before I close my mouth and bite into it, I close my eyes so I can focus fully on the experience.

After the first rush of flavor and sensation, I allow the chocolate to melt in my mouth (not in my hand), and I notice the different flavors and sensations as the texture and temperature of the chocolate begin to change, and how these change as it touches different parts of my hard palate, soft palate, and throat. It's a little like listening to a great musical performance and noticing the subtle variations in tone, pitch, and volume, along with infinitely varying changes in harmonics and overtones.

It can sometimes take several minutes for me to eat a piece of really good chocolate. The experience can be profoundly sensual and gratifying, yet the amount of fat, sugar, and calories is relatively small.

For people who have extensive coronary heart disease and are trying to reverse it, even this amount of chocolate may be unwise. But for most people, having small indulgences like this brings so much pleasure that it makes it easier to eat more healthfully the rest of the time without feeling at all deprived or restricted. Anyway, the first bite is usually the best, the last bite is usually the next best—so if you just have a small amount, you have maximum pleasure with minimum calories.

For me, it's chocolate; for you it might be ice cream, wine, or some other treat such as a wild strawberry. But to the degree that you eat all foods with this heightened awareness, you'll enjoy more and weigh less. Sometimes I eat more than one piece of chocolate at a time, but most of the time, one will do.

Researchers are now finding that consuming dark chocolate in moderation may actually have health benefits. More on this later.

There is a growing awareness among many researchers that foods often have benefits that are not seen when isolated nutrients in these foods are studied. For example, researchers found that people who ate a lot of fruits and vegetables were at lower risk of developing cancer and heart disease. It was presumed that this protective effect was due to beta-carotene, one of the active ingredients in fruits and vegetables.

Since then, there have been a number of studies testing whether taking beta-carotene pills provided the same protection as eating fruits and vegetables.

One study, involving 22,071 physicians, found no statistically significant benefit from the pills after twelve years. Another study tested the effect of beta-carotene in protecting against skin cancer among 1,621 adults. No benefit was found after 4.5 years of treatment.

A Finnish study, testing the effect of beta-carotene among people at high risk of cancer, found that there was an 18 percent *increase* in lung cancer among smokers taking the nutrient compared to smokers who did not. A similar U.S. study found a 28 percent *increase* in lung cancer among men at high risk of the disease who regularly took beta-carotene.

Researchers at Harvard Medical School designed a randomized controlled trial of smokers and gave beta-carotene to almost 20,000 women and an inert placebo to almost 20,000 other women. After four years, they found the same incidence of heart disease and cancer in both groups. However, they found that although beta-carotene was not protective, women smokers who ate five or more carrots per week had a substantially lower risk of developing lung cancer.

Since there are at least 100,000 protective substances in fruits, vegetables, and other foods, it may be that beta-carotene is not the right one to study. However, more likely is that the interaction among these protective substances, in their natural forms, may be what is most beneficial.

In another study, increasing the intake of vitamin E from food sources was shown to reduce the risk of Alzheimer's disease. However, intake of vitamin E from supplements was not significantly associated with the risk of Alzheimer's disease.

In a way, this makes perfect sense. Our bodies have evolved to derive the optimal benefits from foods that occur in their natural, whole, unrefined forms. It's only during the past hundred years or so that food science and technology have made it possible to extract certain nutrients from foods and to process or alter them in new ways, and we may not always be able to predict the outcomes, as these studies are beginning to indicate. Not everything that's natural is good for you, but the chances are much higher that they are.

And what's good for your personal health is also good for the health of our planet. Thanks to former Vice President Al Gore, Lawrence Bender, and others, many people are becoming aware that global warming is a serious concern. However, most people believe that the major cause of global warming is air pollution from cars.

I was surprised to learn that while this is an important factor, according to the U.N. Food and Agriculture Organization's report *Livestock's Long Shadow*, animal-based agribusiness generates more greenhouse gases than all transportation combined. The livestock sector generates more greenhouse gas emissions as measured in carbon dioxide (CO_2) equivalent than does transportation (18 percent versus 13.5 percent). Also, it accounts for 9 percent of CO_2 derived from human-related activities. It generates 65 percent of human-related nitrous oxide, which has 296 times the global warming potential of CO_2. It's also responsible for 37 percent of all human-induced methane, which is twenty-three times more warming than CO_2. Nitrous oxide and methane come mostly from manure. Imagine about 56 billion "food animals" pooping every day.

Also, livestock now use 30 percent of the earth's land surface, mostly for permanent pasture but also including 33 percent of global arable land to produce feed for them. Clearing forests to create new pastures is a major driver of deforestation—some 70 percent of forests in the Amazon have been turned over to grazing.

Eating lower on the food chain is a more efficient way to produce protein. As the earth's population continues to rise and resources decline, eating more foods from the healthier end of the Spectrum frees up more resources to help feed others.

There is more hunger in this country than most people realize. When I learned that one in four children and one in five adults in San Francisco go to bed hungry every night, it really bothered me—especially since this is one of the most affluent cities in the world. So I decided to join the board of directors of the San Francisco Food Bank. I've been very impressed by its dedication and effectiveness in providing food to those who need it most. Every year, it distributes 26 million pounds of food—enough for 55,000 meals per day.

Though giving food to the hungry is important, addressing the underlying causes of hunger is equally significant. It takes many more resources to produce a pound of animal protein than plant-based protein. According to some estimates, it takes sixteen pounds of grain to produce one pound of meat.

Thus, when you help yourself by eating more healthfully, you help the planet as well as those who need it most.

9. Eat less salt.

Your body regulates its concentration of sodium (salt is sodium chloride) very tightly. So if you eat a lot of salt, you can maintain the concentration of sodium in one of two ways.

The first way is to excrete the extra sodium in your urine, which is what most younger people do.

However, especially in someone with long-standing high blood pressure, the kidneys may begin to be slightly damaged, which makes them less efficient at excreting sodium. As a result, if you're eating more sodium than your kidneys can excrete, your body retains water in order to dilute the extra sodium to the same concentration as before. If you retain extra water in a closed system, the pressure begins to rise. As blood pressure rises, the extra force hitting the smaller arteries in the kidneys damages them further, causing them to excrete sodium even less efficiently, and so it continues in a vicious cycle.

If you stop eating more sodium than your body can get rid of, your body will stop retaining extra water, and, as a result, your blood pressure is likely to decrease.

Other factors also regulate blood pressure. Eating more foods containing potassium, or even taking potassium supplements, may help reduce your blood pressure.

In a study of more than three thousand people with slightly elevated blood pressure, Harvard researchers found that those who had significantly reduced their salt intake had a 25 percent lower risk of developing cardiovascular disease than did people who ate their usual diets. Their risk of death from heart disease and stroke was also cut by as much as 20 percent.

Most people in the intervention arm of the studies lowered their sodium intake by 25 to 30 percent, according to Dr. Nancy Cook, Sc.D., of Brigham and Women's Hospital and Harvard Medical School, who conducted the study. "This was not salt restriction, it was salt reduction," said Cook. "These people ate normal diets, but we taught them how to look out for hidden salt and avoid it. Americans consume much more sodium than is necessary, and it comes mostly from processed foods and the foods we eat in restaurants."

Thus, a 25 percent reduction in salt equals a 25 percent reduction in cardiovascular disease.

Last summer, the American Medical Association (AMA) called for a minimum 50 percent reduction in sodium in processed foods, fast foods, and non–fast food restaurant meals within a decade. The group also called on the Food and Drug Administration (FDA) to make greater efforts to educate consumers about the health risks associated with a high-sodium diet.

Dr. James Rohack, who was on the AMA board that issued the directives, says that 150,000 lives could be saved in the United States annually if everyone cut his or her sodium consumption in half. Most people eat much more salt than they realize, he says, because restaurant meals and processed foods have replaced home cooking in much of the American diet.

The American Heart Association recommends that healthy adults should not exceed 2,300 milligrams of sodium a day. This is equal to about one teaspoon of table salt, but sodium is found in many processed and prepackaged foods. According to Dr. Rohack, "The average American is eating three times as much salt as is healthy every day—the equivalent of two to three teaspoons instead of no more than one."

In summary, excessive salt, sugar, meat, and fat may increase your blood pressure, whereas fruits and vegetables may lower it.

Some people are more sensitive to the effects of diet on their blood pressure than others. If you have high blood pressure, try eating less salt, sugar, meat, and fat and more fruits and vegetables. If that's enough to lower your blood pressure, great; if not, make even bigger changes. There's no way to accurately predict who is likely to respond better to reducing salt intake than others, so just try it and see. More on this in the next chapters. Also, experiment with spices as replacements for salt.

10. Drink more tea.

I love coffee. I love the way it smells. I love the way it tastes. (Although I'm so sensitive to caffeine, even a cup of coffee makes me talk as fast as Robin Williams might sound if he were on speed—and, hey, do you have to drive so slowly?) But I drink tea now, most of the time.

Apparently, I'm not alone. Tea is the most widely consumed beverage in the world, other than water. More than 6.6 billion pounds of tea are produced each year. Why? Tea contains a variety—perhaps thousands—of powerful, protective antioxidant substances called polyphenols, especially flavonoids such as catechins, that may help reduce the risk of some of the most common chronic diseases.

For example, a study published in *The Journal of the American Medical Association* followed more than 40,000 Japanese men and women over a seven- to eleven-year period. They found that green tea consumption was associated with a reduced mortality due to all causes except cancer. The more green tea they drank, the lower their risk of dying early. After seven years of follow-up, researchers found that that the overall risk of premature death due to illness was 26 percent lower among those who consumed five or more cups of green tea a day than among those who drank less than one cup per day.

Interestingly, the effects of tea on reducing the risk of cardiovascular disease were caused not only by changes in traditional risk factors such as cholesterol levels or blood pressure; the polyphenols in green tea appear to have powerful antioxidant properties and are scavengers for free radicals that could otherwise damage your cells. These polyphenols may directly and beneficially affect coronary artery blockages (atherosclerosis), dilate arteries, and help reduce the formation of blood clots. Green tea also has significant anti-inflammatory effects. Black tea and oolong teas were found to be less protective than green tea.

This is not surprising. Teas are categorized by their level of fermentation: green tea is unfermented (and so retains the original color of the tea leaves), oolong tea is partially fermented, and black tea is fermented (which makes it dark in color). The process of fermentation reduces the protective activity of the flavonoids, the level of which is highest in green tea, intermediate in oolong tea, and lowest in black tea. On the other hand, the caffeine level is highest in black tea, intermediate in oolong, and lowest in green tea. The caffeine in green tea is also lower than in coffee or caffeinated soft drinks.

Unfortunately, about 77 percent of the tea produced and consumed in the world is black tea, only 21 percent is green tea, and less than 2 percent is oolong tea, according to a recent study in the *International Journal of Cardiology.* The concentration of protective catechins in the blood after drinking green tea is three times higher than after drinking black tea. Still, while green tea is best, all teas have been shown to have health benefits.

Although the Japanese researchers did not find that drinking tea reduced the risk of cancer, other studies have. Animal studies have shown that green tea may inhibit cancer formation in the skin, lung, oral cavity, esophagus, stomach, liver, kidney, prostate, and other organs. In humans, studies suggest that drinking tea may reduce the risk of digestive cancers.

For example, a study of more than 35,000 postmenopausal women in Iowa, published in the *American Journal of Epidemiology* in 1996, found that those who drank more than two cups of tea per day were 32 percent less likely to have cancers throughout their digestive tract, including in the mouth, esophagus, stomach, colon, and rectum than those who did not. Four or more cups of tea per day lowered the risk of such cancers by 63 percent.

Some (but not all) studies with varying degrees of rigor suggest that drinking tea may reduce the risk of early-stage breast, prostate, ovarian, and lung cancers. In one study, green tea extract was found to stimulate prostate cancer cell death. The evidence was strong enough to interest the

National Cancer Institute in conducting a phase II study of green tea extract in men with metastatic prostate cancer, which is now in progress.

Other studies indicate that certain catechins in tea may reduce the risk of skin cancer. Animal studies have tended to show greater value of tea in preventing cancers than in human studies, perhaps because of the differences in diet, environment, and genetics in humans.

In earlier studies, researchers from the Harvard Boston Area Health Study showed that men and women who had consumed one or more cups of green tea per day in the previous year had a 44 percent lower risk of heart attack than those who drank no tea. Other studies indicate that regular drinking of green tea or oolong tea may reduce the risk of developing high blood pressure despite the caffeine, especially when the tea is consumed with meals rather than on an empty stomach. Tea increases the body's production of nitric oxide, which dilates arteries and thereby reduces blood pressure.

Green tea catechins have also been reported to have antibacterial, antiviral, and antifungal activity, especially in early stages of infection. Affected infections include some types of salmonella, *Helicobacter pylori,* influenza virus, herpes simplex, and *Candida albicans.* Also, green tea consumption has been associated with increased bone density and fewer hip fractures.

Some studies suggest that tea may help regulate your blood sugar and may even reduce the risk of diabetes. Flavonoids in tea may have both insulin-like and insulin-enhancing activities. According to Chinese medicine, tea helps control obesity. A classical Chinese pharmaceutical book called *Bencao Shiyi* states, "Drinking tea for a long time will make one live long to stay in good shape without becoming too fat and too heavy." Tea may help reduce obesity by increasing metabolism, reducing fat absorption, activating enzymes, and reducing appetite.

If that's not enough, drinking green tea may reduce your risk of cavities (especially if you don't add sugar) by inhibiting bacterial growth as well as potentially harmful enzymes in your mouth. Also, both green and black teas are natural sources of fluoride, which is why you may find tea as an ingredient in your toothpaste.

Clearly, more research needs to be done. However, coffee does not have the same health benefits as tea. The potential benefits of tea are so great, the side effects relatively small (primarily, the effects of drinking caffeine), and the costs so low that I decided not to wait for more conclusive studies to be conducted and began drinking tea instead of coffee. Most of the time.

In the next chapters, I'll show you how you can make the degree of changes in diet and lifestyle—if any—that you choose to. How much, and to what degree, is up to you. Only you.

YOU ARE UNIQUE

Always remember that you are absolutely unique.
Just like everyone else.

—Margaret Mead

■ ■ ■ ■ ■ ■ ■ ■

You are unique.

In chapter 5, I'll describe the full spectrum of nutrition and lifestyle choices and how you can determine where on this spectrum you currently are and where you may want to be on it.

This approach, sometimes called "personalized medicine," is the medicine of the future, and it's available to you right now.

We're all completely distinctive. We respond differently to changes in diet and lifestyle, and we respond differently to medications.

As I described earlier, foods are neither good nor bad, but some foods are more healthful for you than others. In chapter 5, I've categorized and ranked foods from the most to least healthful according to the criteria described in the previous chapters. If I slip and call them "bad foods" or "good foods," just know that I mean "healthful" or "unhealthful"; there's no moral judgment there. I'll also describe how you can use this information to customize a way of eating and a way of living that's just right for you based on your own needs and preferences.

In simple terms, foods on the healthiest end of the spectrum have the most good stuff and the least bad stuff, whereas foods on the least healthful end of the spectrum have the opposite qualities. These factors include how much and what types of fat, carbohydrates, and protein, as well as the amounts of sugar and salt, nutrient density, calories, fiber, glycemic index/glycemic load, inflammatory properties, and antioxidant effects; the degree of refinement; and the number and amount of other beneficial substances (such as the phytochemicals, bioflavonoids, carotenoids, retinols, isoflavones, genistein, lycopene, polyphenols, sulforaphanes and so on described earlier).

How much you may need to change is a function of how much improvement you want to accomplish. As I'll discuss more fully later in this chapter, our studies showed that the more people changed their diet and lifestyle, the more improvement we measured. This is a very hopeful and empowering message.

If you're trying to stop or even reverse the progression of coronary heart disease, prostate cancer, diabetes, or other serious chronic diseases, you'll probably need to eat most of your foods from the healthiest end of the spectrum. These foods form the basis of what I called the "Reversal Diet" in my earlier books, also known as the "pound of cure." And if you're not interested in making bigger changes, you can consider taking medications—if so, you'll likely need fewer medications and lower doses of them to the degree that you spend most of your time on the healthier end of the Spectrum.

If you're healthy but have certain factors that put you at higher risk of chronic disease, such as elevated cholesterol levels, weight, blood pressure, or blood sugar, you can begin by finding where you are currently on the Spectrum and making more moderate changes in diet and lifestyle. If that's enough to achieve your goals, great; if not, you may want to consider making bigger changes.

Along the same lines, you have a spectrum of choices in how frequently, long, and intensely you exercise and also in how you practice stress-management techniques. For example, the more you exercise, the more fit you become and the more weight you lose, but if you're just trying to stay healthy and reduce your risk of premature death, simply walking twenty to thirty minutes per day—and not necessarily very fast or all at once—may be sufficient. More on this in chapter 8.

This process of customizing a way of eating and living for you is an empirical, iterative process—in other words, you make some changes in your diet and lifestyle based on moving in the healthful direction on the Spectrum, monitor your progress, and then fine-tune these lifestyle modifications based on how well you're responding to the changes you've made so far.

You can monitor changes in a variety of ways—including objective parameters as well as improvements in how you feel—as a way of determining how much further you may need to go, if at all, in a healthy direction on the Spectrum.

If moderate changes in diet and lifestyle are enough to accomplish your goals—e.g., losing a few pounds, lowering your LDL cholesterol a few points, having more energy, etc.—great. That may be all you need to do. If not, you can make progressively bigger changes in your diet and lifestyle by moving further in the healthy direction on the Spectrum.

In our research, we initially focused on proving that the progression of coronary heart disease can often be reversed by making the changes in diet and lifestyle on the most healthful end of the Spectrum. Along the way, we also found that similar changes in nutrition and lifestyle can often cause significant improvements in high blood pressure, diabetes, hypercholesterolemia, obesity, arthritis, depression, prostate cancer (and, by extension, breast cancer), and other chronic diseases.

This approach is consistent not only with our own research but also with many other studies showing, for example, that fruits, vegetables, good carbs, and some good fats may help prevent a wide variety of health problems. They are not disease-specific.

Similarly, chronic stress may be an important factor in contributing to many different types of illnesses. Because Western researchers tend to study specific diseases in isolation from one another, they often miss the patterns of underlying causes that play a role in most illnesses, especially chronic diseases.

Within each condition, I'll give you some suggestions for fine-tuning your place on the Spectrum. For example, if you have high blood pressure, you may want to try eating less salt; if you have diabetes, you may need to be more mindful of your intake of refined carbohydrates than someone else would; if you're trying to lower your LDL cholesterol, you may need to reduce your intake of saturated fat more than others would. More on this in the next chapter. This approach is sometimes called nutritional genomics, or nutrigenomics.

YOUR GENES ARE NOT YOUR DESTINY

Your genes do play a role in a number of conditions. But in most cases, your genes are only a *predisposition* toward various conditions. If your genes make you more likely to have diabetes or heart disease or to gain weight, it just means you may need to go further in a healthy direction on the Spectrum than someone else would in order to prevent or reverse these conditions.

We know, for example, that Pima Indians develop type 2 diabetes at eight times the rate of white Americans. However, Pima Indians who change their diet and lifestyle can often prevent or even reverse their diabetes, so their genetic predisposition can be overcome by making sufficient changes in their diet and lifestyle.

There are at least fifty genes involved in gaining too much weight. Some of these genes influence appetite, others affect your resting metabolic rate (how many calories you burn just sitting still), and yet others play a role in how you deposit fat in your tissues.

For example, some people hold on to fat very efficiently. In earlier times, when food was scarce, this gave them a survival advantage—those who stored calories most efficiently tended to weigh more and live longer during times of famine. Those who did this best were most likely to survive and to pass their genes along to the next generation. Also, when food was scarce, their metabolism would slow down, causing them to burn calories more slowly and to be more likely to survive when food was not very available.

However, in modern times, those same genes may threaten your survival as they predispose you to gain too much weight. Also, this helps explain why losing weight by just consuming fewer calories can be so frustrating. If you reduce your caloric intake by one third, at first you lose weight. But your body may then think you're starving, so these genes kick in and cause your metabolism to slow down by one third so you burn calories more slowly and may stop losing weight even if you keep consuming fewer calories. This is sometimes called the "thrifty genotype hypothesis."

BUGS, DRUGS, AND SLUGS

Some intriguing new studies raise the possibility that the microorganisms in your gut may also affect how much you weigh. As I described in the previous chapter, there are literally trillions of microbes in your intestinal tract. When the balance of these is not disrupted by antibiotics, stress, or other factors, these microbes have a number of helpful functions in your body: they produce some vitamins, provide enzymes that help with digestion, and help metabolize cholesterol.

These microbes also affect how efficiently your body absorbs the calories in your diet. For example, mice that have been raised in germ-free laboratories and had no intestinal microbes had 60 percent less body fat than real-world mice, even though they ate more food.

It may be that variations in the number of microbes in different people's intestinal tracts may account for part of their differences in weight. Two people may eat foods with exactly the same number of calories, but one may be more efficient at absorbing those calories than the other due to differences in their intestinal microbes.

In related studies, some intriguing research by Drs. Richard Atkinson and Nikhil Dhurandhar found that infecting animals with a type of virus called the Ad-36 adenovirus caused them to gain weight. When they studied humans, they found that people who had antibodies to this virus weighed significantly more than those who did not.

They also examined identical twins, in whom one had antibodies to this virus but the other did not. The twin with the antibodies to the virus (in other words, who had had a prior infection with it) had 2 percent more body fat than the other twin, even though their genes were identical.

Dr. Atkinson started a company called Obetech that will test you to see if you have the antibody to the Ad-36 adenovirus (for $450). Those who do are more likely to gain weight, so knowing this may help them become more mindful of their diet and lifestyle.

However, many other factors are involved, not just a virus. One of the most useful tests is also the least expensive and most widely available: standing on a scale each day. If you find that your weight is beginning to increase, move a little closer to the healthy end of the Spectrum, as described in the next chapter.

Some people believe that the inflammation that is often seen with obesity may be caused by a virus and that the virus causes both the obesity and the inflammation. However, obesity causes inflammation even in people who do not have antibodies to the Ad-36 adenovirus, and this inflammation may play an important role in a number of illnesses, as I described in the previous chapter.

Some companies are now emerging with the claim that they can analyze a sample of your DNA from your blood, hair, or tissue and provide you with a tailored recommendation of the diet and lifestyle changes you should be making. Caveat emptor: let the buyer beware. According to Jose Ordovas, Director of the nutrition and genomics laboratory at the U.S. Department of Agriculture Nutrition Research Center at Tufts University in Boston, "We have scientific evidence that the concept is right, that we can provide something along those lines in the future, but we are not there yet."

There *are* credible companies that can do genetic testing for determining whether you're at increased risk for specific illnesses. Now that Dr. Craig Venter had his entire genome decoded, it's only a matter of time before the cost of doing so becomes affordable for most people. As more information becomes available, your predisposition to developing different illnesses will become clearer. If you find that you're at higher risk, then this information may be helpful in motivating you to go further toward the healthy end of the Spectrum than you might otherwise be inclined to do.

For example, the Sciona company in Boulder, Colorado, is offering a DNA test kit for $99 that claims to provide you with personalized diet advice for heart health, bone health, or any of three other areas. Sciona asks people to complete a diet and lifestyle questionnaire and collect their own DNA with a cheek swab to send in for analysis. Current testing focuses on nineteen genes.

Studies show that people with a certain version of a gene called MTHFR tend to have high blood levels of a substance called homocysteine, which has been linked to a higher risk of heart disease and stroke. People with high levels of homocysteine can take more folate and vitamins B_6 and B_{12} to reduce their homocysteine levels. However, homocysteine levels can be measured with a standard blood test at a doctor's office, so the gene testing doesn't really add much, if anything.

Furthermore, according to Gregory Kurtz, who led a probe by the Government Accountability Office, or GAO (the investigative arm of Congress), these tests are of no medical value and can mislead people: "I want to send a message to consumers across the country: Buyer beware."

Investigators bought kits from companies selling through four websites and created fourteen pretend customers. The questionnaires described consumers of different ages and lifestyles but were paired with DNA samples from only two people. The advice the investigators received varied greatly, but mostly contained generalities such as advice not to smoke and that people with bad diets may have a higher risk of developing heart disease.

According to the Associated Press, one company advised three of the fictitious customers to buy a "personalized" dietary supplement blend, costing more than $1,880 a year, that the company claimed could repair damaged DNA. A second company recommended a supplement blend for $1,200 a year that contained the same multivitamins that can be bought in any drugstore for about $35.

"We stop where the science stops," said Rosalynn Gill-Garrison, Chief Science Officer of Sciona. Asked how the company could offer different nutrition advice for the same DNA, Gill-Garrison said that that was to be expected because although there were only two different DNA samples, the health questionnaires varied, and the advice offered was tailored to the questionnaire responses about customers' current diet and health as well as the genomic findings.

There is more evidence for some conditions and some foods than others. For example, as I mentioned in the previous chapter, green tea contains potent antioxidants known to help reduce the risk of coronary heart disease and some types of cancer, but some women who drink tea seem to show less reduction in breast cancer than others. In part, this may be due to a gene that produces an enzyme called COMT, which inactivates some of tea's cancer-suppressing substances. Women who have the gene variant that produces a less-active form of COMT showed the most benefit from tea.

About 10 to 20 percent of the population has a specific genetic variation that makes it harder for their body to absorb calcium in the presence of caffeine, thus increasing the rate of bone loss. If you knew this, then you might be more likely to take a calcium supplement and less likely to drink caffeine.

Another example of where genetic testing may be helpful is the gene for a protein known as apo E, which plays an important role in regulating cholesterol. It has three major variants designated E2, E3, and E4, of which E3 is the most common. People with one or two copies of the E2 variant generally have lower cholesterol levels than usual, but the E4 variant increases the risk of diabetes, raises total cholesterol levels, reverses the usual protective effects of moderate drinking, and substantially increases the risks of smoking.

The good news is that even if you have the E4 variant—seen in about 15 to 30 percent of people—there is an even more compelling reason to make the changes in diet and lifestyle that I describe in the next chapter. If you quit smoking and drinking, maintain a normal body weight, and eat a diet low in trans–fatty acids and saturated fat, you can remove virtually *all* of the increased genetic risk caused by the E4 variant.

While some companies are making claims that go beyond the current state of science, others are much more thoughtful and credible. These include companies such as Navigenics, 23&Me, DNA Direct, deCODE genetics, and others that are actively exploring the extraordinary promise of genomics counseling.

As I wrote in the beginning of this book, awareness is the first step in healing. Genetic testing may play a limited role in highlighting areas in which you may have a genetic predisposition to certain illnesses, which, in turn, may motivate you to make and maintain bigger changes in your diet and lifestyle than you might otherwise. But having an ultrafast CT scan or a 64-slice CT scan to detect early coronary heart disease can be more motivating for many people to change their diet and lifestyle than just learning that they may be at increased risk.

Eventually it may be possible to make precise recommendations for most people based simply on their genetic testing. However, there are more than 25,000 genes in the human genome and more than 3 million common variants within those genes so the challenges are formidable. In addition, foods have thousands of biologically active compounds, so it may be some time before all of these interactions are sorted out.

THE VISION

Because this field is evolving so rapidly, my colleagues and I are developing a website (www.OrnishSpectrum.com) that will offer additional support and resources in personalizing a way of living and eating beyond what this or any book can provide.

Also, genetic testing may progress in the near future to a point that could be very useful. Since your own genetic variability is a factor in where you may want to be on the Spectrum, let's discuss how your genes influence your health.

IT'S *NOT* ALL IN YOUR GENES

Your genes *do* play a role in your health, but they are only part of the story.

For example, two studies recently published in the journal *Science* revealed that three common variations in genes more than doubled the risk of having a heart attack in men who were less than 50 years old and women less than 60 years old.

In the first study, scientists at deCODE genetics in Iceland examined blood samples from more than 17,000 people and compared those who had heart disease with those who did not. They found that there were very small gene variations in those who had heart disease—just single letters of the DNA code, called SNPs (pronounced "snips"), or single-nucleotide polymorphisms. People with this variant on both chromosomes rather than on just one—20 percent of Caucasians—had more than double the risk of developing heart disease at an early age.

In the second study, also published in the same issue of *Science* (it's interesting how different investigators in other parts of the world often make the same discovery at the same time), researchers at the University of Ottawa Heart Institute in Canada looked at DNA changes in more than 28,000 people. They identified another SNP on the same chromosome as the Iceland group that increased the risk of developing early heart disease. People of European descent who had this DNA variant on one chromosome had a 25 percent greater risk of developing heart disease at an early age, and those who had it on both chromosomes had a 40 percent increased risk. In both studies, this increased risk of heart disease was not found in those of African descent.

Another recent study identified seven SNP variants that increase the risk of diabetes. Interestingly, the people who are at highest risk for diabetes may also show the most improvement from making comprehensive lifestyle changes. More research is likely to identify other genes that are associated with an increased risk of illness.

Not surprisingly, genes appear linked to obesity as well. In a recent study, researchers at the University of Oxford found that another common gene variation markedly increased the risk of obesity. Approximately 50 percent of white Europeans have one defective copy of the gene, which increased the risk of obesity by about one third. However, approximately 16 percent of people have two altered copies of the gene, and these people have a 70 percent increased risk of obesity.

These findings are consistent with a classic study of adoptees conducted in Denmark and a study of twins conducted in Sweden. Researchers led by Dr. Albert Stunkard found that there was a strong relation between the weight of adoptees and their biological parents but not between adoptees and their adoptive parents. The Swedish researchers found that the body mass index of twins reared apart was only slightly lower than those reared together, whereas there was more variation in fraternal twins, who share only some of the same genes.

SO WHAT DOES THIS MEAN TO YOU?

Some people may say, "Well, looks like it's all in my genes. There's not much I can do about it." It's tempting to take a nihilistic view since it absolves us of any personal responsibility. But it also means we're powerless, and I don't like feeling that way. Besides, it's not true. Our genes are only part of the story.

I discussed this with Dr. James Hill (Director, Center for Human Nutrition, University of Colorado Health Sciences Center). He replied, "Telling people it's all in their genes is a devastating message. There are a few rare individuals in whom genes are just so bad that the amount of work to maintain a healthy weight is not feasible. But for most people, their genes allow them to maintain a healthy weight if they're willing to make sufficient changes in diet and lifestyle. Some have to work harder than others, and exercise becomes even more important for those who are genetically disadvantaged."

According to Ryan Phelan, Founder and CEO of DNA Direct (a company that offers genetic testing), "It's about putting your genes in context, in perspective—your overall health with the conditions within which you live, including stress, the environment, all of the other lifestyle factors. It's important not to overstate the role of genetics. My hope is that this is really the beginning of personalized medicine for the masses. It's crazy the way our health care system has had to treat us all like we're one and the same person. We're all completely unique. We respond differently to diet, we respond differently to medications, and some small part of that—some people say as much as 20 percent—can be linked to our genetic differences. So to me the challenge is to find where that genetic variance is—to help people use it as a motivational factor, not as a deterrent."

EMPOWER, NOT BLAME

To be responsible is not to blame ourselves, it's to empower us. If we're just victims of our bad genes, bad karma, bad fate, or bad luck, then there's not much we can do about it other than to suffer our destiny. But to the degree that we realize that we *can* do something about it, then we're free to change our fortunes. These new genetic discoveries can help us understand how much we might *need* to change in order to accomplish our goals and to stay healthy and feel good. How much you *want* to change your diet and lifestyle—if at all—is a very personal decision.

Although there is a genetic predisposition to chronic diseases such as coronary heart disease, diabetes, and obesity—and, in all likelihood, to many other illnesses as well—in almost all cases, it is just a predisposition, not a death sentence. For example, even if your mother and father and sister and brother and aunts and uncles died from coronary heart disease, it doesn't mean that you will. However, it probably means that you have to make bigger changes in diet and lifestyle than someone who has better genes.

According to Dr. David Heber (Director, UCLA Center for Human Nutrition), "Genes load the gun, but environment pulls the trigger. The idea that it's all in your genes is nonsense. The human genome changes only one half of one percent every million years. The obesity epidemic is only about thirty years old, so changes in genes do not explain the recent dramatic rise in obesity, not only in this country but also worldwide."

THE MORE PEOPLE CHANGED, THE BETTER THEY BECAME

As I mentioned earlier, during the past thirty years, my colleagues and I at the nonprofit Preventive Medicine Research Institute have conducted a series of randomized controlled trials and demonstration projects documenting, for the first time, that the progression of coronary heart disease may be reversed by making the intensive and comprehensive changes in diet and lifestyle that I recommend. In collaboration with Dr. Peter Carroll (Chair, Department of Urology, School of Medicine, University of California, San Francisco), we found that our program may also slow, stop, or perhaps even reverse the progression of early-stage prostate cancer and, by extension, some types of breast cancer as well.

When I first began conducting these studies, I thought that younger patients with milder heart disease who didn't have a strong family history of heart disease would be more likely to show improvement, but I was wrong. The primary determinant of the degree of improvement was not age, disease severity, or genetics; it was the degree of change in diet and lifestyle. In other words, the more people changed, the more their heart disease improved, both after one year and after five years. Also, the longer they stayed on the program, the more they improved—on average, there was significantly more heart disease reversal after five years than after one year.

We had similar findings with prostate cancer—the more closely people followed our program of nutrition and lifestyle changes, the more improvement we measured in both their PSA levels (a marker for prostate cancer) and their prostate tumor growth.

In short, the more people changed their diet and lifestyle and the longer they maintained these changes, the better they became.

CAN I CHANGE MY GENES BY CHANGING MY DIET AND LIFESTYLE?

Based on these findings, Dr. Carroll and I, along with our colleagues at the Preventive Medicine Research Institute and the School of Medicine, University of California, San Francisco, collaborated on a study to find out if our program of comprehensive changes in diet and lifestyle could affect how genes are expressed in men with prostate cancer.

In this study, we enrolled men with biopsy-proven prostate cancer and asked them to follow the program described in this book from the healthiest end of the Spectrum. After just three months, we repeated their prostate biopsy.

Surprisingly, we found that hundreds of genes were affected—in simple terms, these changes in diet and lifestyle may have "turned on" (upregulated) some of the more beneficial genes and may have "turned off" (downregulated) some of the more harmful ones. For example a gene that promotes inflammation and is elevated in breast cancer was downregulated.

These extraordinary results captured my imagination. We are still trying to understand their full significance, but it's already clear that while you can't change your genes, you may be able to alter, at least to some degree, how your genes are expressed simply by changing your diet and lifestyle.

I find this to be a profoundly hopeful message and an antidote to genetic nihilism. It's *not* all in your genes.

In a related study, described more fully in chapter 6, we found that these comprehensive lifestyle changes were able to significantly increase the DNA-repairing enzyme telomerase in only three months.

A recent study by investigators in Finland randomly assigned men and women with metabolic syndrome (which includes elevated blood sugar, obesity, and high blood pressure) to a rye-pasta diet (with a low insulin response) or an oat-wheat-potato diet (with a high insulin response).

After twelve weeks, those in the low-insulin-response group had seventy-one genes showing decreased expression and none showing increased expression. In the high-insulin-response group, sixty-two genes showed increased expression and none showed decreased expression. Some of these genes were related to diet and disease.

An editorial accompanying this article stated:

> Molecular pathways involved in hormone action have been the target of a multibillion-dollar pharmaceutical research effort. However, many of these pathways may normally be under dietary regulation. The results of the present study emphasize the age-old wisdom to "use food as medicine"—in this case, for the targeted prevention and treatment of obesity, diabetes, and heart disease.

These research results resonate with the basic theme of this book: what you choose to eat, and how you choose to live each day, may make a powerful difference in your health and well-being, and you have a spectrum of choices. It's not always easy to change your diet and lifestyle, but knowing that these changes are likely to make a big difference in your health and well-being can be a persuasive motivator.

These research findings provide yet another series of mechanisms to help explain why changes in diet and lifestyle affect our health and well-being—for better and for worse.

When I first began conducting research thirty years ago, the idea that heart disease could be reversed by anything was considered impossible, but especially not just by changing diet and lifestyle, and definitely not in only thirty days. After all, coronary artery blockages take decades to build up, so how could they show any measurable improvement in only a month?

Yet we showed that coronary heart disease *did* begin to reverse in the patients we studied in only a month. We knew *that* they were getting better, but we didn't have a clue *why* they were improving, especially in such a short time.

Over the next decades, the mechanisms that cause coronary heart disease became increasingly well understood. For example, your arteries are not rigid pipes in which rust builds up over time. They are flexible and are lined with what's called smooth muscle, which causes them to constrict or dilate.

It turns out that a diet high in fat and cholesterol makes your arteries more likely to constrict. So do too much sugar and other refined carbohydrates (bad carbs). So does nicotine. So does cocaine. So does a lack of exercise. So does emotional stress.

We're at a similar place now—just as we found in our earlier research that chronic diseases such as heart disease, diabetes, and prostate cancer were much more dynamic and modifiable than had previously been realized, we're finding that the same may be true with your genes as well.

Though you can't change your genes, it appears that you *may* be able to alter how they are expressed—for better and for worse—just by changing your diet and lifestyle. These changes may also help explain why we were able to bring about such major improvements in a relatively short time. We're just beginning to understand the significance of these findings. The emerging field of nutritional genomics, or nutrigenomics, is based on these concepts.

As we gain a greater understanding of the mechanisms by which comprehensive lifestyle changes affect our health and well-being, we have more reasons to explain why these changes play such a powerful role in health and illness and how to tailor a program.

In short, you have a spectrum of nutrition and lifestyle choices. Your genes are only one factor in determining where you are on this continuum.

Your genes *do* play an important role in health and well-being, more so for some people than for others. However, in most cases, diet and lifestyle modifications override genetics if you're willing to make big enough changes. Those with a strong family history of a disease may have to make bigger changes in diet and lifestyle than others who have better genes. Most of the time, nurture trumps nature, but it's not always easy. However, it may be easier than you think.

5

THE NUTRITION SPECTRUM

Food is an important part of a balanced diet.

—Fran Lebowitz

■ ■ ■ ■ ■ ■ ■ ■ ▪ ▫

Foods are neither good nor bad, but some are more healthful for you than others.

This chapter outlines the nutrition spectrum. Based on the latest science, while recognizing the limitations of research, I have categorized foods from the most healthful (Group 1) to the least healthful (Group 5).

I started to say "most indulgent" to describe Group 5, but that's part of the problem. Whether or not a food is healthful is not the primary determinant of how good it tastes. How fresh are the ingredients? Where was it grown? Was it grown locally? Is it organic? How processed is it? How skillfully was it prepared?

As the gifted chef Art Smith's recipes show, you can make Group 1 and Group 2 foods that are good for you and also taste great and feel indulgent. (Conversely, less-skillful chefs can make Group 5 foods unappealing if they're not well prepared.)

Most of Art's recipes begin with ingredients from Group 1. I also asked him to offer variations of most of his recipes that include ingredients from other groups so you can customize each meal based on your own desires, needs, and preferences. The only exception is that some of his desserts include butter and sugar, so these ingredients put these recipes in a higher group category and should be considered special treats, and are only for those who do not have serious health or weight problems.

I've worked with many chefs over the years, and Art is truly extraordinary. He uses just the right balance of foods that are delicious and nutritious, in recipes that are sophisticated yet easy to prepare. Even I can make them! (Well, most of them . . .)

I want to emphasize again what I've been saying all along in this book: what matters most is your *overall* way of eating. I am not saying that you should never consume foods from Group 5 (unless you have a serious health condition). If you indulge yourself one day by eating foods from Group 4 or 5, spend a little more time in Groups 1 and 2 the next day.

If you go *on* a diet, chances are that you'll go *off* it. Sooner or later. For most people, being on a diet—*any* diet—is not sustainable.

Even the word "diet" conjures up feeling restricted, deprived, controlled—all the manipulative, fascist feelings I described in chapter 2.

In contrast, the Spectrum approach is all about freedom and choice. There is no diet to get on and no diet to get off. Nothing is forbidden. No "Thou Shalt Nots," no "You Better!" No guilt, no shame; no right, no wrong.

The Spectrum is based on love, not willpower. It's about feeling good, not just avoiding feeling bad. Joy of living, not fear of dying. Losing weight and gaining health.

Okay, here's how it works.

First, find your place on the Spectrum based on the foods you tend to eat most of the time. Then, according to your own needs and preferences, decide how far, and how quickly, you want to move in a more healthful direction (if at all). In general, the further you move toward the Group 1 end of the Spectrum and the faster you move there, the more benefits you're likely to gain and the more quickly you'll experience them.

It's not all or nothing.

In the chapters that follow, I describe how you can use the Spectrum for specific conditions—to lose weight, lower your blood pressure, decrease your cholesterol level, and help prevent or even reverse the progression of diabetes, prostate cancer, breast cancer, and heart disease. Of course, the health benefits of making these changes are not limited to these illnesses; rather, these are examples of how powerful these changes may be.

In general, if you're healthy and just want to stay that way, you may not need or want to make very many changes at all. If you're trying to reverse heart disease, you probably need to make much bigger changes than otherwise.

Foods in Group 1 are, in general, the most healthful. As Michael Pollan writes in the opening of one of his essays, "Eat food. Not too much. Mostly plants." This is a good example of what I mentioned in chapter 1—someone who is able to distill a complex subject to its most important essence.

Group 1 foods are predominantly fruits, vegetables, whole grains, legumes, soy products, nonfat dairy products, and egg whites in their natural forms, as well as some good fats that contain omega-3 fatty acids. As I mentioned in chapter 3, these are the foods that are rich in good carbs, good fats, good proteins, and other protective substances. There are at least 100,000 substances in these foods that have powerful anticancer, anti–heart disease, and antiaging properties.

Group 2 foods are also predominantly plant-based but somewhat higher in fat (predominantly monosaturated fat and polyunsaturated fat) such as avocados, seeds, and nuts. Oils are included but in small amounts, since they are so dense in calories. Canola oil is a better choice than olive oil, as previously noted, since canola oil contains some of the good omega-3 fatty acids and a better ratio of omega-6 fatty acids to omega-3 fatty acids. Group 2 also includes foods canned in water (rather than sugary syrup), canned vegetables (if their sodium content is not too high), low-fat (1%) dairy products, decaffeinated beverages, low-sodium soy sauce, and so on.

Group 3 includes some fish and seafood, some refined carbohydrates and concentrated sweeteners (in moderation), some oils that are higher in saturated fat, oils that have a higher ratio of omega-6 fatty acids to omega-3 fatty acids, some reduced-fat (2%) dairy products, margarines free of trans–fatty acids, sweeteners containing high-fructose corn syrup, and foods containing more sodium.

In Group 3, I have given preference to fish and seafood that are higher in omega-3 fatty acids, such as salmon. Anchovies are high in omega-3 fatty acids but also high in fat if packed in oil. Wild salmon tends to be lower in bad stuff (mercury, dioxin, PCBs) than is farmed salmon, which should especially be avoided by pregnant and nursing women (although pregnant and nursing women should be sure to take omega-3 fatty acid supplements each day, which may make their babies smarter and healthier). The tables on pages 94 and 95 are a guide to the content of omega-3 fatty acids in various fish, recognizing that there will be some variability.

Remember, you don't have to eat fish to consume omega-3 fatty acids. Three grams per day of most fish oil capsules contain about one gram of DHA plus EPA, which is all that most people require. If you take fish oil capsules in which the bad stuff has been removed, you receive the benefits of the omega-3 fatty acids without the potential toxicity. Also, vegetarian sources of omega-3 fatty acids are now available.

Group 4 foods contain additional fat, higher-fat animal protein, and fewer protective nutrients. These include poultry, fish that are higher in mercury, whole milk and whole-milk dairy products, margarine, mayonnaise, doughnuts, fried rice, pastries, cakes, cookies, and pies.

Group 5 foods are, in general, the least-healthful foods. They are the lowest in protective substances and the highest in "bad fats" (especially trans–fatty acids and saturated fat). Group 5 foods include red meat in its various forms, egg yolks, fried poultry, fried fish, hot dogs, organ meats, butter, cream, and tropical oils.

If you're consuming red meat, look for organic meat from animals that have been raised and slaughtered in ways designed to minimize their suffering. Sometimes this information is on the label; other times you may need to go to a company's website to find out. Compared with natural grass-fed animals, meat from grain-fed animals raised in feedlots contains more total fat, saturated fat, cholesterol, and calories. It also has less vitamin E, beta-carotene, vitamin C, and omega-3 fatty acids.

I put "bad carbs" in Group 3 and "bad fats" in Group 5 because the harmful effects of bad carbs can be offset by consuming them in a meal along with good carbs and other high-fiber foods that have a low glycemic index and glycemic load. In contrast, the unhealthful effects of too much saturated fat and trans–fatty acids are not mitigated as much by consuming them with more-healthful foods. Eating too many "bad carbs" on an empty stomach puts them into Group 5.

The Spectrum of Food Choices table in this chapter is just a guide. Other factors can change a food's category, including the type of food, the amount of it, and other foods it's consumed with.

For example, you can turn a healthy food into an unhealthy one if you eat too much of it. A little olive oil belongs in Group 2, but pouring it freely over your pasta and dipping your bread in it will move it to Group 3 or even Group 4 due to the excessive calories, saturated fat, and omega-6 fatty acids from eating so much of it. Margarine made from canola oil is healthier than margarine made from oils high in trans–fatty acids and saturated fat. Eating a little dark chocolate every day may lower your blood pressure, but eating a lot of it will give you a large amount of sugar, calories, and saturated fat. A tiny sliver of butter may be healthier than a large scoop of margarine. You may want to explore alternatives to both.

In general, choose smaller portion sizes if you're trying to lose weight, lower your cholesterol or blood pressure, or reverse the progression of a chronic disease than if you just want to continue to stay healthy. If you're going to eat more-indulgent foods, have them with healthier ones. More on this in the next few chapters.

As I've said, it's not all or nothing. When we eat more of our foods on the healthier end of the Spectrum, it makes us feel better. It also does less harm to animals, helps reduce global warming (as I described in chapter 3), and frees up more arable land to grow food for those who most need it. In short, it's the healthiest way to eat both for us and for our planet.

We all need to find our place on the Spectrum that's comfortable and congruent with our own personal values as well as with our health needs. And it may evolve or devolve over time. The point of the Spectrum is to provide you with information that you can use to make informed and intelligent choices.

But this I know for sure: only you can decide what's right for you. Only then is it sustainable.

Selected Fish and Their Omega-3 Fatty Acid Content (2 grams and above per serving)

FISH HIGH IN OMEGA-3 FATTY ACIDS	AVERAGE GRAMS OF OMEGA-3 FATTY ACIDS per 6-ounce portion
Anchovy, European, canned in oil	3.4 g
Wild salmon	3.2 g
Pacific and jack mackerel	3.2 g
Sablefish	3.0 g
Whitefish	3.0 g
Pacific sardine	2.8 g
Bluefin tuna	2.8 g
Atlantic herring	2.4 g
Atlantic mackerel	2.0 g
Rainbow trout	2.0 g

Source: www.med.umich.edu/umim/clinical/pyramid/fish.htm.

Selected Fish and Seafood with Moderate Omega-3 Fatty Acid Content
(less than 2 grams per serving)

COMMON FINFISH	AVERAGE GRAMS OF OMEGA-3 FATTY ACIDS per 6-ounce portion	COMMON SEAFOOD	AVERAGE GRAMS OF OMEGA-3 FATTY ACIDS per 6-ounce portion
Tuna, white albacore, canned in water	1.4 g	Mussel	1.4 g
Halibut	0.8 g	Wild eastern oyster	1.0 g
Pollock	0.8 g	Farmed eastern oyster	0.8 g
Ocean perch	0.4 g	Blue crab or Alaskan king crab	0.8 g
Tuna, light, canned in water	0.4 g	Shrimp	0.6 g
Yellowfin tuna	0.4 g	Scallop	0.6 g
Cod	0.2 g	Clam	0.4 g
		Lobster	0.2 g
		Crayfish	0.2 g

Source: www.med.umich.edu/umim/clinical/pyramid/fish.htm.

ENJOY THE HOLIDAYS WITHOUT PIGGING OUT

When the Pilgrims enjoyed that first Thanksgiving, they were worried about having enough food to survive the winter. Today we have a different challenge—how to survive Thanksgiving dinner without feeling more stuffed than a twenty-four-pound turkey and without gaining unwanted pounds. The whole holiday season can feel like a minefield of overindulgence.

But it doesn't have to be that way. It's actually not very difficult to enjoy the bounty of the holidays without bloating up as big as the Mayflower.

Prepare to Indulge Before the Holidays

During the holidays, it's virtually impossible not to eat more than we want to. I'm pretty disciplined about my diet, yet at holiday parties and dinners, like everyone else, I find myself reaching for that extra cookie or brownie. After all, it's the holidays, the time of year to eat, drink, and be merry.

Knowing that you're going to indulge yourself during the holidays makes it easier to eat a little more mindfully in the weeks before Thanksgiving. You know what to do: cut back on fat, refined carbohydrates, and calories, and exercise more.

How to Indulge During the Holidays

- Eat something beforehand. If you don't eat all day, you may arrive at holiday meals and parties ravenous and lose control. Have a low-calorie but filling snack beforehand: an apple, a whole-grain bagel, a small bowl of soup, or whole-grain cereal.
- Put 20 percent fewer high-calorie foods and 20 percent more fruits and vegetables on your plate. Studies show that you probably won't notice the difference.
- Eat the healthier foods first—they will fill you up somewhat, so you'll be less likely to overeat the more-indulgent foods.
- Choose foods that leave evidence—e.g., keep the shrimp tails and chicken wing bones on your plate after you've eaten them. Studies show that if you have cues to see how much you've eaten, you'll eat less.
- Try not to put more than two or three items on your plate at one time. We eat more when food is in front of us.
- Eat more slowly. The faster we eat, the more we eat. It takes up to twenty minutes after eating for the brain to realize that we're full. Sip water between bites. Holiday meals last longer than typical meals. If you wolf down your food, your plate may be clean while others are still eating, which will lead to seconds. If you take a sip of water after every bite or two, it slows you down. You don't eat as much and you don't get uncomfortably stuffed.

- If you have a choice, use a smaller plate. A study found that people ate more popcorn when it was in a large container than in a medium-size one—even if the popcorn was five days old and stale! The smaller the dish, the less you take and the less you eat.
- If you're at someone's home, try to serve yourself instead of allowing your sister-in-law to heap your plate full.
- Arrive a little late and make a grand entrance. More of the indulgent foods will be gone by then.
- If you go to a restaurant, ask your server not to put bread on the table beforehand. If it's there, you'll probably eat it. You can have bread anytime; leave more room for your favorite holiday foods instead.
- Substitute cranberry sauce for gravy, which is usually high in fat and calories. Cranberry sauce is nutritious and loaded with antioxidants.
- If you eat baked potatoes and yams, avoid toppings such as butter, cheese, bacon, and sour cream. If possible, substitute low-fat yogurt or nonfat sour cream.
- Watch the alcohol, which is high in calories (almost 200 calories per ounce) and slows down your metabolism. Also, too much alcohol impairs judgment, so the more you drink, the more you're likely to eat.
- Close your eyes and savor the food periodically during the meal. You'll consume fewer calories and experience more pleasure.
- Have just a few bites of dessert. The first and last bites are always the best, anyway.
- Take a walk after dinner. You don't have to hike five miles. A stroll around the block is a good start. Walking not only burns calories, it also helps relieve bloating and prevent heartburn.

In his wonderful book *Mindless Eating*, food psychologist Brian Wansink describes how becoming more mindful of cues that affect our eating allows us to make different choices based on awareness rather than simply willpower.

The Spectrum of Food Choices

(A Representative but Not Exhaustive List)

	GROUP 1	GROUP 2	GROUP 3	GROUP 4	GROUP 5
	Most-Healthful Choices	More-Healthful Choices	Intermediate Choices	Less-Healthful Choices	Least-Healthful Choices
FRUITS	Fresh; choose locally grown fresh fruit when available Apples Bananas Berries Cherries Cranberries Currants Figs Grapes Guava Kiwi Lemon Lime Litchi nuts Mango Melon Oranges Papaya Persimmons Pomegranates	Frozen and canned (packed in water or its own juice, no added sugar) Avocados Olives	Canned fruit packed in syrup Dried fruit with added sugar		

	GROUP 1 Most-Healthful Choices	GROUP 2 More-Healthful Choices	GROUP 3 Intermediate Choices	GROUP 4 Less-Healthful Choices	GROUP 5 Least-Healthful Choices
FRUITS (cont.)	Quinces Rhubarb Star fruit Tangerines Watermelon Winter melons Zapote Dried fruit, without added sugar: Cherries Cranberries Dates Mango Papaya Raisins				
VEGETABLES	Fresh, frozen, or low-sodium canned; choose locally grown fresh vegetables when available Artichokes Arugula	Canned vegetables, regular sodium			

The Spectrum of Food Choices (cont.)

	GROUP 1	GROUP 2	GROUP 3	GROUP 4	GROUP 5
	Most-Healthful Choices	More-Healthful Choices	Intermediate Choices	Less-Healthful Choices	Least-Healthful Choices
VEGETABLES *(cont.)*	Asparagus Bamboo shoots Bell peppers; red, green, yellow, or orange Bok choy Broccoli Cabbage Carrots Cauliflower Celery Chilies Chinese celery Corn Cucumber Dandelion greens Edamame (soy beans) Eggplant Escarole Fennel Garlic Grape leaves Green beans				

	GROUP 1	GROUP 2	GROUP 3	GROUP 4	GROUP 5
	Most-Healthful Choices	More-Healthful Choices	Intermediate Choices	Less-Healthful Choices	Least-Healthful Choices
VEGETABLES (cont.)	Green leafy vegetables Jicama Kale Leeks Lettuce Mushrooms Mustard greens Napa or Chinese cabbage Okra Onions Parsnips Pickles Potatoes Radicchio Scallions Seaweed Shallots Spinach Squash, summer and winter Sundried tomatoes, not in oil Swiss chard				

The Spectrum of Food Choices (cont.) ▪▪▪▪▪▪▪▪

	GROUP 1 Most-Healthful Choices	GROUP 2 More-Healthful Choices	GROUP 3 Intermediate Choices	GROUP 4 Less-Healthful Choices	GROUP 5 Least-Healthful Choices
VEGETABLES (cont.)	Tomatoes Tomato paste Tomato sauce Water chestnuts Watercress Yams				
GRAINS AND CEREALS	100 percent whole-grain bread, bagels, English muffins, pita bread 100 percent whole-grain low-fat crackers (Woven Wheat, Finn Crisp, Wasa) Amaranth Barley Brown rice Buckwheat		Angel food cake Fat-free biscuit mix Regular-fat flour tortillas Rice crackers, white rice White bread, bagels, pita bread, English muffins White pasta White flour		Biscuits Cakes Cookies Croissants Doughnuts Fried breads Fried desserts Fried noodles Fried rice Fried tortillas Pastries Pies

	GROUP 1	GROUP 2	GROUP 3	GROUP 4	GROUP 5
	Most-Healthful Choices	More-Healthful Choices	Intermediate Choices	Less-Healthful Choices	Least-Healthful Choices
GRAINS AND CEREALS (cont.)	Bulgur Corn Corn tortillas (not fried) Couscous, whole wheat Faro High-fiber whole-grain cereals (containing at least 4 grams fiber per 100 calories and less than 5 grams sugar) Hominy grits made without fat, butter, or bacon Kasha Millet Oatmeal Oats Pasta made from whole grain Polenta Polvillo				

The Spectrum of Food Choices (cont.)

	GROUP 1 Most-Healthful Choices	GROUP 2 More-Healthful Choices	GROUP 3 Intermediate Choices	GROUP 4 Less-Healthful Choices	GROUP 5 Least-Healthful Choices
GRAINS AND CEREALS *(cont.)*	Quinoa Rice crackers, whole grain Rye Soba noodles Spelt Sweet potatoes Tabouli salad made without oil Tortillas, fat-free Udon noodles Wheat Wheat berries Wheat tortillas, fat-free Wild rice				
LEGUMES	Fresh, dried, frozen, canned (no added salt), jarred (no added salt), vacuum sealed (no added salt)	Regular-sodium canned, jarred, or vacuum-sealed beans and lentils Baked beans			Pork and beans

	GROUP 1 Most-Healthful Choices	GROUP 2 More-Healthful Choices	GROUP 3 Intermediate Choices	GROUP 4 Less-Healthful Choices	GROUP 5 Least-Healthful Choices
LEGUMES (cont.)	Black beans Black-eyed peas Cannellini or butter beans Chickpeas (garbanzo beans) Fava beans Great northern beans Italian white beans Lentils Lima beans Mung beans Navy beans Peas Pinto beans Red beans (kidney beans) Sprouted beans Wax (yellow) beans				
PROTEIN	Egg whites or liquid egg substitutes Hummus made without oil or tahini	Salmon, wild Alaska and Pacific	Anchovies, fresh Arctic char Butterfish Catfish Caviar	Poultry, chicken, turkey	Bacon Bacon bits Beef Bison Bologna

The Spectrum of Food Choices (cont.)

	GROUP 1	GROUP 2	GROUP 3	GROUP 4	GROUP 5
	Most-Healthful Choices	More-Healthful Choices	Intermediate Choices	Less-Healthful Choices	Least-Healthful Choices
PROTEIN (cont.)	Soy and soy alternatives: Edamame Natto Soy fat-free sausage Soy hot dogs Tempeh Tofu Veggie burgers		Clams Cod Crab Crawfish Flounder Halibut Herring Lobster Mahimahi Monkfish Mussels Orange roughy Pacific flounder Pacific sole Pollock Sand dabs Sardines, not packed in oil Scallops Sea bass Shrimp Snapper Squid (calamari) Striped bass Sturgeon	Products made from light chicken and turkey, such as poultry-based luncheon meats, poultry-based sausage, poultry-based hot dogs Deli sliced turkey Albacore tuna Anchovies in oil Oysters *Fish high in mercury:* King mackerel Shark Swordfish Tilefish (golden snapper)	Deli sliced ham, pastrami, roast beef Deviled eggs Egg salad sandwich Egg yolks Elk Fried chicken Fried fish or shellfish Ham Head cheese Hot dogs made from pork or beef Lamb Organ meats Pork Sausage made from pork or beef Venison

	GROUP 1 Most-Healthful Choices	GROUP 2 More-Healthful Choices	GROUP 3 Intermediate Choices	GROUP 4 Less-Healthful Choices	GROUP 5 Least-Healthful Choices
PROTEIN (cont.)			Tilapia Trout Tuna, fresh or canned light		
DAIRY AND DAIRY SUBSTITUTES	Enriched oat milk Enriched rice milk Enriched soy milk Fat-free buttermilk Fat-free cottage cheese Fat-free cream cheese Fat-free or skim milk Fat-free sour cream Fat-free yogurt Canned evaporated milk Coconut water Fat-free milk (skim) Fat-free dry milk powder	Low-fat (1%) dairy products Sweetened nonfat and 1 percent yogurt Fat-free frozen yogurt Fat-free puddings and sweets (up to two servings daily) Parmesan cheese as a flavor enhancer	Reduced-fat (2%) canned evaporated milk Reduced-fat (2%) cheese Reduced-fat (2%) dairy products Nondairy creamer (1 tablespoon)	Full-fat dairy products (4%) Full-fat goat milk Light coconut milk Nondairy whipped cream	All other full-fat cheeses Butter Coconut milk Half-and-half Heavy cream

The Spectrum of Food Choices (cont.)

	GROUP 1 Most-Healthful Choices	GROUP 2 More-Healthful Choices	GROUP 3 Intermediate Choices	GROUP 4 Less-Healthful Choices	GROUP 5 Least-Healthful Choices
FATS/OILS	Canola oil Fat-free margarine spreads Fat-free nondairy salad dressings Fish oil (omega-3 fatty acids) Flaxseed oil Nonstick cooking spray	Olive oil Safflower oil Nuts and nut butters: Almonds, unsalted Sunflower seeds, unsalted Walnuts	Light or reduced-fat margarines free of trans fats Low-fat mayonnaise Corn oil Peanut oil Sesame oil Soybean oil Nuts and nut butters: Cashews, unsalted Mixed nuts, unsalted Peanuts, unsalted Pecans, unsalted Pumpkin seeds, unsalted Sesame seeds	Margarine, regular Mayonnaise, regular	Trans fats Tropical oils: Palm kernel oil Palm oil

	GROUP 1 Most-Healthful Choices	GROUP 2 More-Healthful Choices	GROUP 3 Intermediate Choices	GROUP 4 Less-Healthful Choices	GROUP 5 Least-Healthful Choices
HERBS, SPICES, AND OTHER FLAVOR ADDITIVES	Bonito flakes Brewer's yeast Broth, vegetable, mushroom Capers Chili flakes Chutneys Fennel seeds Flaxseeds Fresh or dried herbs and spices, such as allspice, basil, cinnamon, coriander, cumin, curry powder oregano, parsley, etc. Garlic Ginger Green chiles, canned Hoisin sauce and plum sauce Malt powder Miso Mustard Natural vanilla Pepper	Barbecue sauce Bouillon cubes/ granules, vegetable (low sodium) Dark chocolate (small amounts) Rice wine vinegar, regular-sodium Sesame seeds Sofrito (see page 326) Soy sauce (low sodium)	Bouillon cubes/ granules, vegetable, (regular-sodium) Table salt	Chicken broth	Beef broth

The Spectrum of Food Choices (cont.)

	GROUP 1	GROUP 2	GROUP 3	GROUP 4	GROUP 5
	Most-Healthful Choices	More-Healthful Choices	Intermediate Choices	Less-Healthful Choices	Least-Healthful Choices
HERBS, SPICES, AND OTHER FLAVOR ADDITIVES (cont.)	Poppy seeds Rice wine vinegar, low sodium Salsa or picante sauce Vinegars, plain and flavored Wheat germ Yeast				
SWEETENERS	Stevia	Splenda Unsweetened jam, jelly, or preserves	Corn syrup High-fructose corn syrup Honey Maple syrup Molasses Sweetened jam, jelly, or preserves White, brown, or raw sugar or syrup		

	GROUP 1	GROUP 2	GROUP 3	GROUP 4	GROUP 5
	Most-Healthful Choices	More-Healthful Choices	Intermediate Choices	Less-Healthful Choices	Least-Healthful Choices
BEVERAGES	Beer (12 ounces daily) Caffeine-free herbal teas, iced or hot Fruit juice (up to 8 ounces daily) Green tea, iced or hot Hard alcohol (1.5 ounces) Mirin Sake Wine (6 ounces daily)	Black tea Caffeine-free, sugar-free colas and other sodas (sweetened with stevia or Splenda) Decaffeinated coffee Decaffeinated tea	Coffee Regular colas and soda		

Oils and Fats

TYPE	SATURATED	MONOUNSATURATED	POLYUNSATURATED	SMOKE POINT	USES
Butter	66%	30%	4%	150° C (302° F)	Cooking, baking, as condiment, sauces, as flavoring
Canola oil	6%	62%	32%	238° C (460° F)	Frying, baking, in salad dressing
Coconut oil	92%	6%	2%	177° C (350° F)	In commercial baked goods, candy and sweets, whipped toppings, nondairy coffee creamers, shortening
Corn oil	13%	25%	62%	236° C (457° F)	Frying, baking, in salad dressing, margarine, shortening
Cottonseed oil	24%	26%	50%	216° C (420° F)	In margarine, shortening, salad dressing, commercially fried products
Diacylglycerol (DAG) oil	3.5%	37%	59%	215° C (420° F)	Frying, baking, salad oil

TYPE	SATURATED	MONOUNSATURATED	POLYUNSATURATED	SMOKE POINT	USES
Ghee (clarified butter)	65%	32%	3%	190° C (374° F)	Deep-frying, cooking, sautéing, as condiment, as flavoring
Grapeseed oil	12%	17%	71%	204° C (400° F)	Cooking, in salad dressing, margarine
Lard	41%	47%	12%	138–201° C (280–395° F)	Baking, frying
Margarine, hard	70%	14%	16%	150–160° C (300–320° F)	Cooking, baking, as condiment
Margarine, soft	20%	47%	33%	150–160° C (300–320° F)	Cooking, baking, as condiment
Olive oil, extra light	14%	73%	13%	242° C (468° F)	Sautéing, stir-frying, frying, cooking, salad oil, in margarine
Olive oil, extra virgin	14%	73%	13%	207° C (406° F)	Cooking, salad oil, in margarine
Olive oil, refined	14%	73%	13%	225° C (438° F)	Sautéing, stir-frying, cooking, salad oil, in margarine
Olive oil, virgin	14%	73%	13%	215° C (420° F)	Cooking, salad oil, in margarine

Oils and Fats (cont.)

TYPE	SATURATED	MONOUNSATURATED	POLYUNSATURATED	SMOKE POINT	USES
Palm oil	52%	38%	10%	230° C (446° F)	Cooking, flavoring, shortening
Peanut oil	18%	49%	33%	231° C (448° F)	Frying, cooking, salad oil, margarine
Safflower oil	10%	13%	77%	265° C (509° F)	Cooking, in salad dressing, margarine
Sesame oil, semirefined	14%	43%	43%	232° C (450° F)	Cooking, deep-frying
Sesame oil, unrefined	14%	43%	43%	177° C (350° F)	Cooking, deep-frying
Soybean oil	15%	24%	61%	241° C (466° F)	Cooking, in salad dressing, margarine, shortening
Sunflower oil	11%	20%	69%	246° C (475° F)	Cooking, in salad dressing, margarine, shortening

Source: http://en.wikipedia.org/wiki/Cooking_oil, July 11, 2007.

6

THE STRESS-MANAGEMENT SPECTRUM

The greatest weapon against stress is our ability to choose one thought over another.

—William James

Always forgive your enemies—nothing annoys them so much.

—Oscar Wilde

■ ■ ■ ■ ■ ■ ■ ■ ■ ■

When I was in the midst of my internship at Harvard Medical School's Massachusetts General Hospital, one of the attending physicians—who was world-famous in his field—started giving me a hard time for believing that emotional stress played a significant role in any illnesses. That was in 1981, not so long ago.

Since then, there has been an explosion in the number of well-conducted scientific studies showing the powerful connection between our emotions and our health—for better and for worse. In the meantime, unfortunately, many people are finding that life seems to have become even more stressful.

We now know that emotional stress is an important factor in the vast majority of illnesses, both directly and indirectly. The mechanisms by which this occurs are becoming increasingly well understood.

Stress can have a negative impact on just about every part of your body. It can suppress your immune function, cause a heart attack or stroke, increase your risk of cancer, delay wound healing, promote inflammation, cause you to gain weight, impair your memory, cause depression, exacerbate diabetes, and worsen your sexual function. Just for starters.

Stress also makes you age faster even at a genetic and cellular level. If you've ever compared photographs of any of the past U.S. presidents at the beginning and at the end of their term, you can see how quickly chronic stress accelerates aging.

Telomeres are DNA at the end of your chromosomes that directly affect how quickly your cells age. As they become shorter and as their structural integrity gets weakened, then cells age and die more quickly.

In simple terms, as your telomeres get shorter, your life gets shorter.

Chronic emotional stress may cause your cells to age more quickly. My colleagues Drs. Elissa Epel and Elizabeth Blackburn of the University of California, San Francisco, School of Medicine, conducted a pioneering study of mothers who were caring for a child with a chronic illness. Using biochemical techniques, they studied their telomeres as well as telomerase, your natural enzyme that repairs damaged telomeres.

They found that the longer the stress, and the more stress the women reported, the shorter their telomere length and the lower their telomerase level. Women with the highest levels of perceived stress had telomeres shorter, on average, by the equivalent of at least one decade of additional aging compared to low-stress women.

I wondered: If chronic stress can decrease telomerase and cause telomeres to age more quickly, could healthy lifestyle changes prevent this from occurring?

To address this question, my colleagues and I recently conducted a study with Dr. Blackburn, Dr. Peter Carroll, and others to see if the program of comprehensive lifestyle changes described in *The Spectrum*, including stress-management techniques and support groups, might help prevent accelerated aging.

We think it did.

Participants were asked to eat and live on the healthiest end of the Spectrum for three months. They were tested at the beginning and again after three months. We found that their telomerase level (which repairs telomeres) actually increased significantly.

This appears to be the first study showing that comprehensive lifestyle changes may prevent or even reverse stress-induced damage to DNA telomeres. These results are very encouraging. Like all studies, these findings need to be replicated in larger studies with a randomized control group.

MELTDOWN

A lot of people are feeling that life is increasingly difficult as our world seems to be spiraling out of control. We watch helplessly as parts of our globe descend into madness and terrorism, and our governments seem increasingly unresponsive to individual needs.

Middle East meltdown. Global warming meltdown. Nuclear meltdown. Stock market meltdown. Emotional meltdown.

Fortunately, while we can't always change what's going on in the world, there is a lot we can do about how it affects us.

Stress comes not only from what's going in your life but, even more important, from how you *react* to it. When you practice some simple stress-management techniques on a regular basis, you can be in the same job, the same environment, even the same family but react in more constructive and healthful ways.

One of the most interesting findings in the Epel/Blackburn study was that the mothers' *perceptions* of stress were more important than what was objectively occurring in their lives. The researchers gave the women a questionnaire and asked them to rate on a three-point scale how stressed they felt each day and how out of control their lives felt to them.

The women who perceived that they were under heavy stress also had significantly shortened and damaged telomeres compared with those who felt more relaxed. Conversely, some of the women who felt relaxed despite raising a disabled child had more normal-appearing telomeres.

In other words, if you *feel* stressed, you *are* stressed.

A recent study showed that chronic loneliness affects the expression of several genes in ways that may increase the risk of developing a number of diseases. Once again, it was the *perception* of loneliness and stress that was strongly correlated with adverse changes in genes, independent of how many friends and acquaintances someone actually had.

These researchers found that those who were the loneliest had alterations in specific genes that caused high levels of chronic inflammation. As I described in chapter 3, chronic inflammation may lead to a variety of illnesses. Chronic loneliness also caused changes in genes that affect immune function, causing an impairment in the body's ability to fight invading bacteria and viruses.

One of the keys to managing stress well is to be able to turn it off sometimes. Techniques like yoga and meditation give you a break from chronic stress, providing an internal oasis that you can experience anywhere. Stress is most likely to cause disease when it's chronic and unrelenting. Even your heart, which beats steadily, rests in between contractions.

Some people thrive on stress, and it doesn't cause them to get sick. Studies have found that they can turn it on when needed, but they can also turn it off.

They have appropriately elevated levels of stress hormones at work during the day, but their stress hormones drop sharply at night. In other words, they can turn it off. In contrast, people who feel chronically stressed and anxious have stress hormones that remain elevated, and this predisposes them to a wide variety of illnesses.

Stress-management techniques can help you turn it off. They are not about withdrawing from the world; rather, they enable you to embrace it more fully and effectively. When you're feeling less stressed, you can think more clearly and creatively, making it easier to find constructive solutions. When you're less desperate, you're more empowered.

People who thrive on stress tend to see challenges as opportunities. As an analogy, when people are first learning how to surf, even a small wave is stressful and can knock them over. After they practice for a while, they begin to seek out bigger waves, because they're more fun.

Scientists are beginning to be able to identify changes in your genes that may predispose you to stress and depression and may help explain, at least in part, why stressful experiences lead to depression in some people but not in others.

For example, a study in the journal *Science* found that people with a variation in a region of a single gene called 5-HTT were more likely to be diagnosed as depressed or even to commit suicide later in life. This gene helps regulate serotonin, one of the neurotransmitters affected by antidepressants such as Prozac.

In a related study, researchers found that monkeys who had this genetic variation and were reared with both parents in a healthy family environment did not show abnormalities, whereas a comparable group of monkeys raised without their parents in a depressed and stressful environment did. Thus, even though all of these monkeys were genetically predisposed to depression, being reared in a warm, nurturing environment protected them from exhibiting signs of being depressed.

This is another wonderful example of how genes can affect our predisposition to certain conditions but can often be altered if we're willing to make bigger changes in what we eat and how we live—in other words, to go further toward the healthy end of the Spectrum. As I wrote at the end of chapter 4, nurture can trump nature, but you may have to go further toward the healthier end of the Spectrum if you're genetically predisposed to conditions such as depression.

Having more control over your life helps reduce the harmful effects of stress. One of the reasons why social class is such a powerful predictor of health and illness is that, in general, more affluent people generally have more control over their lives. For example, musicians who play in orchestras often report feeling more stressed than those who play in chamber quartets, because those in an orchestra are under the complete control of the conductor, whereas those in a smaller quartet have more autonomy.

While it's good to have more power, affluence, and control in our lives, sometimes it's not possible. However, part of the value of stress-management techniques is that they help us realize that we have more power and control than we may have thought. We can't always control external events, no matter how much power we may have. The president of the United States may be the most powerful person in the world, but even the president can't always get Congress to do what he or she wants, much less control events and leaders in the rest of the world.

Fortunately, practicing meditation and other stress-management techniques on a regular basis gives us more power to control how we *react* to these external events. As a patient once said to me after learning meditation and yoga, "Well, the situation didn't change, but *I* did."

As I described in chapter 2, I always try to give my son, Lucas, as much control and choice as possible within the bounds of what's appropriate. What do you feel like doing today? What do you want for lunch? What movie would you like to see? This way, he feels empowered and less stressed than he otherwise would, and he gets used to making decisions for himself. Also, when I do set limits, he is more likely to respect them because he knows they're not arbitrary, and I always explain the reasons for my actions.

Many doctors, even those who are interested in nutrition and exercise, view stress-management techniques as less important than other factors. They believe that nutrition is important. Also, you have to eat every day; it's just a question of what you consume, so it's in your awareness. Most people know and appreciate the importance of exercise—and exercise looks productive, as if you're really *doing* something.

However, stress-management techniques are not part of most people's daily routine; until they are, it may take some effort to remind yourself to do them. Also, to the untrained observer, sitting with your eyes closed looks as though you're not doing very much.

In fact, these approaches are very powerful, as many research studies are documenting. Meditation, for example, is about focusing your mental energy. Focusing energy increases its power. When you can concentrate better, you can perform better—in school, in business, in sports. Whatever you do, you can do it more effectively and with less stress.

As with nutrition and exercise, you have a spectrum of choices when it comes to practicing stress-management techniques; it's not all or nothing. The longer and more frequently you practice these techniques, the more benefits you receive.

How much you need to do depends on what you're trying to accomplish.

For reversing heart disease, our research indicated that those who spent at least one hour per day on the stress-management techniques used in these studies (including yoga-based stretching, breathing techniques, meditation, and imagery, and participation in the support group) showed the greatest amount of improvement in their coronary artery disease.

However, you may not need to spend as much time practicing stress-management techniques if you're just trying to stay healthy or lose a few pounds. Even practicing a few minutes a day has benefits.

Surprisingly, given the limitations of self-reported data, we found a direct dose-response correlation with the frequency and duration of practicing stress-management techniques and changes in coronary artery blockages. We found this after one year and again after five years. Again, the more people changed, the more improvements we measured. The improvements in coronary artery blockages due to stress-management techniques appear to be independent of changes in diet.

In my experience, consistency is more important than duration—more is better, but even a minute of meditation each day can make a meaningful difference. Sometimes, when I'm really busy and pressed for time, I'm tempted to skip doing the meditation. Of course, the times I'm busiest are usually the times I need it the most. As Sydney Harris once wrote, "The time to relax is when you don't have time for it."

Instead, I play a little game with myself. I'll ask, "Do I have just one minute to meditate?" If I don't, then I have to admit to myself that my life is so out of balance that it's easier to just go ahead and meditate for one minute.

Getting started is always the hardest part for me. Once I've overcome the inertia and I'm meditating, chances are that I'll do it for more than just a minute anyway.

Now, even a minute of meditation has value. Have you ever listened to a song on the radio and found yourself humming it later in the day? It's like that with meditation—you continue to meditate subconsciously throughout the day.

In summary, if you have a serious illness, try to practice stress-management techniques for at least an hour a day. If you can't do that much, do what you can, knowing that more is better. If you are just trying to stay healthy, you have a much wider spectrum of choices. In other chapters, I recommend how much stress management is optimal for each condition. Anne and I offer these stress-management techniques more fully in the next chapter and in the guided meditations DVD that accompanies this book. Others are available at www.ornish.com and www.OrnishSpectrum.com.

WHAT CAN YOU DO TO MANAGE STRESS MORE EFFECTIVELY?

Breathe. Your breath is the link between your mind and your body. It both *reflects* and *affects* your level of stress. In other words, your mind affects your body, and your body affects your mind.

When you're relaxed, you tend to breathe more slowly and deeply. When you're feeling stressed, your breath becomes more rapid and shallower, so it can be a way of letting you know when you're feeling stressed.

When you become aware that you're stressed, remind yourself to take some slow, deep breaths, which will reduce your stress level almost immediately. You breathe slowly and deeply when you're feeling relaxed, and forcing yourself to breathe slowly and deeply can cause you to feel relaxed.

Besides connecting your mind and body, breathing is a bridge between your sympathetic and parasympathetic systems, which are your neurological yin and yang. During times of emotional stress, your sympathetic nervous system becomes stimulated; after the danger has passed, your parasympathetic nervous system is activated.

Emotional stress causes the "fight-or-flight" response, in which your body goes through a series of physiological changes that prepare you to fight or run. Your pupils dilate so you can see better, your muscles contract to fortify your "body armor" in case you have to go into combat, your heart rate and blood pressure increase to provide you more energy, and your arteries constrict and your blood clots faster to stop bleeding more quickly in case you're injured in battle.

If stresses become chronic, as they often do in modern life, the same mechanisms that are supposed to protect us may lead to illness and even premature death.

For example, when your muscles are chronically contracted, over time this may cause back pain and muscle dysfunction. Chronic stress may cause the arteries in your heart to constrict and your blood to clot too vigorously, leading to a heart attack or stroke.

Your parasympathetic nervous system has the opposite effects. Taking a deep breath when you're feeling stressed helps break the stress cycle and rebalance your sympathetic and parasympathetic nervous systems, calming you down. Even when you can't control a situation, you can always direct your breathing and thus help change your reaction to those circumstances.

Meditate. Meditation is the practice of paying attention. There are two basic ways of doing this.

1. Focus on something peaceful.

You can meditate on almost anything—a sound, a word, a prayer, a song, an image, or your breathing.

Interestingly, different cultures meditate on words that sound very similiar—beginning with an "ah" or "oh" and ending with an "m" or "n," like a parent humming to a baby. Om. Shalom. Salaam. Amen. Ameen. These words are often translated as meaning "peace" because they help you experience it.

Choose a word, sound, or image that's comfortable for you. The word "One" works just as well, if you prefer something that sounds more secular (although "One" may actually be the most spiritual of all words).

To meditate, sit in a comfortable position in a chair or on the floor with your back straight. Close your eyes, take a breath, and say the word out loud, emphasizing the humming sound at the end. When you come to the end of the breath, take another breath and say the word again. And so on.

When your mind wanders, just bring it back to the meditation, without judging or berating yourself. Everyone's mind wanders. Everyone, even the Dalai Lama's, although probably not as much as yours or mine.

When you focus your mind in this way, a number of good things begin to happen:

- *You get better at focusing your awareness.* When you can concentrate better, you can accomplish more—in school, at work, and in athletics. In that context, meditation gives you a competitive advantage.

- *You enjoy what you're doing more fully.* Although meditation is sometimes viewed erroneously as an ascetic experience, it's actually profoundly sensual. When you pay attention to something—food, sex, music, art, massage—you enjoy it more fully, and you don't need as much of it to experience the same level of pleasure. As I described in chapter 2, when you pay attention to what you're eating, you receive more pleasure with fewer calories. In Tantric yoga, making love becomes a form of meditation, with full awareness and intention, and it can go on for hours. Listening to music in this way can become a form of meditation as you become one with the music.

- *Your mind quiets down, so you feel more peaceful.* Your mind quiets down, and you begin to experience an inner sense of peace and well-being. You realize that this state of inner calm is always available to you, at any moment, not just when you meditate. Meditation didn't *bring* you peace; it simply helped you to stop disturbing what was there already, at least temporarily.

- *You can access your inner wisdom more easily.* Have you ever awakened in the middle of the night and figured out the answer to a problem that had been troubling you? All spiritual traditions describe a "still, small voice within," a voice that speaks very clearly but very quietly. It's easily drowned out by the chatter and business of everyday life. For many people, the only time their mind is quiet enough to hear their inner voice is when they wake up in the middle of the night. Sometimes it says, "Listen up, pay attention, I have something important to tell you."

  Meditation can help you access your inner wisdom more intentionally. At the end of a meditation session—whether it's been one minute or one hour—your mind is much quieter and calmer, so you can hear your still, small voice within more clearly. I ask myself, "What am I not paying attention to that I need to hear?" And then I wait—and listen. Over time, I've learned to trust and recognize my inner voice. So can you. When we practice listening to our inner voice in quiet moments, we can learn to access it at the stressful times when we most need it.

  If we pay attention to our inner wisdom, we can often recognize problems in their earlier stages when they are easier to rectify. As Oprah Winfrey once said, "Listen to the whisper before it becomes a scream."

- *You can directly experience a transcendent state.* On one level, we're all separate and apart from one another. You're you, and I'm me. On another level, meditation, taken deeply enough, allows us to experience that we're all a part of everyone and everything. When we can maintain that "double vision"—the duality and the underlying unity—we can enjoy life more fully and accomplish even more without so much suffering and stress, from a place of wholeness rather than lacking, from a feeling of interconnectedness rather than separateness and isolation.

2. Mindfulness meditation.

Everything we do can become a form of meditation if we do it with awareness.

One of the leading proponents of mindfulness meditation, Dr. Jon Kabat-Zinn, describes it this way:

> Mindfulness is about living fully in the present moment, observing ourselves, our feelings, others and our surroundings without judging them. Mindfulness meditation is moment to moment awareness. It is being fully awake. It involves being here for the moments of our lives, without striving or judging.
>
> Mindfulness is coming home to yourself, to live your own life, as you are, in the only moment that you have to live—this moment.

Another renowned teacher of mindfulness meditation is Jack Kornfield:

> Mindfulness is an innate human capacity to deliberately pay full attention to where we are, to our actual experience, and to learn from it.
>
> Much of our day we spend on automatic pilot. People know the experience of driving somewhere, pulling up to the curb and all of a sudden realizing, "Wow, I was hardly aware I was even driving. How did I get here?" When we pay attention, it is gracious, which means that there is space for our joys and sorrows, our pain and losses, all to be held in a peaceful way. . . .

Some Practical Points about Cultivating Mindfulness and Either Beginning or Deepening a Personal Meditation Practice, by Jon Kabat-Zinn, Ph.D.

1. The real meditation is how you live your life.
2. In order to live life fully, you have to be present for it.
3. To be present, it helps to purposefully bring awareness to your moments—otherwise you may miss many of them.
4. You do that by paying attention on purpose, in the present moment, and nonjudgmentally to whatever is arising inwardly and outwardly.
5. This requires a great deal of kindness toward yourself, which you deserve.

6. It helps to keep in mind that good or bad, pleasant or unpleasant, the present moment is the only time any of us are alive in—and therefore the only time to learn, grow, see what is really going on, find some degree of balance, feel and express emotions such as love and appreciation, and do what we need to do to take care of ourselves—in other words, embody our intrinsic strength and beauty and wisdom—even in the face of pain and suffering.

7. So a gentle love affair with the present moment is important.

8. We do that through learning to rest in awareness of what is happening inwardly and outwardly moment by moment by moment—it is more a *"being"* than a *"doing."*

9. Formal and informal meditation practices are specific ways in which you can ground, deepen, and accelerate this process, so it is useful to carve out some time for formal practice on a regular daily basis—maybe waking up fifteen or twenty minutes earlier than you ordinarily would to catch some time for ourselves.

10. We bring awareness to our moments only as best we can.

11. We are not trying to create a special feeling or experience— simply to realize that this moment is already very special— because you are alive and awake in it.

12. This is hard, but well worth it.

13. It takes a lot of practice.

14. Lots of practice.

15. But you have a lot of moments—and we can treat each one as a new beginning.

16. So there are always new moments to open up to if we miss some.

17. We do all this with a huge amount of self-compassion.

18. And remember, you are not your thoughts or opinions, your likes or dislikes. They are more like weather patterns in your mind that you can be aware of—like clouds moving across the sky—and so don't have to be imprisoned by.

19. Befriending yourself in this way is the adventure of a lifetime, and hugely empowering

20. Try it for a few weeks—it grows on you.

For more information and resources: www.jonkabat-zinn.com.

Practice yoga. Gentle hatha yoga stretches can relax chronically tensed muscle groups and increase both physical and mental flexibility. Just as your mind affects your body, so does your body affect your mind. When your body is more relaxed, your mind feels less stressed. (For more on yoga and meditation, please consult *Dr. Dean Ornish's Program for Reversing Heart Disease* as well as www.OrnishSpectrum.com.)

Reduce your exposure to stimulants (both physical and mental). Caffeine, found in sodas, "energy" drinks, coffee, tea, and many medications, potentiates stress—that is, it shortens your fuse and makes you more reactive to stress. In other words, it does the opposite of meditation.

Caffeine and other stimulants don't give you energy; rather, you borrow it from yourself. You get an initial rush of energy, followed later by feeling really tired. There's a good fix for that feeling—more caffeine. And so it goes in a vicious cycle.

If you don't think you're addicted to caffeine, just try to stop drinking it; your body goes into withdrawal, you may get headaches and may feel tired, irritable, and fuzzy. It's not pretty.

Slowly reduce your intake of caffeine. Also, re-experience what it feels like to live without the constant stimulation of the television, radio, or iPod being on 24/7. While it's important to stay informed, give yourself a break from the news continually droning on about disasters.

Exercise. In addition to the physical benefits described in chapter 8, physical exercise is a great way to discharge the stressful feelings that accumulate during the day. Just walking for twenty to thirty minutes a day makes you feel better and look better. Incorporate exercise into your daily life: park a little farther from your destination, take the stairs, have more vigorous sex. More on this in chapter 8.

Enhance your social support. When you're depressed, it's easy to feel as if you're the only person who feels that way since it's not something that most people talk about.

You're not. The most commonly prescribed drugs in this country are antidepressants. Last year, more than 120 million prescriptions were written for these drugs. Adults' use of antidepressants almost tripled between the periods 1988–1994 and 1999–2000. Between 1995 and 2002, the use of these drugs rose by almost 50 percent, according to the Centers for Disease Control and Prevention.

That's a lot of depressed people. People who feel lonely, depressed, and isolated—the silent epidemic in this country—are many times more likely to get sick and to die prematurely than those who have a strong sense of connection and community.

Call a friend. Get a pet. Volunteer somewhere. Find a therapist. Talk with your minister or counselor. Make love with your spouse or significant other. Go to church or synagogue. Have dinner with your family.

Practice forgiveness, altruism, compassion, and service. Chronic hostility and hatred are among the most toxic forms of stress. When you are really angry with someone, you empower the person you hate to make you stressed out or even sick. That's not smart.

When you forgive someone, it doesn't excuse their actions; it frees you from your own stress and suffering. This is true for nations as well as individuals. Otherwise, the cycle of violence continues and escalates from country to country and from generation to generation, fighting in the name of peace.

It takes strength and courage to forgive; those who are afraid to look weak often preach vengeance and violence. We remember and respect those who had the courage to be nonviolent, whose lives inspired lasting change for the better: Mahatma Gandhi, Martin Luther King, Jr., and other giants. Similarly, altruism and compassion are powerful ways of reducing stress and transforming our lives.

Like many people, I have been inspired by Nelson Mandela. If he could forgive those who kept him in jail for more than ten thousand days in the prime of his life, I can let go of my petty grievances. I had the privilege of meeting him in Davos, Switzerland, several years ago, and I was struck by the gentle yet profound strength that he embodied. I treasure the copy of his autobiography, *Long Walk to Freedom,* that he sent me. In it, he wrote:

> It was during those long and lonely years that my hunger for the freedom of my own people became a hunger for the freedom of all people, white and black. I knew as well as I knew anything that the oppressor must be liberated just as surely as the oppressed. A man who takes away another man's freedom is a prisoner of hatred, he is locked behind the bars of prejudice and narrow-mindedness. I am not truly free if I am taking away someone else's freedom, just as surely as I am not free when my freedom is taken from me. The oppressed and the oppressor alike are robbed of their humanity.
>
> When I walked out of prison, that was my mission, to liberate the oppressed and the oppressor both. Some say that has now been achieved. But I know that that is not the case. The truth is that we are not yet free; we have merely achieved the freedom to be free, the right

not to be oppressed. We have not taken the final step of our journey, but the first step on a longer and even more difficult road. For to be free is not merely to cast off one's chains, but to live in a way that respects and enhances the freedom of others. The true test of our devotion to freedom is just beginning.

Echoing these feelings, when President Bill Clinton addressed the Nigerian parliament in 2002, he said:

Some things you just have to forgive and let go. That's one thing I learned from my friend Mandela. I asked him, "When you were taking your last walk for freedom, didn't you hate your oppressors again?" Walking out the last time. He said, "I did for a while, after all. Look, they kept me for twenty-seven years. I didn't get to see my children grow up. I felt hatred, and I was afraid. I hadn't been free in so long." And then he smiled at me and he said, "If I still hated them when I got outside the prison gate, I would still be their prisoner." He said, "I wanted to be free, and so I let it go."

One of the advantages of practicing stress-management techniques is that they reduce anger. In our research, participants showed striking reductions in self-reported measurements of chronic anger and hostility. Also, yoga has been shown to significantly reduce anger, depression, and anxiety in a recent study.

One of the most exciting emerging findings in neurosciences in the past decade has been the discovery of what are called "mirror neurons." These parts of the brain fire when doing an action or observing an action performed by another person.

For example, if a monkey performs a certain task, neurons become activated in a specific part of its brain. However, if a monkey merely watches another monkey perform the same task, neurons in the same part of the brain fire in the monkey who is watching, just as if it were doing the same action.

This may be one of the mechanisms by which visualization and guided imagery work. If you close your eyes and imagine something stressful, your body reacts as though something stressful is actually occurring—i.e., your arteries constrict, blood pressure increases, blood clots more quickly, muscles tense, breathing rate increases, and so on. If you close your eyes and imagine something healing occurring instead, then healing tends to happen as well. It's not wishful thinking; it's something that occurs on a physiological level.

This may also help explain why compassion and forgiveness are so powerful—not only for the recipient but also for the giver. In this context, it helps redefine the false choice between taking care of yourself ("selfish") versus looking out for others ("unselfish"). When we act in ways that are loving, compassionate, and altruistic, it helps us as well as others.

Mirror neurons also help explain on a physiological level "what goes around, comes around" or what Dan Goleman calls "emotional contagion," the tendency of one person to catch the feelings of another, particularly if strongly expressed.

Our emotions resonate with those of other people—for better and for worse. If I'm with a close friend, my anger may raise his blood pressure as well as mine. Conversely, my loving feelings may lower my wife's blood pressure as well as my own.

So the most "selfish" thing we can do for ourselves may be to act toward others in ways that are loving, forgiving, altruistic, compassionate, and nurturing, for that is what helps free us from suffering, disease, and premature death. When we help others, we also help ourselves.

In short, we are hardwired to help each other. This has helped us survive for the past several hundred thousand years. When we forget this, we often suffer needlessly.

These are not new ideas. "Health" comes from a root meaning "to make whole." The word "yoga" derives from the Sanskrit for "to yoke," to bring together. Science is helping document the wisdom of ancient traditions.

The values of community, compassion, forgiveness, altruism, and service are part of almost all religious and spiritual traditions as well as many secular ones—what the German philosopher Gottfried Wilhelm Leibniz called "the perennial philosophy." It was later popularized by Aldous Huxley in a book of the same name: the common, eternal underpinnings of all religions once you get past the rituals and forms that are all too often used to divide rather than unify.

Prayer and meditation can provide the direct experience of the interconnectedness of life—on one level, we're separate and isolated, but on another level, we are a part of something much larger. Altruism may be healing for both the giver and the recipient because giving to others with an open heart helps heal the isolation that separates us from one another.

This is true in helping us survive on a global level as well as an individual one. As the Dalai Lama said when he was awarded the Nobel Peace Prize, "The realization that we are all basically the same human beings, who seek happiness and try to avoid suffering, is very helpful in developing a sense of brotherhood and sisterhood—a warm feeling of love and compassion for others. This, in turn, is essential if we are to survive in this ever-shrinking world we live in. For if we each selfishly pursue only what we believe to be in our own interest, without caring about the needs of others, we may end up harming not only others but also ourselves."

All divisions are man-made. In an era in which war and terrorism are often based on religious and ethnic differences, rediscovering the wisdom of love and compassion may help us increase our survival both as individuals and as a species at a time when the increasingly divided world so badly needs it.

The stress-management techniques and teachings described in this chapter are part of all cultures and all religions in one form or another. The ancient swamis and rabbis, monks and nuns, mullahs and maharishis didn't use these approaches simply as powerful stress-management techniques, although they are. They are also powerful tools for transformation and transcendence, providing a direct experience of what it means to be happy and peaceful if we simply stop disturbing our natural state of inner peace.

These techniques do not *bring* peace and happiness; they simply help us experience and rediscover the inner peace that is there already, once we stop disturbing it. As the ecumenical spiritual teacher Swami Satchudananda often said, "I'm not a Hindu; I'm an Un-do."

In a way, this is a radically different perspective from the messages we often receive in our culture, especially via advertising: that we are supposed to get happiness and peace of mind from outside ourselves by getting more, buying more, doing more. If we just acquire more possessions, achieve more accomplishments, and get more stuff—money, power, beauty, whatever—*then* we'll feel peaceful and happy.

Paradoxically, when we are more inwardly defined—i.e., when we realize that peace is our natural state until we disturb it—then we can go out in the world and accomplish even more, without getting so stressed and sick in the process.

People have power over you only if they have something you think you need. The more you experience inner peace, the less you need and the more power you retain.

Sometimes the most successful and powerful people are the unhappiest. It's hard to tell yourself that if you could just go from having $2 billion to having $3 billion, *then* you'd be happy. Before, at least, they had the myth that success brings happiness. Now they know better.

This dis-illusionment can be the beginning of real transformation. So can suffering in any form if we can reframe it into this context, as a powerful catalyst for transforming our lives for the better. Not that we seek out suffering, but, all too often, there it is. When we use our suffering to help us transform our lives, it helps bring meaning to our suffering, as I described in chapter 2.

When you embody peace, people around you feel it—maybe it's the mirror neurons in action. You become an example for others to emulate. When you meet hatred with love, fear with hope, it transforms yourself as well as those around you. As Gandhi wrote, "Be the change you want to see in the world."

Here's a poem about the transformative power of forgiveness from my favorite poet, Hafiz, who lived in Persia almost seven hundred years ago:

Forgiveness Is the Cash

Forgiveness
Is the cash you need.

All the other kinds of silver really buy
Just strange things.

Everything has its music.
Everything has genes of God inside.

But learn from those courageous addicted lovers
Of glands and opium and gold—

Look,
They cannot jump high or laugh long
When they are whirling.

And the moon and the stars become sad
When their tender light is used for
Night wars.

Forgiveness is part of the treasure you need
To craft your falcon wings
And return

To your true realm of
Divine freedom.

7

GUIDED MEDITATIONS

If you judge people, you have no time to love them.

—Mother Teresa

■ ■ ■ ■ ■ ■ ■ ■ ■

These guided meditations are a powerful way of helping to rediscover your inner sources of peace, joy, and healing. Remember, these guided meditations do not bring them to you; rather, they help quiet down your mind and body, thereby enabling you to experience what is there already.

These meditations were written by Anne Ornish, who is Vice President of the nonprofit Preventive Medicine Research Institute, where she directs all activities related to stress-management training. Although I am happily biased since Anne and I are married and have worked together for more than ten years, she is one of the most gifted yoga and meditation teachers anywhere.

A DVD of these guided meditations is included with this book. Some of these guided meditations are also available for free in streaming video at www.webmd.com.

Alternatively, you can ask someone to read them to you so you can participate with your eyes closed. Or you may want to read them into a tape recorder and play them back whenever you want. Choose the ones that appeal to you the most, in whatever order you desire. Here they are:

Breath Alignment

Your breath is the perfect, natural object of meditation—it's the most readily accessible and powerful tool we have—awareness of your breathing serves as a bridge between mind and body, consciousness and unconsciousness—which furthers the goal of increasing your field of overall awareness, or, in other words, "As is the breath, so is the mind and body." Our breathing rate powerfully corresponds with our pulse and heart rate. By practicing slow, rhythmic breathing, we can better regulate a steady heart rate and a more serene mind and relaxed body. By cultivating greater awareness of the breath, we support an ever-expanding and all-encompassing moment to moment attunement with our thoughts, feelings, and behaviors.

Steady and Grounded

Let's get steady and grounded through our center: Start by establishing a comfortable sitting position that's evenly aligned—so that the ears float above the shoulders and the shoulders float above the hips—this should support a tall, spacious spine—completely at ease. Reaching and extending your arms out to the sides, breathe in a full-body breath as you float your arms upward and turn your hands so that your palms come together above your head. Releasing the breath out, draw your palms down in front of you through your central axis, pausing at your heart center. Gently press your palms into each other as you expel any residual breath—it's while pausing here, empty of breath, that you can feel your body release and relax its weight into its stable contact with the earth.

- Breathe in and rise up; breathe out and root down; each time, enjoy a resting pause, empty of breath.

- Breathe in, wide awake; breathe out, fully supported by gravity's cushion.

- Breathe in, hugely open-hearted; breathe out, basking in the steadiness of your entire being.

Repeat three times.

Energy Boost

Let's give ourselves a boost of invigorating energy. First, enliven your body by lengthening your spine upward from a comfortable position that's evenly aligned in your seat. This exercise moves breath in and out rapidly through your nose, while keeping your mouth gently closed. Your inhalation and exhalation should be of equal length and as short as comfortably possible, producing a lively movement of the diaphragm. This is called "bellows breathing." You may want to first observe the way it looks and sounds—then we can practice it together with greater ease. (Practice bellows breathing for approximately 20 seconds.) Resuming natural easy breathing . . . notice that you're ready to reenter your day, feeling enlivened and refreshed.

Let It All Go

Let's lighten our load of everyday stress. Sit comfortably, evenly aligned in your seat, and tall in your spine. Let your arms rest naturally down along the sides of your body, palms open to the front of you. Breathing in, feel yourself clench all of your stress and tension into tighter and tighter fists, and suspend the breath in as you shrug your shoulders up toward your ears. Then, slowly, release the tension as you release the breath, release your shoulders, soften and reopen your fists. Finally, shake your hands out from the wrists, feeling the tension ease and unwind from your being.

- Breathing in, clench and consolidate all stress into your fists—then, with a swooshing out-breath, soften and reopen your fists and shake it all out.

- Breathing in, shrug your shoulders upward—then, with a sweeping out-breath, roll the shoulders back and down and shake it all out— feel yourself looser, lighter, and letting it all go.

Repeat two times.

Tranquillity of the Senses
Let's revel inwardly in the sumptuousness of our senses. Gently, yet briskly, rub the palms of your hands together, generating some heat. Then place one palm over your heart and the other over your belly so that you can feel your full body breathing. Now turn your attention inwardly to the quality of your breathing: feel the silky texture of your breath as it coats your throat, lungs, and belly; sense its tidelike rhythm as it naturally rises and falls away; and listen to the lapping sounds as it washes in and washes out from the shore of your body. Feel yourself as part of this life-giving breath. It can be especially powerful to practice this when you're in a noisy, bustling environment by simply plugging your ears to quickly and powerfully regarner your inner quiet and calm. For now, simply bask in the sensual pleasures of escorting your breath with full awareness—notice the heightened sensitivity and awe of being alive by fully inhabiting your body with breath.

The Equilibrium Advantage
Let's realign our mind and body with this ancient, balanced nostril-breathing technique. Our two nostrils function separately via two different nerve currents, which correlate with the right and left hemispheres of our brains. When there's equilibrium between these two entities, we feel more balanced.

To begin:

1. Exhale through both nostrils, clearing any residue.
2. Using your right thumb, seal the right nostril by pressing on it, and inhale through the left (for a count of 4).
3. Using your right ring finger, seal the left nostril by pressing on it, and exhale through the right (for a count of 4).
4. Keeping the left nostril sealed, inhale through the right (for a count of 4).
5. Seal the right nostril, and exhale through the the left (for a count of 4).
6. Keeping the right nostril sealed, inhale through left (for a count of 4). Repeat three times. Switch nostrils after each inhalation—in other words: exhale, inhale, switch nostrils, exhale, inhale, switch nostrils, end with an exhale through your right nostril.

Finally, as you resume your natural, easy breathing, notice a sense of inner spaciousness, a realignment with your natural inner symmetry and balance.

Greet a Great Day

Begin each day as the author of your life! Because if not you, then who? By imbuing attention with intention, you can effectively manifest the vision for your day, every day. As Winston Churchill said, "You create your own universe as you go along." Begin by becoming as clear and specific as possible about how you'd like your day to go. Script your day unfolding—just so—from morning through lunch, all afternoon, and into the evening. Believe that it is possible, as if it has already happened—go there in your mind's eye, feel it on a cellular level: feel vibrantly healthy, feel prosperous, feel confident, feel all the conditions that you're recruiting to support you today, and you will go there in your body. Take a moment now to cast the feeling tone and vision for your day. What begins to happen is that your predominant feelings will manifest, and circumstances and people will correspond to and cooperate with the nature of your intention, because they sense that it is powerfully imbued. Now remember that life can and will throw you some curveballs, so be prepared to regarner your focus, your desired intention and feeling tone, while going with the flow. When you align your thoughts and feelings internally, you're more readily able to manifest your reality externally—all will naturally flow forth from the inside out.

Reframe Frustration

Whenever you feel frazzled with frustration, remind yourself that you can always reclaim your sense of peace by the simple yet transformative practice of gratitude. When you are grateful, fear disappears and abundance appears, or, as one anonymous quote says, "Gratitude can reframe the past, bring peace for today, and create a vision for tomorrow." When things seem to be getting out of control around you, take a moment to reflect inwardly. Just like the axis of a wheel, when you return to your center, you find stillness. Take a moment to catch your breath here. Place one palm over your heart and rest your attention there as you take a series of deep full-body breaths. Now give yourself permission to open your heart to all that you're grateful for in your life. Identify three things for which you're grateful, that give you inspiration, guidance, and support. Feel them one by one. Practicing gratitude provides a doorway to a much deeper part of who you are: from here love blooms naturally, inspiration flows automatically, creativity bubbles up, and compassion emanates. Giving yourself a few minutes to practice gratitude can help you see your circumstances from a new angle, one with grace and abundant opportunities. It is from this inner locus that we can reframe, recalibrate, and regain our calmness and vigor to persevere. So remember, when frustration and despair arise, invoke the attitude of gratitude. Gratitude is the bottomless well within you and all around you.

Seek Haven

Sometimes, it can feel like a jungle outside. Fortunately, your own private sanctuary awaits you inside, and it is only a few breaths away. Let's begin by adopting any posture you like that's essentially at ease, supported, and relaxed. Take a moment to get completely comfortable throughout your entire being. From here, turn your senses inward by anchoring your awareness on the free flow of your breath—feeling it flow slowly, fully, naturally, and rhythmically. Begin to hold a space for stillness and inner quiet by visualizing a place in your mind's eye that's beautiful, safe, serene, and special to you. Once you've unveiled it, fully inhabit this haven within you with a genuine curiosity. Enjoy the clear "blue-sky mind" that's fresh, open, and naturally available while you inhabit this private sanctuary of yours. Attend inwardly to your heart softening and opening itself like an exotic flower that shows its full petals only when conditions are just right. Invite a pure, loving light to shine down upon you, infusing each cell with such luminosity that you feel it radiating from within you and all around you. Having bathed in your inner brilliance, you can now reemerge feeling brighter and deeply connected to your source, knowing that this private sanctuary always awaits you within, whenever you wish.

Eating with Ecstasy

Let's relish the ecstasy of eating with our five phenomenal senses. Before taking a bite, take a moment to imagine that you have never tasted or even seen food before. Examine the food you're about to eat with an inspired curiosity. Touch it, feel it—how does it feel, smell, and look? Lick it—how does it feel on your tongue and how does it taste? Now go ahead and put it into your mouth, enveloping it with all of your senses, but don't chew yet. Notice as you roll it around the different areas of your tongue how it feels and tastes. Now fully explore the sensations of your teeth sinking into the food as you slowly begin to chew, trying to chew until you no longer can, until only liquid flavors are left, then swallow. Maintaining this inspired curiosity and rapture, continue to take slow, conscious bites, intimately observing first the food's shape, its color, and how it feels in your hands, then the smell, textures, and tastes inside your mouth, down your throat, and finally nourishing your entire being.

Reveal Personal Insight

What's *in* the way *is* the way. It can be helpful to remind ourselves that the "stumbling" stone along life's path is often also the "stepping" stone. Although stress and suffering are inevitable parts of the human experience, how we relate and respond to the "potholes" of life is our choice. At one time or another, we've all experienced that despite changing our job, our relationship, even where we live, the same pesky patterns of discontent tend to emerge again. Why is that? It's actually quite liberating to recognize that the one common denominator is typically—you! Let's experiment now with a mindfulness practice designed to reveal this insight. Let's begin by coming back into your body. Establish a comfortable sitting position that's tall in the spine yet grants overall ease and support. Fully inhabit your body with a genuine curiosity. Allow your breath to flow slowly, fully, naturally, and rhythmically for the duration of this practice. Hold a space for stillness and inner quiet. In the beginning, you're likely to notice the inevitable and incessant tides of thoughts and feelings that come and go for a while. No matter how savory, simply witness them and let them pass as if you're simply an objective observer. You may make a peripheral "note to self" for later if that helps you clear your thinking mind. Sift, settle, and let it all go. For now, allow yourself to soften into your essence here without judgments, and invite the presence of your most wise and loving self that lies within you to emerge and expand. Eventually, after allowing the mind to settle, a mirror reflection of your true self will be revealed. Ask this presence to bring to light what shift you can make in your life that will result in a sustainable, deeply meaningful manner. Take a moment to ask yourself, "What am I not paying attention to that I need to understand?" Honesty, patience, and trust are required. Your reward, when the blind spots are removed, is a less-encumbered, more-empowered you! Source here as often as you like; the presence of your essence is always available, all knowing, and omnipotent.

Relax Deeply and Progressively

This exercise is designed to relax the body and promote healing. To support yourself in relaxing deeply and progressively, you can choose to lie on your back or sit in a chair. You can keep your eyes closed or open for the duration of this practice.

Situate yourself so you feel comfortably at ease in whatever position feels good to you. You may want to place pillows under your knees and head for more comfort.

If you want a pendulum to go to one side, you first pull it to the other side and let it go. The same is true for your body—to fully relax your muscles, it can be helpful to begin by tensing them first.

• Begin by inhaling as you gently tense the muscles of your right leg. Exhale as you relax. Do the same with the left leg. Inhale and gently tense your right arm. Exhale as you relax. Do the same with your left arm.

• Now inhale and tense the muscles of your buttocks. Exhale as you relax.

• Inhale and expand your abdomen. Then let your abdomen relax completely as you exhale through your mouth.

• Leaving your arms relaxed at your sides, inhale, bring your shoulders up toward your ears, and exhale as you relax. Inhale, then bring your shoulders toward each other in front of your chest. Exhale. Relax. Inhale and push your shoulders toward your feet. Exhale as you relax.

• Slowly roll your head from side to side and allow your neck to relax. Inhale and gently squeeze together all your facial muscles, including your jaw, mouth, eyes, and forehead. Squint and blink your eyes so as to soften the small muscles around your eyes, releasing any tension in your jaw, allowing it to hang slightly open.

- Exhale and relax.

- Using your mind, go through your body, mentally allowing each part of it to relax even more. You're not actively *trying* to relax your body; you're just *allowing* it to relax.

- Allow your feet, legs, and hips to relax.

- Allow your hands, arms, and shoulders to relax.

- Allow your buttocks, abdomen, chest, heart, and throat to relax.

- Allow your spine and all the muscles in your back and neck to relax.

- Allow all the muscles of your face and head to relax.

- Now bring the awareness to your breathing. Without trying to change your breathing pattern, observe or feel the gentle flow of air as it comes in and out as your body and mind begin to quiet down (about 1 minute).

- Observe what is happening in your mind. Simply notice whatever thoughts or feelings come up; let them pass without trying to judge, suppress, or control them. Allow a few minutes of silence to fully enjoy the experience of deep relaxation.

- Now ask your inner wisdom, your inner teacher, to make itself known to you in some way. It's a voice that speaks clearly but quietly. Silently express your appreciation to it for guiding you. Ask it if there is anything you need to pay attention to that you may have been ignoring. This inner teacher may communicate to you in words, images, symbols, or other ways. Listen.

- Gradually allow your inhalations to become a little deeper with each breath. Imagine that you are breathing in light and healing energy as well as oxygen that is revitalizing and recharging your body and mind. Allow this energy to come in through your head, down your back, spine, and the front of your body, your arms to your hands, and your legs to your feet.

- After a few minutes, slowly move your fingers and toes, hands and feet. Then gently roll your arms and legs back and forth.

- When you are ready, slowly roll over onto one side, bend your knees, and then come to a seated position (if you're not already sitting), feeling refreshed and rejuvenated.

- Quietly listen to what is there to be heard, dwelling within with the feeling tone of any sensations that are there to be felt, honoring inhabiting your body as a precious temple enshrining your existence, as a divine mirror keeping you alive, alert, and informed. Continue to follow your breath as it merges with the currents of energy moving from head to toe, enlivening the experience of your body as a whole.

THE EXERCISE SPECTRUM

Go pump some neurons! Expand your craniums!
—Robin Williams in the movie *Mrs. Doubtfire*

■ ■ ■ ■ ■ ■ ■ ■ ■

You don't need to read this chapter to know that exercise is good for you. You probably already know that regular, moderate exercise is one of the best things you can do for your health and well-being.

What you may not know is that new research is showing that exercise beneficially affects your genes, helps reverse the aging process at a cellular level, gives you more energy, makes you smarter, and may even help you grow so many new brain cells (a process called neurogenesis) that your brain actually gets bigger.

Really.

YOUR GENES ARE NOT YOUR FATE

Here again is another demonstration of the theme of this book: your genes are not your fate. The choices you make each day in your diet and lifestyle have a direct influence on how your genetic predisposition is expressed—for better and for worse. You're only as old as your genes, but how your genes are expressed may be modified by exercise, diet, and lifestyle choices much more than had previously been believed—and more quickly.

For example, Finnish scientists reported in a recent study that increased moderate to vigorous physical activity modified two genes involved in type 2 diabetes and reduced the risk of developing the disease, independent of changes in weight or diet.

ENERGY EFFICIENCY

One of the reasons that many people feel less energy as they get older is that their mitochondria work less efficiently with age. Your mitochondria are the "energy generators" of your body.

A recent study compared mitochondria from muscle biopsies of older and younger men and women. The investigators found that mitochondrial function declined markedly with age, and was affected by more than three hundred genes.

Then the investigators put the older men and women through a six-month exercise program that involved strength training for one hour two days per week using the types of weight machines found in most gyms. The resistance exercise for each session consisted of three sets of ten repetitions of leg press, chest press, leg extension, leg flexion, shoulder press, lat pull-down, seated row, calf raise, abdominal crunch, and back extension and ten repetitions of arm flexion and arm extension.

After six months, there were dramatic changes at the genetic level. According to Dr. Simon Melov, Director of Genomics at the Buck Institute in Novato, California, and coauthor of the study, "The genetic fingerprint [of the elderly participants] was reversed to that of younger people—not entirely, but enough to say that their genetic profile was more like that of young people than old people."

In other words, the mitochondrial impairment and muscle weakness often seen as you get older can be at least partially reversed by only six months of strength training. This is amazing stuff.

If the mitochondria in these participants improved—remember, mitochondria are the "power plants" inside your cells—you'd think that they would feel more energetic. Well, that's just what happened.

Objectively, their strength improved by 50 percent. And according to Dr. Mark Tarnopolsky, one of the study's lead authors, "Anecdotally, some reported that before the training, they had a hard time picking up their grandchildren. Afterward, they could pick them up." Others said that it became easier to carry heavy grocery bags or run up the stairs.

BIGGER BRAINS

Equally exciting is new research showing that regular exercise may cause your brain to grow new neurons. Until about nine years ago, it was thought that you were born with a certain number of neurons (brain cells) and they decreased in number as you got older. The best you could hope to do was to slow the rate at which you lost brain cells.

Fortunately, this is not true. Researchers at the Salk Institute for Biological Studies showed that older adults continue to generate new neurons at virtually any age. More recently, these researchers found that just walking for three hours per week for only three months caused so many new neurons to grow that the size of people's brains actually increased.

Best of all, the region of the brain that grew the most was the hippocampus, the one most involved with memory and cognition. After only three months, those who exercised had brain volumes typical of people three years younger! Also, the new neurons tend to find their way to well-established existing connections and replace ones that were damaged or nonfunctioning.

The authors concluded, "These results suggest that cardiovascular fitness is associated with the sparing of brain tissue in aging humans. Furthermore, these results suggest a strong biological basis for the role of aerobic fitness in maintaining and enhancing central nervous system health and cognitive functioning in older adults." According to the study's senior author, Dr. Arthur Kramer, "It's not just a matter of slowing down the aging process. It's a matter of reversing it."

Nutrition also affects your neurons—for better and for worse. A diet high in sugar and saturated fat diminishes neurogenesis, whereas other foods increase it, including chocolate (in moderate amounts), tea, and blackberries, which contain a substance called epicatechin that improves memory. Small amounts of alcohol increase neurogenesis, whereas larger amounts decrease it. Chronic emotional stress decreases neurogenesis, but stress-management techniques increase it. Drugs such as nicotine, opiates, and cocaine decrease neurogenesis, whereas a study published in the *Journal of Clinical Investigation* in 1995 showed that cannabinoids (found in marijuana) may increase it, at least in rats. (Uh, what were we just talking about?)

Also, regular, moderate exercise (along with healthier eating and stress-management techniques) reduces inflammation throughout your body, including in your brain, and also reduces the incidence of tiny strokes that can impair your ability to think clearly. In addition, levels of beneficial neurotransmitters such as dopamine, serotonin, and norepinephrine are higher in those who exercise. These, in turn, may help reduce depression, elevate mood, and help you focus better.

EXERCISE MAKES YOU SMARTER

Other studies have shown that older adults who exercise regularly have better memory, are better at going from one mental task to another, and can focus and concentrate better than those who are sedentary.

In other words, exercise makes older people smarter.

Exercise makes younger people smarter, too. Kids who exercise have fewer problems with attention deficit disorder and learn faster. Studies have shown that physical education in schools improves academic performance as well as physical fitness.

For example, a study by the California Department of Education of more than 350,000 fifth-grade students found a direct correlation between physical fitness and subsequent SAT scores. Those who were most physically fit were in the seventy-first percentile, while the least fit were in the thirty-sixth percentile—almost half as much. When they looked at 322,000 seventh-grade students, they found an even bigger gap—the most fit scored in the sixty-sixth percentile on their subsequent SAT tests, whereas the least fit scored in the twenty-eighth percentile.

These findings are consistent with a recent article published in *The Journal of Pediatrics.* Dr. Jennifer Miller and her colleagues reported that kids with early-onset morbid obesity had significantly lower cognitive function and more behavioral problems than those with no history of childhood obesity, due to the abnormal hormones and metabolism found in obese kids.

Given these findings and the research showing the direct beneficial effects of exercise on the brain, you'd think that exercise would be an important part of every child's education.

Not.

I was shocked to learn that only one state in the country—Illinois—mandates physical education in schools. That's pitiful.

I called Dr. Kenneth Cooper, one of the pioneers of preventive medicine, who coined the term "aerobics," and asked him why. "When we went to school many years ago, ninety percent of us had physical education," he said. "Now it's just reversed—only ten percent of schools have physical education. Why can't we change this? One of the single most important things that America could do to reverse this trend is to put physical education back in schools and mandate it for all students."

I also spoke with Jim Whitehead, who is Vice President of the American College of Sports Medicine and is serving this year as President of the National Coalition for Promoting Physical Activity. I asked him, "Why can't we pass laws that mandate physical education in every school? What would have more public support than something that's proven to prevent something really awful in kids?"

NO CHILD'S BIG BEHIND

According to Whitehead, one of the unintended consequences of the No Child Left Behind Act was to significantly reduce the number of schools offering physical education. Schools are rewarded or punished based on the results of standardized tests, so many schools are cutting physical education out of the curriculum in order to spend more time teaching students to do well on these tests. "The physical fitness of students is not one of the metrics used to incentivize schools," he said, "so it worsens the trend of getting physical activity out of the school systems on a national basis."

Most people know that exercise is good for them, even if they aren't familiar with the latest research. Why, then, do only 25 percent of Americans exercise at the minimum level suggested by the surgeon general? And why is it that almost 40 percent of the adult population is physically inactive?

For all the reasons you probably already know. Kids play computer games instead of sports or even hide-and-seek. It's not always safe for kids to play outside as previous generations did. For adults, modern technological conveniences have replaced a great deal of physical labor. Remote controls. Automatic garage door openers. Electric golf carts. Such conveniences are great for everything except our health.

In addition, more people have long commutes to work and spend more time working. If you spend an hour traveling each way, that's two hours out of your day, ten hours a week, which leaves less time for exercise.

Also, too many Americans have bought into the idea that for exercise to be health-enhancing, it has to hurt. No pain, no gain. Go for the burn. Join a gym, sweat buckets, and run marathons.

Exercise should be fun, not painful. If you don't enjoy it, you won't do it. At least not for long. If it's fun, it's sustainable. A little goes a long way.

Fitness and health are not the same. As I wrote in chapter 4, the more you exercise, the fitter you become and the more weight you lose, but if you're just trying to stay healthy and reduce your risk of illness and premature death, just walking twenty to thirty minutes per day may be sufficient. And not even all that fast or even all at once.

If you want to compete in the Olympics, you have to get into peak aerobic condition. But if your goal is to lose weight, sleep better, feel happier, enjoy sex more, suffer less constipation, lower your cholesterol level and blood pressure, and reduce your risk of developing diabetes, arthritis, heart disease, and many cancers, you can do that with just thirty minutes of brisk walking a day—or any other type of physical activity you enjoy: biking, dancing, swimming, gardening, you name it.

BENEFITS OF REGULAR PHYSICAL ACTIVITY

- Controls weight. Exercise raises your metabolic rate so you burn more calories. Regular exercisers even burn more calories while resting.
- Makes you feel happier. Elevates mood. Lessens the risk of depression.
- Makes you feel less hostility and anger.
- Makes you feel more resilient and better able to cope with life stresses.
- Makes you feel more self-confident; you enjoy greater self-esteem and a general sense of well-being.
- You have more energy for both work and play.
- Your joints are healthier, so you can move more easily and comfortably with less pain.
- Improves your sleep.
- Lowers your blood pressure; you may be able to get off medication.
- Lowers total cholesterol. Lowers LDL ("bad") cholesterol. Lowers triglycerides. Increases HDL ("good") cholesterol. Reduces the need for drugs.
- Increases your strength.
- Increases your flexibility.
- Increases your stamina.
- Improves your heart function. More blood is pumped per beat, carrying more oxygen to all cells.
- Improves muscle efficiency; your muscles work better.
- Lowers blood sugar, reducing the risk of diabetes.
- Reduces the risk of heart attack and of developing blood clots that trigger heart attack.
- Reduces the risk of stroke. Most strokes are caused by blood clots in the brain.
- Increases bone density so there is less risk of osteoporosis and fractures.
- Improves balance so there is less risk of falls and fractures.
- Decreases body fat and increases lean tissue/muscle mass.

EASY DOES IT

Exercise isn't complicated. I've outlined a lot of information on exercise in this chapter, but it can be distilled to this:

Do what you enjoy, make it fun, and do it regularly. That's it.

To gain all the health benefits of regular exercise, you don't have to join a gym, hire a personal trainer, or organize your life around 10-Ks. In the Women's Health Study, a major ongoing research project involving tens of thousands of women, those who walked briskly for just sixty to ninety minutes a week—just fifteen minutes a day—cut their risk of death from heart attack and stroke in half.

What if you want more than just health benefits? What if you want increased fitness? A recent study in *The Journal of the American Medical Association* showed that the same amount of exercise—sixty to ninety minutes a week—improved fitness quickly in people who were very unfit: overweight, sedentary, and with borderline high blood pressure.

The belief that exercise means superstrenuous workouts is a key reason that more than half the people who start an exercise program quit, usually within six months. I'd quit, too, if I thought I had to spend hours a day on a stair machine.

Park a little farther from work or the mall and walk a bit more? That can give you ten minutes of exercise a day. Enjoy dancing, yoga, swimming, biking, or gardening? They all count as exercise. So does making love with your beloved, "horizontal aerobics," which has the added benefit of love and intimacy. If you incorporate any physical activity you enjoy into your daily life, it doesn't take much to gain the physical and emotional benefits of exercise.

When people ask me what I do for exercise, I explain that I use an elliptical trainer (low-impact aerobics) and weight machines on a regular basis. I also practice yoga, enjoy tennis, hike, and take karate classes with Anne and Lucas.

For those who want more detailed information on exercise, here it is.

THE EXERCISE SPECTRUM

There are three components of exercise:

- Stamina, often called aerobics, endurance, or cardiopulmonary conditioning
- Strength, often called resistance training
- Flexibility

A good exercise program includes all three. Keep them in mind as you consider how to customize an exercise program that works for you.

The Stamina/Aerobics Spectrum

Exercise that enhances stamina is important for the prevention and reversal of most chronic diseases. It conditions the heart, lungs, and muscles, as well as the circulatory, digestive, nervous, and hormonal systems. In a nutshell, aerobic exercise uses the large muscles in your body—arms and legs—in a repetitive, continuous way at an intensity that challenges your personal comfort level without exhausting you or turning you off to regular exercise.

Exercise physiologists like to use the acronym FITT—Frequency, Intensity, Time, Type—to describe the aerobic exercise spectrum.

Frequency: At least three times per week if possible.

Intensity: Here's a handy rule of thumb: exercise hard enough so that you can talk while doing it but not feel able to sing. Or, as exercise physiologists say, exercise at 40 to 80 percent of the maximum heart rate recommended for your age group.

Time: Thirty to sixty-plus minutes per day. It doesn't have to be all at once. Feel free to break it up into ten- to fifteen-minute chunks, for example, a fifteen-minute walk at lunch.

Type: Continuous activity that uses large muscles: walking, swimming, cycling, dancing, running, tennis.

If you are not currently doing any aerobic exercise, start easy, for example, with a walk around the block every other day. Over a few weeks, work up to a daily walk around the block. Then a walk at lunch and after work, and so on. Over a few months, see if you can work up to thirty minutes at a time every day.

Then reassess your goals. Are you feeling happier, more resilient, and less stressed? Are you losing weight at a pace that feels right? Is your blood pressure coming down? If so, great; just stick to what you're doing or experiment with similar activities that you enjoy (called cross-training). If not, gradually increase the frequency and duration of your exercise until you reach your goal. Just be careful about increasing exercise intensity. Always increase the frequency and duration of exercise before the intensity to decrease the risk of overuse injuries.

The Strength/Resistance Training Spectrum

Strength training is about being able to lift your suitcase comfortably while traveling, not how big your muscles are. Again, you don't have to join a gym or invest in barbells or an elaborate weight machine, although they can be fun. Even repetitively lifting a can of food while talking on the phone has value. The benefits of strength training include:

Loss of fat and weight	Increased metabolism
Less arthritis pain	Improved bone density
Lower blood pressure	Lower cholesterol
Feeling happier; less depression	Less risk of diabetes
Improved self-confidence	Less constipation

Like aerobic exercise, resistance training is based on the "overload principle": if you regularly coax your muscles, including your heart, to work a bit harder than usual, they will adapt to the minor overload and, over time, become stronger and more efficient.

Safety and injury prevention are crucial. Don't overdo it. Customize your strength training based on your own individual situation, your health needs, and your specific goals. Good form (e.g., keeping your back straight and your knees slightly bent) helps prevent injuries. Exhale when lifting, pushing, or pulling. Inhale as you release. If you can afford it, a few sessions with an exercise professional will help you get off on the right foot (no pun intended).

The Strength/Resistance Training Spectrum looks like this:

Frequency: Two to five days per week.
Intensity: As before, exercise so you can talk while doing it, but not feel able to sing. Exercise at 40 to 80 percent of maximal capacity or a perceived exertion of very light to hard (vigorous).
Time: Eight to ten different exercises, each with one to three sets. Each set will require ten to fifteen repetitions, and you'll rest for one to three minutes between sets.
Type: You may want to invest in a set of free weights or elastic bands, but you can get the same benefit by using canned food or plastic bottles of water.

If you want to build muscle mass, do fewer repetitions with heavier weights. If you want to increase your muscle tone, go for more repetitions with lighter weights.

If you are just starting to strength train, pick a weight light enough that you can complete one set of eight repetitions, with the last repetition feeling a little difficult. Over several weeks, slowly increase the weight and the number of repetitions (reps). Increase the load slowly, by just 2 to 10 percent. Water bottles are good for this. Start with a large bottle only partly filled. Then, over time, slowly fill it.

Progression Spectrum to Increase Muscular Strength

Frail or older adult	1 set	10–15 repetitions	2–3 days/week
Healthy adult—beginner	1 set	8–12 repetitions	2–3 days/week
Novice—after three to four months of training	1–3 sets	8–12 repetitions	2–3 days/week
Intermediate	1–3 sets	1–12 repetitions	2–3 days/week
Advanced	1–3 sets	1–6 repetitions	4–5 days/week

Source: Adapted from American College of Sports Medicine, "Position Stand on Progression Models in Resistance Training for Healthy Adults," *Medicine and Science in Sports and Exercise* 34, no. 2 (2002): pp. 364–380.

Tips for strength training:

- Exercise larger muscles before smaller ones—for example, thighs before calves.
- Do exercises that involve multiple joints before single ones—for example, do overhead lifts before wrist curls.
- Do harder exercises before easier ones.
- It's better to exercise the same muscle groups on alternate days.

The Flexibility Exercise Spectrum

Are your muscles and joints stiff? Do you think that's a normal part of getting older? Aging brings some natural loss of muscle and joint tone, but the major reason why Americans feel muscle and joint stiffness is that they neglect flexibility exercise. To most Americans, "exercise" means building strength and stamina. These are important, of course, but so is flexibility, typically the forgotten element in exercise. Good flexibility enhances your ability to do just about everything. Not only that, it also decreases stress, improves your mood and posture, and decreases the risk of injury and falls.

One of the best ways to gain flexibility is to practice hatha yoga on a regular basis. Learn a style that suits your temperament from a teacher you trust.

Exercise Spectrum for Flexibility Exercise

	GENERAL POPULATION	AGING/FRAIL
Frequency	Minimum 2–3 times/week	Minimum 2–3 times/week
Intensity	To a point of mild discomfort	Mild discomfort with no pain
Time/Repetitions	10–30 seconds, 3–4 reps per stretch	10–30 seconds, minimum of 4 reps per muscle group
Type	Static stretches to the major muscle groups	Static stretches to the major muscle groups

Now let's determine how much you need to exercise. In the following chapters, I describe an exercise spectrum for preventing or reversing each of the chronic diseases.

Exercise for health and illness prevention. As stated earlier, if you are healthy and want to stay that way, you really don't have to do very much. Just accumulate thirty minutes of moderate aerobic exercise about three times a week. You don't even need to do it all at once. Try to include at least two sessions per week of some type of strength training, and stretch a couple times a week.

Exercise for fitness. The more frequently, intensely, and longer you exercise, the fitter you become. If you exercise more than walking, do it consistently. Being a "weekend warrior" increases your risk of injury.

Here is a summary of basic principles of sustainable exercise:

1. Choose activities that you enjoy.

What brought you joy when you were a child? Jumping rope? Using a pogo stick? What would bring you joy now? You will be much more likely to be consistent with your physical activity and exercise if you enjoy it.

Do you enjoy gardening more than softball? Then garden. Do you love rollerblading but hate treadmills? Then buy some nice Rollerblades and use them.

2. Listen to your body.

Don't overdo it. As mentioned earlier, you should be able to talk while you exercise. Focus on the difference between pain and soreness. If you experience any sharp or burning pain while exercising, stop what you're doing immediately, apply an ice pack to the injury, and perhaps take an over-the-counter anti-inflammatory drug (aspirin, ibuprofen, naproxen). If it hurts, stop doing it.

However, it's normal—in fact, good—to feel some achy soreness the day after exercise, especially if you're new to working out. Soreness means you've pushed your muscles just a bit beyond their comfort level. It means you're getting stronger.

If pain persists or gets worse after a few days, see your doctor.

3. Be consistent.

When exercising for health, consistency is more important than duration or intensity. It's better to exercise a little every day than to be a "weekend warrior" and go overboard one or two days a week.

4. Be flexible.

If you aren't able to exercise one day, do a little more the next. Stuff happens.

Keep a pair of walking shoes and sweats in the car in case an appointment is canceled and you find yourself with some unexpected free time.

5. Exercise your core.

Your core is the area around your navel. It's also your center of gravity, where all large-muscle movements originate. By strengthening your core, you gain several benefits: protection against back pain, improved posture, and greater abdominal muscle tone.

6. The easiest way to increase physical activity is to make it part of your daily routine.

- Instead of driving, walk or bicycle to work or to the store. If that's not practical, park a little farther away (where parking places are usually easier to find, thereby also reducing your stress level).

- Take the stairs instead of an elevator, especially if you're going only one or two floors.
- If you use the moving sidewalks at airports, don't just stand there—walk!
- Get off the bus or subway a stop or two early and then walk the rest of the way.
- If you play golf, walk instead of using an electric cart.
- Exercise with family or friends to provide social support, for more motivation and a double benefit.
- On a vacation, walk rather than driving to see and experience the sights.

7. Invest in a good pair of shoes.

A good pair of shoes makes it more fun to walk. In addition, proper exercise clothing that wicks moisture away from the skin is important for regulating body temperature.

8. Walk your dog, whether you have one or not.

Pet ownership is associated with many health benefits: greater resilience, more self-esteem, lower blood pressure, and, in the case of dogs, more exercise because you have to walk them. If you don't want a dog, connect with friends who have them and ask to walk *their* dogs or join them when they walk their pets.

9. Collaborate with your doctor.

If you are a man under the age of 45 or a woman under the age of 55 and do not have a chronic disease or significant risk factors for cardiovascular disease (smoking, obesity, high blood pressure, high cholesterol), it's not essential to see your doctor before starting an exercise program, but it's useful to talk with him or her about exercise in the context of your overall health, especially if you've been sedentary for a while.

The following chapters describe how to use the Exercise Spectrum to customize just the right amount of activity for you.

LOWERING YOUR CHOLESTEROL
LEVEL USING THE SPECTRUM

It is a scientific fact that your body will not absorb cholesterol if you take it from another person's plate.

—Dave Barry

■ ■ ■ ■ ■ ■ ■ ▪ ░

TESTIMONIAL:
Wesley Miller, Clarksburg, West Virginia

A year ago, I didn't think I'd still be here. It's been quite an adventure.

In November 2001, I had a wake-up call with unstable angina, ended up in the ICU, and got some alarming news from my cardiologist. He said, "Your bypass grafts are totally occluded, and your vessels are too small and diseased to bypass again or to angioplasty." Any further surgical intervention was discouraged.

Well, that didn't give me a whole lot of choices. I thought that I had been doing most everything right for my coronary artery disease since my bypass surgery in 1994, but now I was convinced that I was going to die.

While visiting me in the ICU, my family practice physician informed me that I had been diagnosed with diabetes mellitus, type 2, and that he had also referred me to a new lifestyle-modification program that was soon to be offered by the United Hospital Center. When I heard the phrase "reversing heart disease," I was interested. It's been a wonderful, rewarding experience. We live in a partially hydrogenated world. When I began changing my diet and lifestyle, I began to see some amazing physical transformations. This program has done more for me than I imagined possible.

Because of my angina, walking was difficult and I often needed a cane or wheelchair. My physical condition was already less than desirable due to chronic back pain caused by three ruptured disks and spondylolisthesis with neuropathy in both legs and feet. I had trouble getting to my mailbox without experiencing chest pain.

In November 2001, I was using a cane to walk with, and I had the humiliating experience of riding a wheelchair around Wal-Mart. Now, I didn't like that. I wasn't going to settle for that. I knew there had to be a better way, and thank God I found a better way.

By the seventh week of the program, my angina had disappeared. I no longer had any chest pain at rest or during exercise. I thought that was a little too good to be true, but it was real. I used to get chest pain after walking seventy-five feet; now I can walk more than two miles without any pain at all. I can ride a stationary bike from eight to ten miles a day without any angina or other pains. I feel like the Energizer Bunny.

I no longer use a cane or a wheelchair.

After being in Dr. Ornish's program:

- My cholesterol decreased from 243 to 110 mg/dl.
- My triglycerides came down from 819 to 93 mg/dl.
- My HDL is up from 27 to 38 mg/dl.
- I lost 50 pounds—anyone looking for an inexpensive wardrobe, let me know.
- My heart's ejection fraction increased from 45 percent to 61 percent.
- My PSA (prostate-specific antigen) decreased from 4.5 to 3.3 ng/ml.
- I no longer have to take my diabetes medications.
- My doctor has discontinued or reduced my other medications by 75 percent.

Now, these statistics are fine, and I have certainly worked hard to get to this point. But the most wonderful part of the program is the quality of life that I'm able to enjoy now that I thought I'd never be able to again. Instead of a fear of dying, it's been replaced by a gratitude of living. I have made a permanent lifestyle change.

The program did not give me self-discipline; rather, it awakened my discovery of the self-discipline that I thought I never had. It uncovered my need to exercise my power of choice instead of reacting to the dictates of my default mode, as I had been doing for most of my life. This, in turn, uncovered my need for the exercise of the rest of my body, soul, and spirit.

I am not alone. Each of us is a participant in our individual and mutual healing. I am my brother's keeper. We see each other as the persons that we have been designed to be, not who we have been told we are or, as victims, have allowed ourselves to become.

The German poet Goethe said, "Treat people as if they were what they ought to be, and you help them to become what they are capable of being."

This is an emotional thing. It's not something to take lightly. And I am so thankful that I'm a part of this program. It's certainly been a lifesaver for me.

Am I going to die? Someday, but not today. I have too much life to live. To me, the Ornish lifestyle-modification program has given a whole new meaning to "heartfelt thanks."

THE NUTRITION SPECTRUM

How efficiently—or inefficiently—your body is able to metabolize and get rid of dietary saturated fat and cholesterol in your diet is regulated, in part, by your genes.

So let's say you decide to have your cholesterol level checked, since you know that reducing LDL cholesterol saves lives. Maybe even yours. So you go to your doctor, get some blood drawn, and return for a follow-up visit a few weeks later.

All too often, the doctor says, "Well, it looks like your cholesterol level is too high. I imagine that you aren't going to change your diet or lifestyle very much. So don't worry about doing that; I can just give you a statin cholesterol-lowering drug, and that'll do it."

The diagnosis is right, but the prescription is incomplete: not surprisingly, many people just take the drug and do not change their diet and lifestyle.

Our health care system—really, a disease care system—is set up to make it difficult for doctors to counsel patients about alternatives to drugs and surgery. This system is enormously frustrating for both doctors and patients. Usually, the doctor has only about five minutes to meet with you, and besides, we doctors learn very little about nutrition and comprehensive lifestyle changes as part of our medical training. Drugs and surgical procedures are reimbursable, but diet and lifestyle training are usually not (although my colleagues and I have been working hard with Medicare and many insurance companies to help change that).

"Well, I really would like to try changing my diet and lifestyle first," you might say to your doctor, who may be likely to reply, "Okay, just change your diet moderately—a little less red meat, more fish and chicken, four eggs a week, fewer doughnuts."

So you do. When you go back to the doctor a month later to get your blood checked, your cholesterol level probably hasn't budged very much. Now the doctor says, "I'm sorry, your diet failed; now we have to put you on a statin drug like Lipitor for the rest of your life."

In fact, though, your diet didn't fail; just that particular type of diet. You have a spectrum of choices. Whether or not you want to try alternative approaches is, of course, up to you, but I do think it's important to know your options so that you can make informed and intelligent choices.

The first option, and usually the best one, is to make progressively bigger changes in your diet and lifestyle. For some people, the moderate changes in diet recommended by the American Heart Association and the National Cholesterol Education Program are enough to lower their cholesterol levels sufficiently, but not for many. Studies show that most people achieve only a 5 percent reduction in their LDL cholesterol level from making these moderate changes in diet.

However, bigger changes in your diet and lifestyle usually result in larger improvements in your cholesterol levels. In our research, which was a randomized controlled trial published in *The Journal of the American Medical Association,* we found that there was a *40 percent average reduction in LDL cholesterol* after one year in a free-living group of men and women, none of whom was taking cholesterol-lowering drugs. This is comparable to what can be achieved with statin drugs such as Lipitor but without the costs and potential side effects, such as liver and muscle damage. But these people made bigger changes in diet and lifestyle than most doctors have been recommending.

There is a genetic variability in how efficiently people can metabolize dietary fat and cholesterol. The Nobel Prize in Medicine was awarded to Drs. Michael Brown and Joseph Goldstein for discovering what are called cholesterol receptors. These receptors, on the surface of your cells, bind and remove cholesterol from your blood. The more receptors you have, the more efficiently your body can metabolize (get rid of) the saturated fat and cholesterol in your diet.

Some people are genetically lucky. They have a lot of cholesterol receptors; because of this, they are so efficient at getting rid of fat and cholesterol in their diet that they can eat almost anything yet their cholesterol levels remain low—sometimes referred to as the Winston Churchill effect, since he lived to ninety despite a reputed diet of marrow bones, champagne, and cigars. Other people have fewer cholesterol receptors, so they just look at butter and their cholesterol level rises. In the middle of this spectrum is most everyone else.

The good news is that even if you're on the inefficient, or "unlucky," end of the spectrum because you don't have very many cholesterol receptors, you are still likely to improve significantly if you make bigger changes in your diet and lifestyle than otherwise. In other words, it doesn't matter so much if you're not very efficient at metabolizing dietary saturated fat and cholesterol if you're not eating very much of it.

This provides a genetic basis for the concept of a spectrum of choices. Begin by making moderate changes in your diet; if that's enough to achieve your goals, great. If not, you can make progressively bigger changes until you do. Even if you're not genetically very efficient, continuing to reduce your consumption of saturated fat and cholesterol will usually cause your cholesterol level to decrease even more.

You don't need to actually measure the number of your cholesterol receptors; you can just make progressively bigger changes until you achieve the reduction you want to accomplish. If your cholesterol level decreases in response to moderate changes in your diet and lifestyle, chances are you have a larger number of cholesterol receptors than most people do.

But it's not necessary to know that; all you need to do is to go further and further toward the healthy end of the Spectrum until you respond. This is an example of the empirical, iterative process I described in chapter 4.

Statin drugs are effective ways of lowering cholesterol levels. Several large-scale randomized controlled trials have demonstrated that statin drugs can reduce cardiac events and premature death, and they may have additional anti-inflammatory benefits. Some people, only half facetiously, talk about adding them to the water supply. I prescribe them for patients when indicated.

Although statins are beneficial, I just don't think that these drugs are the best first choice for most patients, since all medications have costs and side effects, both known and unknown. Last year, billions of dollars were spent on statin drugs, most of which could have been avoided by making bigger changes in diet and lifestyle, and the only side effects of diet and lifestyle changes are good ones.

Now, whether or not anyone wants to change his or her diet and lifestyle is a personal decision. I don't even tell my own patients to change. Instead, we go through the various options, including drugs, and the risks, costs, benefits, and side effects of each. I support whatever action they choose.

Most doctors believe that taking a pill is easy but changing a lifestyle is really difficult, if not impossible. It turns out that the conventional wisdom is wrong—two thirds of patients who are prescribed statin drugs are not taking them just twelve months later, according to a 2002 study published in *The Journal of the American Medical Association*.

Why? Because cholesterol-lowering drugs don't make you feel better. So you're asked to take a pill today that doesn't make you feel any better in order to help prevent something really awful like a heart attack or stroke that's really too scary to think about—so you don't.

In contrast, most people who make comprehensive lifestyle changes feel so much better so quickly that it reframes the reason for changing from fear of dying to joy of living. As I wrote in chapter 2, for many people, these are choices worth making—not only to live longer but also to feel better.

So here's a summary of how to use the proven approach of the Nutrition Spectrum to improve your cholesterol level and lipid profile, some of which I discussed in more detail in earlier chapters:

- **Eat less saturated fat,** which is found predominantly in animal products such as red meat, butter, and cream and in tropical oils. Your liver uses saturated fat to make LDL cholesterol.

- **Eat fewer foods containing trans–fatty acids,** which are found in most fried foods and processed foods such as cakes, cookies, and snack foods. If the label says "hydrogenated" or "partially hydrogenated," avoid it.

- **Eat fewer simple carbohydrates** such as sugar, white flour, white rice, and high-fructose corn syrup, which can markedly increase your triglycerides.

- **Eat more unrefined, complex carbohydrates** such as fruits, vegetables, whole grains, legumes, and soy products.

- **Lose weight,** which will help lower your cholesterol level as well as your blood sugar level.

- **Take 3 grams per day of fish oil,** which provides omega-3 fatty acids—preferably brands in which the bad stuff (mercury, PCBs, dioxin, etc.) has been removed. Besides their other significant health benefits, such as reducing your risk of sudden cardiac death by up to 80 percent, the omega-3 fatty acids may significantly lower your triglycerides and reduce inflammation.

- **Add soluble fiber to your diet;** this binds cholesterol in the intestinal tract and increases its elimination from the body, thereby reducing your LDL cholesterol. Food sources of soluble fiber include oat bran, flaxseeds, barley, psyllium husk, citrus fruits such as oranges and apples, and vegetables such as carrots, beans, and peas.

- **Curcumin** is the active ingredient of the Indian curry spice turmeric, as I mentioned in chapter 3. According to the latest research, curcumin may reduce cholesterol by interfering with intestinal cholesterol uptake, increasing the conversion of cholesterol into bile acids, and increasing the excretion of these bile acids. Curcumin has powerful antioxidant and anti-inflammatory properties and may help prevent the oxidation of LDL cholesterol to a more dangerous form that is more likely to end up in your arteries.

- **Red rice yeast extract** contains the same ingredient found in statin drugs. Some experts believe that red rice yeast extract has fewer side effects than statin drugs due to other substances present in the yeast, but this is controversial. It's best to take this under a doctor's supervision, given the potential side effects.

- **Niacin** is a B vitamin that is often given at much higher doses to effectively lower cholesterol. At these doses, niacin should be considered a cholesterol-lowering drug, even though it is available over the counter. It is best taken under a doctor's supervision, as niacin may cause flushing and even liver toxicity in some patients.

There are also some other alternative treatments, for which the evidence is more controversial:

- **Garlic.** Some studies show that garlic lowers cholesterol. However, the Agency for Healthcare Research and Quality, part of the U.S. Department of Health and Human Services, has concluded that these studies are inconclusive. In addition to reducing your cholesterol, too much garlic may also reduce your social support.

- **Guggul** is a yellowish resin produced by the mukul mirth tree, a small, thorny plant that grows throughout northern India. Guggulipid is extracted from guggul and contains chemicals called plant sterols. Several studies published before 2003 suggested that guggul and guggulipid may lower cholesterol levels in people with high cholesterol. However, more recent, well-designed research reports no improvements in cholesterol levels. Guggul may cause stomach discomfort or allergic rash as well as other serious side effects and interactions. It should be avoided by pregnant or breast-feeding women and by children.

- **Beta-sitosterol** is a plant sterol that may block absorption of cholesterol. It is one of several plant sterols found in almost all plants, especially in soybeans, rice bran, and wheat germ. It is also used to reduce symptoms of benign prostatic hypertrophy. Benecol is a margarine that uses a similar plant sterol to reduce cholesterol levels by blocking its absorption.

- **Policosanol** is derived from the waxy portion of Cuban sugarcane. In one well-designed study from Havana, policosanol lowered LDL cholesterol by 27 percent and raised HDL cholesterol by 17 percent. However, a randomized controlled trial study from Germany published in *The Journal of the American Medical Association* earlier this year did not find policosanol to reduce cholesterol levels more than a placebo did.

- **Pantethine** is formed in your body from pantothenic acid, a B vitamin that is found in a wide variety of foods. Pantethine is converted to coenzyme A, which has an important role in metabolism. Several studies suggest that pantethine may effectively lower cholesterol levels with few side effects.

- **Chocolate** may reduce oxidative modification of LDL cholesterol, thereby helping to keep it from ending up in your arteries. In addition, small amounts of dark chocolate may reduce your body's production of substances called leukotrienes that promote inflammation. However, large amounts of chocolate may increase your cholesterol levels.

THE EXERCISE SPECTRUM

A study in *The New England Journal of Medicine* reported that those who exercised in addition to changing their diet showed greater reductions in their LDL cholesterol ("bad cholesterol") than those who only modified their diet.

Also, research indicates that those who exercise have less oxidation of their LDL cholesterol molecules than those who are sedentary. When LDL cholesterol is oxidized, it's more likely to end up in your arteries, so exercise may help prevent this from happening.

Just as exercise helps lower your LDL cholesterol levels, lowering your cholesterol levels improves your ability to exercise normally. Researchers in Brazil found that there was a 75 percent reduction in the number of abnormal exercise stress tests after sixteen weeks in those who lowered their cholesterol levels compared with only 13 percent in those who did not.

In addition to lowering your LDL cholesterol, another study in *The New England Journal of Medicine* found that regular exercise improved eleven different types of cholesterol (lipoproteins) in beneficial ways. It significantly decreased the concentration of small, dense LDL and LDL particles, both of which are particularly harmful to your arteries, as well as other types of harmful cholesterol lipoproteins and triglycerides. Exercise also increased the concentration of total HDL ("good") cholesterol and other protective cholesterol lipoproteins.

The second major finding of this study was that the *amount* of exercise appeared to have a greater effect on harmful cholesterol levels than the *intensity* of exercise did. Those who exercised for a longer period of time (running seventeen to eighteen miles per week at a moderate pace) showed more improvement than those who exercised intensively but for a shorter time. So choose an exercise you enjoy, such as walking, that you can do on a regular basis. Those who exercised more intensively were more fit, but they didn't have more improvement in their cholesterol levels. This study provides greater evidence for the Exercise Spectrum: more is better, but even moderate changes have benefits.

THE STRESS-MANAGEMENT SPECTRUM

Stress can raise your cholesterol level independently of diet, whereas stress-management techniques may help lower it.

In our research, we found (not surprisingly) that the more people changed their diet, the more improvement we measured in their cholesterol levels. We also found that stress-management techniques decreased triglycerides and improved the ratio of total cholesterol to HDL cholesterol. The more people practiced stress-management techniques, the more impact it had on their cholesterol levels.

Besides lowering your cholesterol levels, meditation has been shown to reduce the oxidation of cholesterol. Meditation also helps prevent oxidized LDL cholesterol from ending up in your arteries.

Begin by practicing at least a few minutes a day of the stress-management techniques described in chapters 6 and 7 along with changes in a healthier direction on the Nutrition Spectrum and Exercise Spectrum.

SUMMARY

You can lower your cholesterol levels by moving in the healthier direction on the Spectrum. Start by making moderate changes in your diet: eat a little less saturated fat, trans fats, dietary cholesterol, and refined carbohydrates; exercise a little more; practice a few minutes a day of some stress-management techniques; and spend a little more time with your friends, family, and other loved ones.

If that's enough to get your cholesterol level down far enough, great; if not, you can make progressively bigger changes until you achieve your goal. Or you can start taking cholesterol-lowering drugs such as Lipitor. You can also try some combination of both. The further you go in the healthy direction on the Spectrum, the fewer medications you are likely to require, if any.

I suggest that you consult with your doctor to find the options that are best for you. If your doctor is unwilling to discuss all of the treatment options, consider consulting with another one who is. After all, it's *your* life.

Let's apply the Spectrum approach to preventing and reversing other conditions in the following chapters.

10

LOSING WEIGHT USING THE SPECTRUM

One word frees us of all the weight and pain in life. That word is love.

—Sophocles

■ ■ ■ ■ ■ ■ ■ ■ ■

TESTIMONIAL:
Gary Scales, San Francisco

In April 1993, I weighed 305 pounds. I wasn't fat; I was clinically obese. I was huge.

Not only was I fat, I was taking daily medication for hypertension. I was taking medicine for insomnia, and also for panic attacks, and anxiety attacks. I had a herniated disk, and was a borderline diabetic. I was really a physical and mental wreck. I was a walking time bomb at that time.

In the course of the next twelve months, I lost 100 pounds. My waist went from fifty to thirty-four inches, my blood pressure went from 150/100 to between 110/70 and 120/80. My total cholesterol went from 275 to 175, my HDL went from 35 to 72, and my LDL dropped from 150 to about 100.

My body fat content dropped from about 35 percent to 18 percent, and at the same time, my percentage of calories from fat dropped from 40 percent to 15 percent. It was fascinating to see the ratio between my body fat and the percent of fat that I was consuming. Indeed, I was what I ate, or I am what I'm eating.

My resting heart rate went from 76 to 55. I thought about that for a while, and I realized that in the course of one year, my heart will beat 11 million times less. Over the next ten years, my heart will beat 110 million fewer times. And I think of how when I started, my heart was going like this *(thump-thump-thump-thump)* and now it goes *thump* . . . thank you . . . *thump* . . . thank you . . . *thump*. . . .

How did this happen, and, more important, why did it happen? How important this program has been to me, how it has helped me, and how it has become part of my life.

I think it's interesting to understand that there is the "how" of weight loss, but there is also the "why." Anytime any of us is faced with decisions to change our lifestyle or change what we're doing about things, there are really two parts of the process. And it is the "how" that most of us know in weight loss. It's all pretty simple: if you eat less food and you exercise, you're going to lose weight.

But there's also the "why" of it. The "how" was the mechanics; the "why" was the dynamics of it.

When I started losing weight, people would often say, "What are you doing differently?" or "What's going on? You must have changed your lifestyle." When we talk of lifestyle, we're often just looking at the physical, the exterior. I did change my lifestyle, which meant that I ate different foods and I exercised more and I did certain things on the exterior, but really what happened and what made it successful, and what I hope will make it permanent, is that I had a *values change*, a *priority change* within.

Like me, you have an opportunity to sit down and examine what you're doing and how it affects you, to see where your priorities are, and to set out a game plan of where you want to go with it.

I knew I had a problem, and I knew I needed to do something about it. I was in my early fifties, and two-thirds of my life had passed. I was concerned not so much with the quantity of my remaining life but with the quality; not my fear of death but the loss of potential life.

Looking back at all the times I tried to lose weight—I've been in every diet program, I was one of the first males in Weight Watchers, twenty years ago in San Francisco, and none of them worked.

Over the previous thirty years, I gained almost 100 pounds. I tried to apply business principles to it, and I first defined the problem. Well, I had gained 100 pounds in thirty years, which is about 3⅓ pounds a year. And I asked myself, what does that really represent?

It's about 3⅓ pounds a year, which translates to about 12,000 calories a year, which, when I divided it by 365, meant that my body had consumed 35 calories a day more than it had expended, and in thirty years, I had gained 100 pounds.

Had I only known, I wouldn't have had that extra half of an Oreo cookie; I would have exercised for ten minutes—all of us would! It was such a revelation to me, and I was mad at myself, but really that was the key to reverse the process.

I said, "If I eat thirty-five fewer calories a day, in thirty years I'll lose a hundred pounds. The problem is, I'll be in my eighties." But then I said, "What difference does that make?" In the first year, I'd lose 3½ pounds, ten years, 35 pounds, that wasn't too bad at all.

And I started working with that, because I knew I could do that. And then I said, if I make three 50-calorie decisions a day and walk for thirty minutes, I'd lose 35 pounds in a year.

I committed myself for one year; I knew I could do it for one year. At age 50, one year represented 2 percent of my life to date. And really what I was going to say was, if I had twenty-five years left to go, with a seventy-five-year average life, each of those years, my future years, represented 4 percent of my remaining life. And the real question came down to—it was so basic, and it was so obvious to me—Was I willing to spend 4 percent of my remaining life to dramatically increase the odds and the percentage that for the remaining 96 percent I had an opportunity to improve not only the quantity but also the quality? That was a clear choice.

I had basically figured out the "how"—diet and exercise. But the "why" is what was so important and what Dean introduced and showed me—the support group and the stress reduction.

I ate a little red meat, some fish and chicken, mostly fruits and vegetables and whole grains. I just ate healthy foods. I did have indulgences. I never forgot what Dean said about chocolate ice cream—eat the best chocolate ice cream and savor a spoonful of it and that's all. That made so much sense to me. I won't eat junk food, but I will eat a bite or two of good ice cream; I will have one or two bites of cake—I won't eat the whole thing; and I get just as much satisfaction from it as if I had eaten all of it.

I eat fruit and yogurt for breakfast; I eat raw vegetables and sprouted wheat bread for lunch; and for dinner, fish or chicken or vegetables and fruit for dessert. I'll have half a cookie for dessert.

We were in Argentina in February for three weeks, and I had some wonderful steak there. But I didn't eat all of it, and I enjoyed it while I was there and I knew that when I came back I would eat more healthfully. When I indulge myself, I try to eat more healthfully the next few days. I tend to avoid cheese, animal fat, butter, ice cream, fried foods, desserts. I avoid refined carbohydrates in general, but I don't completely rule them out. I may have them occasionally along with high-fiber foods, but I do try to avoid them.

I don't know about most of you, but the idea of revealing my inner thoughts, feelings, emotions, and attitudes to other people—particularly strangers—was not something that I did easily or do easily. But the more I did it, the more I began understanding the emotions and the attitudes that I had about myself and about other people.

I had read a book years ago by a Jesuit philosopher by the name of John Powell. The name of the book was *Why Am I Afraid to Tell You Who I Am?* When I addressed that question for myself, the answer was really pretty simple: I'm afraid to tell you who I am because if I really open myself up to you, you might not like me. And then what would I do?

Instead I put on masks. I put on a mask for my parents, I put on a mask for my teachers, I tried to relate to what I thought you wanted me to be. The support groups allowed me to take off the masks that I wore and be authentic.

Food was a way for me to try to mask stress. Food was my emotional outlet. I knew what I was doing, but I just ate anyway, and it was out of dissatisfaction with myself, I think, more than anything else.

I've also significantly reduced my alcohol intake, which is just tons more calories. I'll have two glasses of wine in the evening, whereas I used to have two cocktails and two glasses of wine at a minimum. It was my way of coping with stress.

I'm the one who caused my feelings of stress. A lot of it was caused by a negative outlook I had of myself; it was a self-fulfilling prophecy.

Now I'm very happy with myself, with who I am. When I started to have little successes in losing a little weight, it gave me self-confidence in many other areas as well—a positive self-fulfilling prophecy. Meditation gives me insight. I am much more nonjudgmental and patient, really appreciating myself and others. I could be more compassionate with myself and view myself with more loving-kindness, which enabled me to do that with others as well.

I now look at things as challenges and opportunities and ways to learn rather than as I did before, as things that used to cause me a lot of emotional tangles. I love tension in my life; I think tension is good for us. I enjoy working. I enjoy being involved in things because I think tension gives us structure and keeps us together.

But rather than eating a lot of fattening foods, I'll go home this afternoon and munch on a couple of carrots or I'll eat an apple, rather than having a big piece of cheese or things like that. Or I'll go out and exercise for an hour, and that replaces time when I used to be eating.

It finally came to me; it was as simple as ABC. The "A" part of it was Accepting myself, not where I had been, not where I wanted to go, but where I was right now, right here. "B" was Be myself, take the mask off, just be who I am. "C" was see myself, see myself as who I was, what I was doing, what I was trying to do. When I looked at that as the "why" of what I was accomplishing or trying to accomplish, it made an awful lot of sense.

An attitude is really how we look at something. It's a filter. We all have different attitudes, we all see things differently, and as a result of our attitudes, our emotions come out. We all know it, whether it's anger, whether it's stress, whether it's frustration, whether it's lack of self-esteem, and I really started digging back through, like unpeeling the layers of an onion. Sometimes I found things I didn't particularly like about myself, and I just dragged them out, like pulling weeds. Once they were out in the daylight and I could see them and share them with other people, the problems went away.

Then I really started to appreciate the "why" of what I was doing. And it really made a lot of sense, and it made a difference.

When I told my family that I was going to take yoga and meditation classes, I am sure they thought I was turning into a left-wing, vegetarian mystic. And I assure you, that didn't occur. But when I started to understand that yoga and stress reduction are a lot more than just poses and breathing, I really started to learn more again about the "why."

And what I really saw, when I looked through it more, was that there is an interdependence, there is a connection, there is a total involvement between our physical self, our mental self, our emotional self, and our spiritual self. That realization didn't come overnight, but in time as I saw it and started to appreciate it, it made an awful lot of sense to me.

I realized that this was my one and only being, this was my one and only body, and I—and I alone—am responsible for its care and its maintenance.

I accept the responsibility, I embrace the responsibility that my health, my happiness, and my well-being are a direct result of what I do and that I have the main control of it.

I enjoy life. One of my goals is to dance with my wife at our fiftieth anniversary to "If You Were the Only Girl in the World (and I Was the Only Boy)." This summer, we will celebrate our forty-fifth anniversary. We have seven grandchildren now, and I know I said that I wanted to teach them the stars in the sky and how to fly-fish for rainbow trout.

When I started, my first goal was to lose 100 pounds. I did that, and I've kept it off now for more than twelve years. It's permanent. Then it evolved to where it is now: I want to live the rest of my life as a fully alive and fully aware human being.

As you know by now, obesity is a major health problem. The obesity epidemic is real.

If you want to see something really scary, go to the website of the Centers for Disease Control and Prevention in Atlanta (www.cdc.gov/nccdphp/dnpa/obesity/trend/maps/), which has been tracking the rise in obesity. You can see the obesity epidemic spreading like cancer metastasizing across the country from 1985 until now. It looks as if an alien force or a conquering army were taking over the United States, state by state, year by year.

Almost two thirds of adults are overweight, of whom one third are obese. Worse, a study in the *Annals of Internal Medicine* that followed 4,000 people over thirty years found that nine out of ten men and seven out of ten women will eventually become overweight.

According to the U.S. Department of Health and Human Services, obesity may account for 300,000 deaths a year, almost as many deaths as from cigarette smoking. People who are obese have a 50 to 100 percent increased risk of premature death from all causes compared to those who are not overweight, including heart disease, diabetes, high blood pressure, gallbladder disease, sleep apnea, osteoarthritis, and some cancers.

And it's not just adults. Since 1970, the percentage of kids who are over-weight or obese has risen almost fourfold, from 4.2 percent to 15.3 per-cent. As a result, this may be the first generation in which kids have·a shorter life span than their parents. According to former Surgeon General Richard Carmona, M.D., "As we look to the future and where childhood obesity will be in 20 years . . . it is every bit as threatening to us as is the terrorist threat we face today. It is the threat from within."

Well, it doesn't have to be this way. Childhood obesity is almost com-pletely preventable. We don't have to wait for a new drug or technology; we just have to put into practice what we already know.

Clearly, genes have changed little, if at all, in the past forty years. If changes in diet and lifestyle during that time caused the obesity epidemic by moving too far to the unhealthy end of the Spectrum, then moving toward the healthy end of the Spectrum can prevent or reverse the obesity epidemic.

In our study of 869 people who went through our program at twenty-two different sites throughout the United States that I mentioned earlier, there was an average weight loss of 12 pounds for men and 9 pounds for women after only three months.

In our earlier study, the Lifestyle Heart Trial, a randomized controlled trial published in *The Lancet* (after one year) and in *The Journal of the American Medical Association* (after five years), my colleagues and I found that people lost an average of 24 pounds during the first year, and they were able to keep off more than half that weight five years later.

There are three aspects of the Spectrum to consider in achieving and maintaining your optimal weight: the Nutrition Spectrum, the Exercise Spectrum, and the Stress-Management Spectrum.

THE NUTRITION SPECTRUM

In our research, we found that there was a direct correlation between intake of dietary fat and changes in weight and also between intake of refined carbohydrates and changes in weight. *Both* are important.

You have much more flexibility in your diet and lifestyle if you're just trying to lose a few pounds than if you're trying to reverse a life-threatening illness such as coronary heart disease (assuming that you're otherwise healthy). Remember, this is not a diet to go on or off of but a way of eating and living that's sustainable indefinitely.

First, find out where you are on the Nutrition Spectrum in chapter 5. How far and how quickly you choose to move in a healthier direction is entirely up to you, and there is a corresponding benefit. The further and more quickly you move in a healthier direction, the more weight you are likely to lose and the faster it will come off. As I described in chapter 3, move your diet in the direction of good carbs, some good fats, plant-based proteins, seafood, and whole foods that are nutrient-dense and away from bad carbs, bad fats, and refined foods.

Remember, what matters most is your *overall* way of eating and living, so you can allow yourself some indulgences as long as you tend to eat more from the healthier end of the Spectrum most of the time.

As I described in chapter 3, if you change the *type* of food you eat, you may not have to worry as much about the *amount* of food you consume. Fat has 9 calories per gram, whereas protein and carbohydrates have only 4 calories per gram. Thus, when you eat less fat, you consume fewer calories even if you eat the same amount of food—because the food is less dense in calories.

Also, the source of calories you consume may also make an important difference. A recent study revealed that trans–fatty acids play an important role in the development of belly fat.

Monkeys fed a diet high in trans fats—comparable to people eating a lot of fried foods—had a 7.2 percent increase in body weight, compared to a 1.8 percent increase in monkeys that ate monounsaturated fats, such as olive oil. What's interesting is that the monkeys were given the same number of total calories and amount of total fat; the only difference was that one group received 8 percent of their calories from trans fats while the other group received the same amount of calories as monounsaturated fat.

All that extra weight went to the abdomen, which is the most dangerous place to store fat. CT scans showed that the monkeys deposited 30 percent more fat in their bellies than the monkeys on the monounsaturated fat even though the monkeys were all given the same number of daily calories, with 35 percent of the calories coming from fat. The number of calories they consumed should have been only enough to maintain their weight, not to increase it.

One of the few interventions that has consistently been shown to prolong life in both animals and humans is calorie restriction. Consuming fewer calories also reduces DNA damage and insulin levels.

You can consume fewer calories by eating less food, but it's hard to sustain because you feel hungry.

A more sustainable way to consume fewer calories is by eating less fat. For example, if you eat foods that are 10 percent fat, you can consume one third fewer calories even if you eat the same amount of food because the food is less dense in calories.

Another important factor is to consume fewer refined carbohydrates, such as sugar. You can consume large amounts of sugar and other refined carbohydrates without feeling full, because the fiber has been removed, as I described in chapter 3.

Therefore, one of the benefits of eating closer to the healthy end of the Spectrum is not only that you lose weight; you're also likely to extend your life span because you're eating fewer calories.

THE EXERCISE SPECTRUM

Again, you have more flexibility here if you're just trying to lose a few pounds than if you're trying to reverse a serious illness. This is the cure of pound, not the pound of cure.

As described in chapter 8, the frequency, intensity, and duration of exercise are the primary determinants of how much weight it causes you to lose and how quickly. The more frequently, intensely, and longer you exercise, the more calories you burn and the more weight you lose. How far you want to go in that direction on the Spectrum is up to you.

One pound equals 3,500 calories. To lose one pound, you have to change your calorie balance by 3,500 calories. You can eliminate some of those calories by eating a lower-fat, higher-fiber diet—more fruits, vegetables, and whole grains and less meat, whole-milk dairy products, fried foods, and junk foods.

But for weight control, regular exercise is also crucial. Regular exercise not only burns calories, it also raises your basal metabolic rate, the number of calories you burn while at rest. Thus, exercise helps you lose weight even when you're not exercising.

If you haven't been exercising, work your way up to 2.5 hours of moderate aerobic and resistance-training exercise a week—just slightly more than twenty minutes a day. If, after a few months, you are not reaching your goal or moving toward it as quickly as you'd like, increase the amount of time you exercise—to thirty to sixty minutes a day of combined aerobic and resistance exercise. This is the level of exercise that appears to be most successful in losing weight and maintaining the weight loss.

Aerobic exercise is helpful in losing weight, and strength training also helps. It burns calories, and it makes you stronger, which makes everyday activities feel easier. It's more fun to do something when you feel strong doing it. And if what you do is fun, you'll be more likely to keep doing it.

And remember: everything counts. Every physical activity, from walking to climbing stairs to unloading your groceries, is exercise that helps you control your weight.

Here is a helpful table published by the American College of Sports Medicine that estimates how long you need to exercise to expend 300 calories.

Minutes of Continuous Activity Necessary to Expend 300 Kcal Based on Body Weight

Body Weight (pounds)

	120	130	140	150	160	170	180	190	200	210	220	230	240	250
Conditioning exercises														
Cycling														
Stationary	66	61	57	53	50	47	44	42	40	38	36	35	33	32
Outdoor (leisure)	83	76	71	66	62	58	55	52	50	47	45	43	41	40
Walking (level)														
2.5 mph	110	102	94	88	83	78	73	70	66	63	60	58	55	53
3.0 mph	94	87	81	76	71	67	63	60	57	54	52	49	47	45
3.5 mph	83	76	71	66	62	58	55	52	50	47	45	43	41	40
Water aerobics	83	76	71	66	62	58	55	52	50	47	45	43	41	40
Lap swimming	41	38	35	33	31	29	28	26	25	24	23	22	21	20
Yoga	83	76	71	66	62	58	55	52	50	47	45	43	41	40
Resistance exercise	55	51	47	44	41	39	37	35	33	31	30	29	28	26
Dancing														
Aerobic dance	55	51	47	44	41	39	37	35	33	31	30	29	28	26
Low-impact aerobic dance	66	61	57	53	50	47	44	42	40	38	36	35	33	32
Ballroom dance (fast)	60	56	52	48	45	42	40	38	36	34	33	31	30	29
Ballroom dance (slow)	110	102	94	88	83	78	73	70	66	63	60	58	55	53
Lifestyle activities														
Golf (walking)	73	68	63	59	55	52	49	46	44	42	40	38	37	35
Raking the lawn	83	76	71	66	62	58	55	52	50	47	45	43	41	40
Lawn mowing														
Walking power mower	73	68	63	59	55	52	49	46	44	42	40	38	37	35
Riding mower	132	122	113	106	99	93	88	84	79	76	72	69	66	63
Vacuuming/sweeping	132	122	113	106	99	93	88	84	79	76	72	69	66	63

Source: "ACSM Position Stand on the Appropriate Intervention Strategies for Weight Loss and Prevention of Weight Regain for Adults," *Medicine and Science in Sports and Exercise* 33, no. 12 (2001): p. 2152.

What I really like about this table is that it shows how many calories can be burned by having fun. Personally, I would rather play forty-nine minutes of golf (walking, no cart) than grind away on a stationary bike for forty-seven minutes in order to expend the same amount of calories. (Notice that compared with people who weigh less, those who weigh more burn more calories doing the same activity.) As I said in chapter 8, if you exercise in ways that you enjoy, you're more likely to do it. If it's fun, it's sustainable.

Find ways of incorporating exercise into your daily life. For example, take the stairs instead of the elevator. Park a little farther from where you're going (which may also reduce your stress level since you can more easily find a place to park—I have to laugh at myself when I find myself getting annoyed if there aren't any parking places close to the gym).

If you're going to do more than moderate exercise, then do it on a regular basis. What gets some people into trouble is when they are "weekend warriors," sedentary couch potatoes during the workweek and playing full-court basketball or shoveling snow on weekends. When you do that, you're increasing your risk of both musculoskeletal injuries as well as sudden cardiac death, whereas regular exercise reduces these risks.

Don't forget flexibility exercises, especially hatha yoga. The combination of stretching and strength training decreases your risk of injury.

Set realistic weight-loss goals. Forget the supermarket tabloids that scream: "Lose 30 pounds in 30 days!" Weight-management experts recommend losing weight at a pace of about two pounds a month—7,500 calories a month, or just 1,875 calories a week. Be realistic and don't expect to lose more than 2 pounds per week.

If you are not losing weight as quickly as you'd like, take a look at how your clothes fit. Are they feeling roomier? Can you tighten your belt an extra notch? Even if you're not losing weight, exercise helps change body composition in a healthier direction—that is, it turns fat into muscle. Maintaining weight while losing a beer belly has been shown to decrease the risk of heart disease.

THE STRESS-MANAGEMENT SPECTRUM

As I described in chapter 3, there's no mystery in how to lose weight: burn more calories and/or eat fewer calories. It's all about energy balance. You lose weight when you burn more calories than you consume.

Calories in, calories out. Energy balance. What you eat and what you do.

However, *how you feel* also determines how much you weigh. Everyone knows that diet and exercise play a role in how much we weigh, but many people are surprised to learn what a powerful role stress has in causing us to gain weight and how stress-management techniques can help us lose it and keep it off.

Chronic emotional stress also causes you to gain weight, in two important ways:

- Many people overeat to cope with feeling stressed, and they often eat foods that are high in fat, salt, and sugar as well.
- Chronic emotional stress stimulates your brain to release hormones that cause you to gain weight, especially around your belly, where it's most harmful.

Since chronic emotional stress promotes weight gain in several ways described earlier, stress-management techniques may play a powerful role in helping you lose weight and keep it off. The psychosocial, emotional, and spiritual issues are as important to address if you want to lose weight and keep it off as the nutrition and exercise ones are.

In our study of 869 patients, the amount of time people spent practicing stress-management techniques was directly correlated with the amount of weight they lost. How much time you want to spend each day on stress-management techniques is up to you; the more time you spend, the more weight you are likely to lose, and in the right places.

Once you've lost the amount of weight you desire, you can experiment with where you want to be on the Spectrum to help you keep it off. More on this can be found in chapter 7.

In addition to energy balance, emotional stress plays a major role in gaining weight. First, as I mentioned above, many people overeat when they're feeling stressed, and they tend to eat foods that are high in fat, salt, and sugar.

Second, chronic stress causes your body to secrete a cascade of hormones from your hypothalamus to your pituitary gland in your brain to other organs in your body (such as your adrenal glands and your thyroid), which, in turn, secrete hormones such as glucocorticoids and insulin, which cause you to gain weight and accumulate fat tissue, especially around your belly, where it's most harmful and least attractive.

Chronic stress also causes stimulation of hormones such as cytokines that promote inflammation. Also, obesity itself causes a low-grade inflammation that, in turn, tends to promote more obesity in a vicious cycle.

As I described in chapter 6, your brain sends messages to your body during times of stress via the sympathetic nervous system. This prepares your body to either fight or run. In the short run, these changes can be beneficial, even lifesaving. But when chronically activated during times of long-term stress, these same mechanisms may be harmful, even fatal.

A study published in the prestigious journal *Nature: Medicine* looked at the effects of stress on weight gain in mice. The investigators reported that chronic emotional stress turns on a peptide (chemical messenger) called neuropeptide Y, which is found in body fat. This hormone increases appetite, especially for carbohydrate-rich foods. It also causes your body to convert these calories into belly fat, a double whammy.

What's especially interesting is that chronic stress alone didn't have much effect on weight gain in only two weeks, nor did a high-fat, high-sugar diet. However, combining the two was especially toxic, and markedly increased abdominal fat deposits in only two weeks.

Over a longer period of time—three months—the high-fat, high-sugar diet caused obesity, but the amount of weight gain increased *threefold* when this same diet was given to mice that were also subjected to chronic stress. It also caused metabolic syndrome (glucose intolerance, which can lead to diabetes, high cholesterol, high blood pressure, and inflammation).

When the researchers blocked the effects of neuropeptide Y, it reduced stress-induced visceral (belly) fat *by 50 percent* "without any discernible effect on food intake, which remained as increased as it was," according to the investigators.

In other words, the mice ate the same amount of food and didn't exercise more, but blocking the effects of neuropeptide Y decreased their belly fat by 50 percent. Amazing.

What about in humans?

In a recent study, the effects of stress on the secretion of hormones such as glucocorticoids that cause belly fat accumulation were intensified by a high-fat diet, at least in rats. So all of these factors on the Spectrum can interact in positive or negative ways. For example, you may eat more fat and sugar when you're feeling stressed to help cope with those feelings, but the high-fat, high-sugar diet causes you to gain more belly fat than would have occurred otherwise.

A major study of almost 7,000 men and 3,500 women over a nineteen-year period found that there was a dose-response relationship between work stress and risk of general obesity (body mass index greater than 30 kg/m^2) and central obesity (waist circumference greater than forty inches in men and thirty-five inches in women, the kind that is the most harmful) that was largely independent of other factors.

In short, *the more stressed people felt, the more belly fat they accumulated.* This was also found in a study of chronic stress in Sweden. Anxiety and depression were also found to increase the risk of obesity. Insulin and blood sugar levels were higher in those who were anxious and depressed.

Neuropeptide Y may also be a common pathway for other chronic diseases, including coronary heart disease and diabetic retinopathy (diseased blood vessels in the eyes, which can lead to blindness). It also stimulates the growth of new blood vessels, called angiogenesis. This is a factor in not only weight gain but also cancer and may help explain the relationship of obesity to increased cancer risk.

How much stress causes your body to secrete neuropeptide Y is, in part, genetically determined. Stress-induced increases in neuropeptide Y are particularly high in people who are of northern European descent and make them especially vulnerable to a greater incidence of atherosclerosis, obesity, and diabetic retinopathy. So if you're of northern European descent, you may want to go a little further in the healthy direction on the Spectrum if you're trying to lose weight.

As you might imagine, the researchers have applied for a patent and begun negotiating with drug companies to make drugs to block neuropeptide Y. It may be years, if ever, before clinical trials in humans are conducted and drugs that affect neuropeptide Y are on the market. In the meantime, stress-management techniques can play a major role in helping you lose weight and keep it off.

As the researchers of neuropeptide Y concluded, "Our findings provide evidence that stress is not 'just in the mind' but rather affects body weight and metabolism by activating neurogenic angiogenesis and fat remodeling."

Therefore, spend some time each day practicing whichever of the stress-management techniques appeal to you the most, as I described in chapter 7. In addition, consciously choosing to increase the amount of love, intimacy, and social support in your life is especially important when trying to lose weight. Ask a friend or family member to join you in this journey, and the support you give each other will make it easier and more fun for both of you.

LOWERING YOUR BLOOD PRESSURE USING THE SPECTRUM

One way to get high blood pressure is to go mountain climbing over molehills.

—Earl Wilson

■ ■ ■ ■ ■ ■ ■ ■ ■

> ### TESTIMONIAL:
> *Bryce Williams, San Francisco*
>
> A series of modest changes over time worked for me.
>
> For most of my adult life, I've had borderline high blood pressure (around 130/88) and for years wrote it off as "white-coat hypertension," meaning that my blood pressure went up when I was having a doctor or nurse measure it. My anxiety and stress about having high blood pressure were creating what I was concerned about!
>
> I said to myself that I'd deal with it if my blood pressure went over the magical 140/90 barrier. Well, a few years back my blood pressure jumped from borderline high to really unhealthy: 156/110 at one point and never lower than 150/94.
>
> Intuitively, I knew this was largely stress-related. At the time, I was chief financial officer of a start-up company that was falling apart. Also, my first child was about to be born, and we had to buy a larger (and, of course, more expensive) house to fit our growing family. I knew I had a spectrum of lifestyle choices (diet, exercise, stress reduction) available to me as well as medication options if I wanted (which I did not).

My doctor never asked me about my diet or lifestyle. I'd get the standard lecture—"blood pressure's called the silent killer"—and an offer of a prescription for antihypertensive drugs. That's all.

My first choice was to look at exercise, as it was something I enjoyed and was likely to succeed at. As I already had a pretty strong aerobic base and didn't have much time (work/family) to add frequency or duration, I focused on adding some interval work periodically and shifted my strength training from primarily weights to more functional, multiple muscle exercises (push-ups, pull-ups, dips, etc.)

Over the next few months, I lost about five pounds. My blood pressure periodically came back down to the borderline high range, but the improvements were transient—one time it would be borderline, the next it would be way too high. I didn't have the time or motivation to exercise more and had to look at other options.

I next tried a few moderate dietary changes—I was already eating a low-fat (probably around 20 percent of total calories from fat), primarily vegetarian diet. My dietary weaknesses included a Dr Pepper habit (picked up from my Texas days—caffeine plus lots of sugar), excess sodium consumption (I have a "salt tooth"—sweets have never been a big draw for me), and eating "on the go," relying too much on processed foods. I chose to eliminate the caffeine and calories associated with my beloved Dr Pepper and other caffeinated beverages.

Net result—I lost a couple more pounds but didn't really see much change in my blood pressure. Salt restriction was something I didn't really feel up to tackling, so I finally decided to start taking a yoga class once a week.

Within a week of adding this once-a-week yoga class (in place of some of my exercise), my blood pressure dropped to a normal range—between 116/74 and 120/80—and it has stayed there ever since without any medication. Since so much of my high blood pressure was due to stress, it's not surprising that the yoga stress-management techniques were so effective for me.

Had this not worked, I don't know what the next step would have been—maybe salt restriction or a touch of medication. Just glad, for now, that I don't have to make that choice.

If you have hypertension, also called high blood pressure, you're at higher risk of having a heart attack, stroke, or kidney disease. Traditionally, normal blood pressure was considered anything less than 120/80, but the latest findings show that an ideal blood pressure is closer to 90/60. In most cases, high blood pressure is not treated with medications until it is consistently about 140/90.

More than 50 million adults in the United States have high blood pressure, and an additional 23 million are in the "borderline" range (between 130/85 and 139/89), accounting for approximately one-third of all U.S. adults. Additionally, more than 50 percent of everyone over the age of 60 in the United States has hypertension.

THE NUTRITION SPECTRUM

As mentioned in chapter 3, too much salt in your diet will raise your blood pressure, and reducing your salt intake will lower it. How much changing your salt intake will affect your blood pressure depends on a number of different factors—how much salt you currently consume, how well your kidneys are working, your race and genetic background, the climate you live in, and a variety of other factors, both known and unknown.

In other words, there is no way to predict with certainty how much you may want or need to reduce your salt intake. That's why the Spectrum approach is useful—you can find the amount that's right for you.

However much salt you're eating, try eating a little less. Check your blood pressure again in a week or so; if that's enough to bring it down to a normal range, great; if not, you have the option of further reducing your salt intake, adding other changes in your diet and lifestyle (outlined below), or taking medications.

One of the other advantages of making gradual changes in your salt intake is that your palate will begin to adapt. Even though salt is one of the four basic tastes (salty, sour, bitter, sweet), if you reduce your intake slowly, at first your food may taste as if it needs a little more salt, but after a week or two it will likely taste just fine. Then, if you go out to dinner and have your usual food, chances are that it will taste too salty. You may find that you begin to prefer the taste of food with less salt on it, which allows the natural flavors of the food to come through more clearly and cleanly.

While dietary salt tends to raise your blood pressure, dietary potassium tends to lower it. This may be one of the reasons that vegetarians have lower blood pressure than those who eat a carnivorous or omnivorous diet, since fruits and vegetables are naturally high in potassium. Studies have shown that the intake of fiber, fruits, and vegetables is inversely associated with systolic and diastolic pressures—in other words, the more fiber, fruits, and vegetables people consumed, the lower was their blood pressure.

Dr. Frank Sacks (a professor of medicine at Harvard Medical School) and I conducted a survey of a vegetarian community many years ago that we published in *The Journal of the American Medical Association*. We found that blood pressure levels in vegetarians were lower than in nonvegetarians of comparable age and risk factors. Subsequent studies of Seventh-Day Adventists and other vegetarian subgroups have shown similar findings.

Dr. Sacks believed that most Americans would not stick to a strict vegetarian diet, so he and his colleagues developed what he called the Dietary Approaches to Stop Hypertension (DASH) diet, which allows a little meat, including poultry and fish, in a diet otherwise rich in fruits and vegetables (approximately ten servings per day) and low-fat dairy products (two servings per day), and low in refined carbohydrates.

When the DASH findings were released, Dr. Sacks said, "This is really groundbreaking. We were very surprised by this data." Researchers said that the reductions seen in the study were so great that some people with hypertension could avoid taking drugs if they just lowered the amount of salt in their diet—and they'd see an even bigger reduction in blood pressure if they followed a low-fat diet, too.

Reduction in Systolic Blood Pressure for Patients with High Blood Pressure and Normal Blood Pressure on Certain Diets

	LOW-FAT DIET	LOW-SALT DIET	LOW-FAT AND LOW-SALT DIET
High blood pressure	3 mm	8.3 mm	11.5 mm
Normal blood pressure	5 mm	6.7 mm	7.1 mm

Also, this study found that a diet rich in fruits and vegetables and low in meat and sugar can not only help lower blood pressure but can also reduce levels of homocysteine, a substance that promotes inflammation. Other studies have confirmed these findings.

Minerals in our diet may play an important role in regulating blood pressure. The healthy end of the Nutrition Spectrum provides plenty of fruits and vegetables, which are good sources of potassium, calcium, and magnesium, and these are consistently associated with lower blood pressure.

THE EXERCISE SPECTRUM

In our study of 869 coronary heart disease patients that I described earlier, there were significant reductions in only three months in systolic blood pressure (down an average of 12 points in men and 9 points in women). These reductions were especially remarkable considering that their blood pressures were already reasonably well controlled at baseline—from an average of 132/78 to 120/71 in men and from an average of 131/76 to 122/71 in women.

For most people, this amount of blood pressure reduction was the difference between needing to be on antihypertensive medications for the rest of their lives and not needing them at all. (Of course, it's important to check with your doctor or nurse before making any changes in any of your medications.)

People who exercise regularly are less likely to develop high blood pressure. Regular physical activity decreases blood pressure, and both aerobic and resistance-training exercise have the ability to lower blood pressure, effects that are largely independent of weight loss. Just walking three or four days per week for at least half an hour per day has been shown to significantly lower blood pressure in hypertensive patients.

A study of the Pritikin combined lifestyle-modification program (which is similar to the healthy end of the Spectrum) found that 83 percent of people with high blood pressure were able to safely discontinue taking their antihypertensive medications after only three weeks of changing their diet and exercise. Other combined nutrition and lifestyle interventions have documented similar reductions in blood pressure.

A single exercise session can lower your blood pressure by 5 to 7 mm/Hg, which may persist for as long as twenty-two hours. However, the blood pressure benefits of exercise are reduced after only one to two weeks of returning to the couch, so regular exercise is important to sustain the reductions in blood pressure.

Aerobic exercise is more effective than strength training for reducing blood pressure. But strength training still helps. So does flexibility training, especially activities such as yoga, which also contain a meditative component.

The Exercise Spectrum for people who want to lower their blood pressure is very similar to the general Spectrum. Here are a few ways that it can be customized for greatest benefit:

- Exercise daily, or at least every other day.
- If you are just starting an exercise program, begin with twenty minutes a day and, over several months, progress to sixty minutes per day.

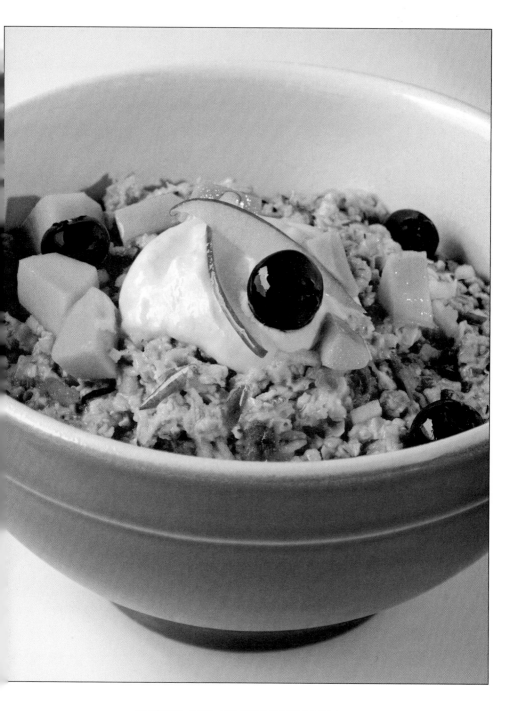

MANGO AND BLUEBERRY MUESLI

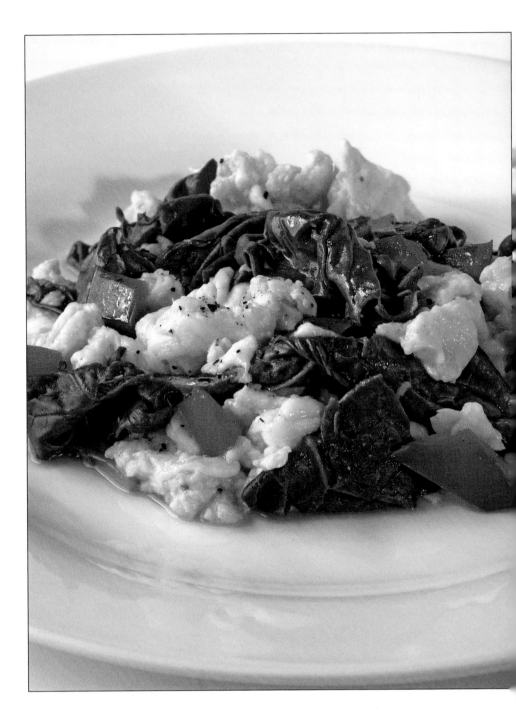

1-2-3 TASTY MORNING SCRAMBLE

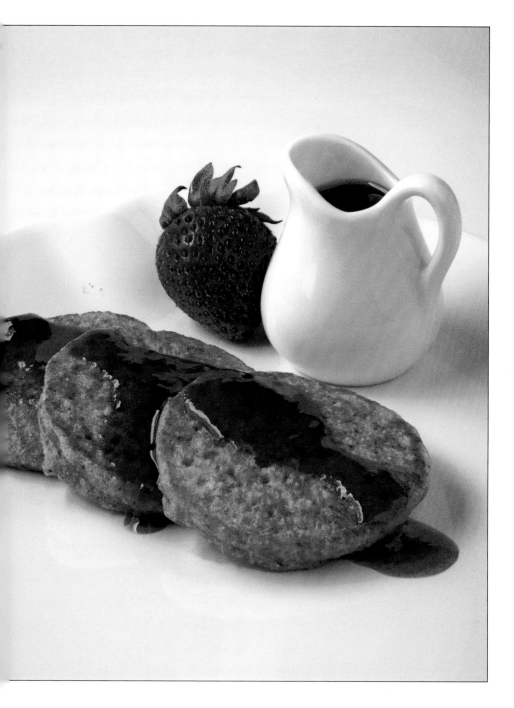

MULTIGRAIN PANCAKES WITH STRAWBERRY "SYRUP"

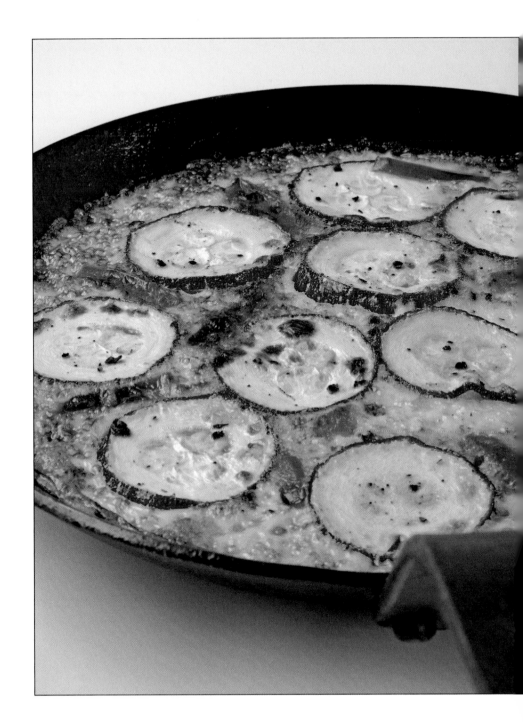

ZUCCHINI FRITTATA

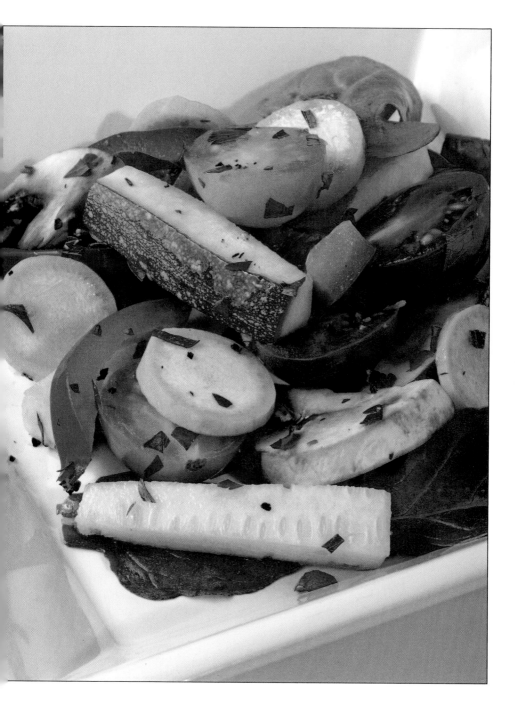

MARINATED VEGETABLE SALAD

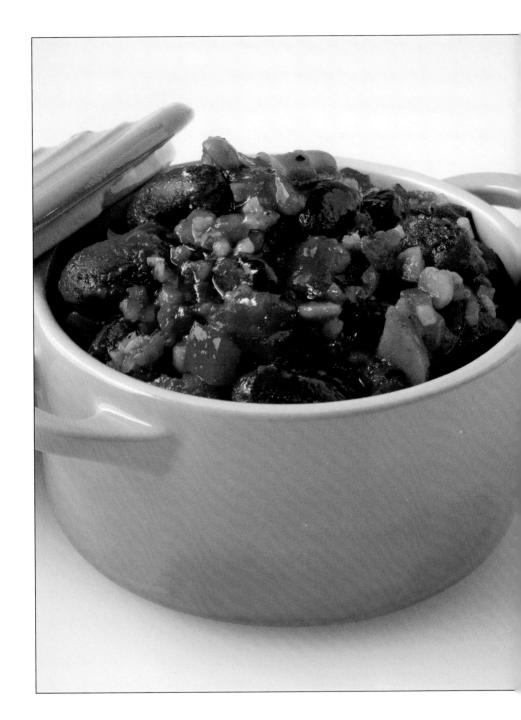

VEGETARIAN CHILI

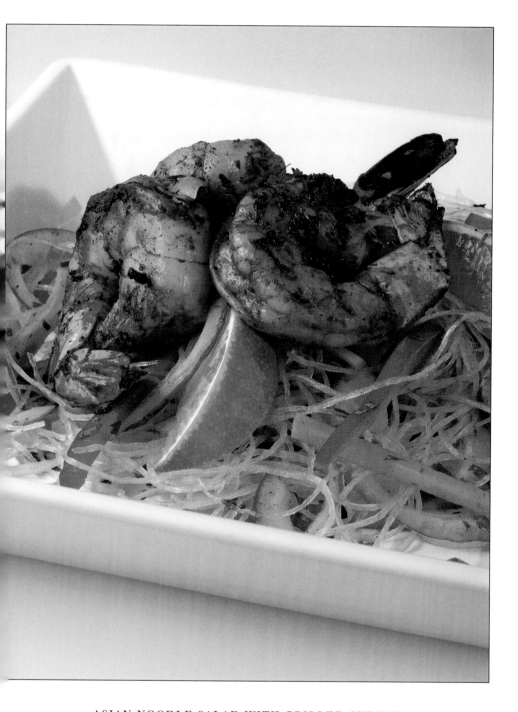

ASIAN NOODLE SALAD WITH GRILLED SHRIMP

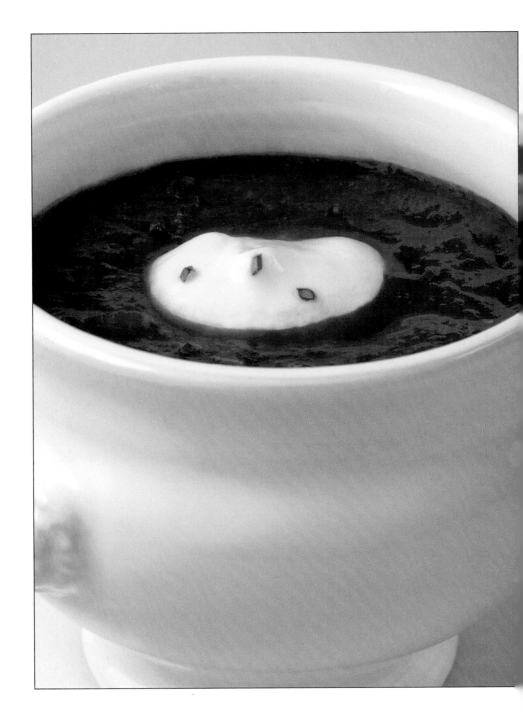

ROASTED TOMATO SOUP

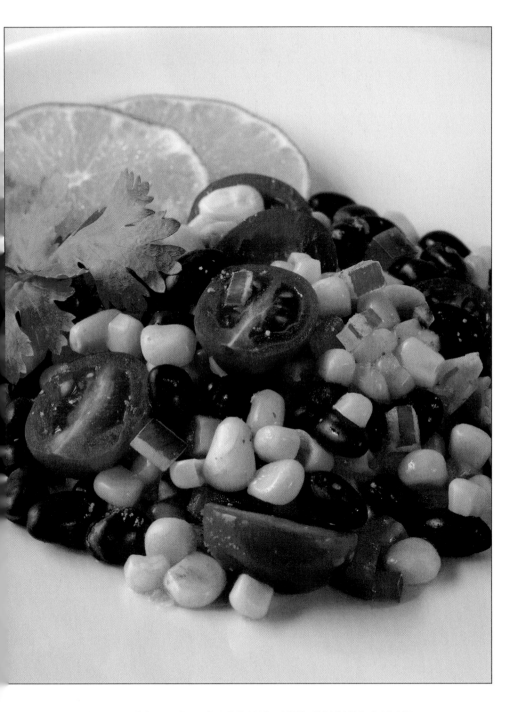

SWEET CORN, BLACK BEANS, AND TOMATO SALAD

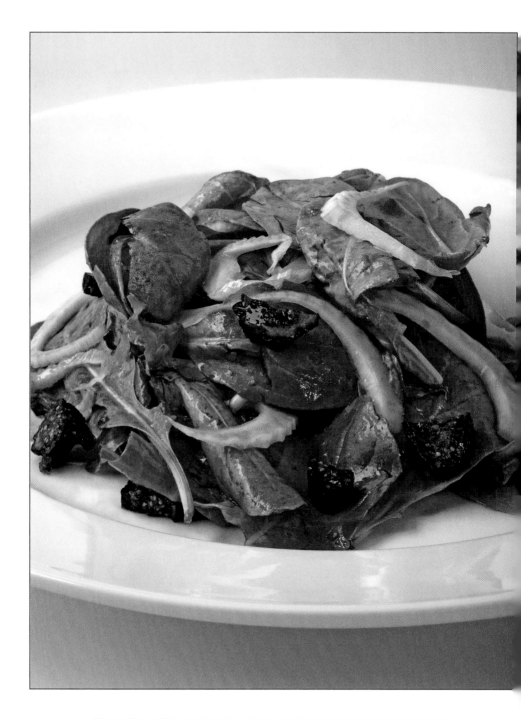

FENNEL AND ARUGULA SALAD WITH FIG VINAIGRETTE

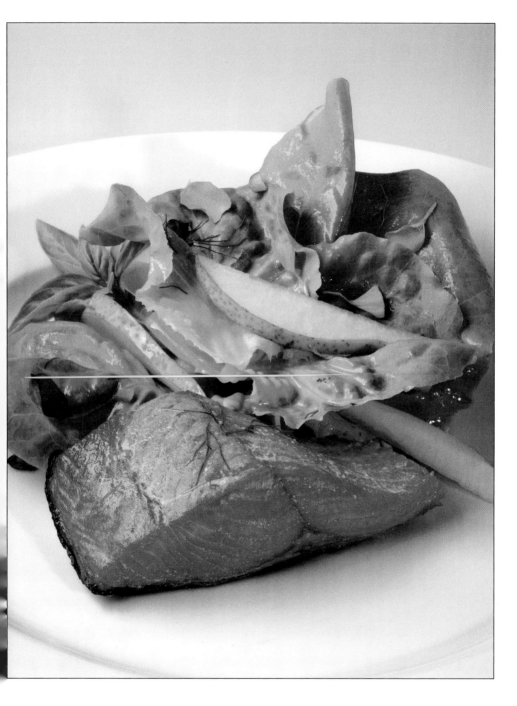

WILD SALMON WITH PEAR, BUTTER LETTUCE, AND FRESH
HERBS WITH A HONEY-INFUSED VINAIGRETTE

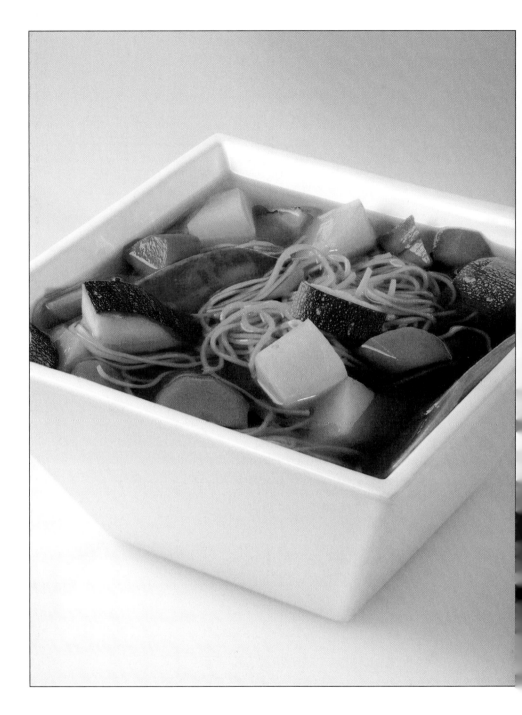

CURRIED VEGETABLE HOT POT

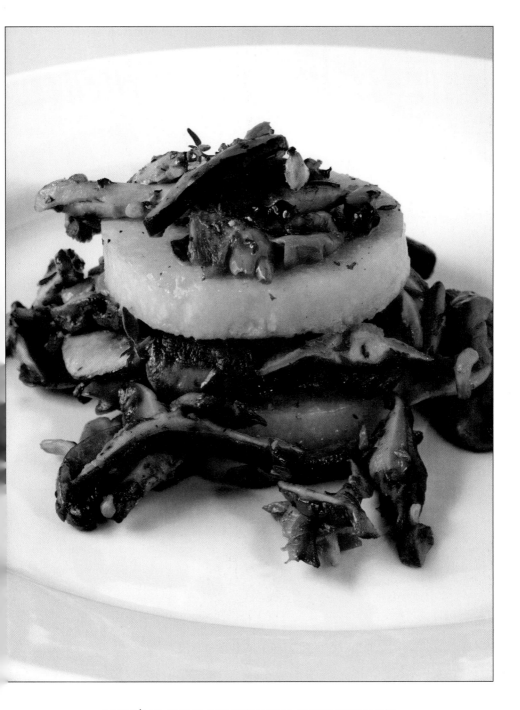

SAUTÉED WILD MUSHROOMS WITH POLENTA

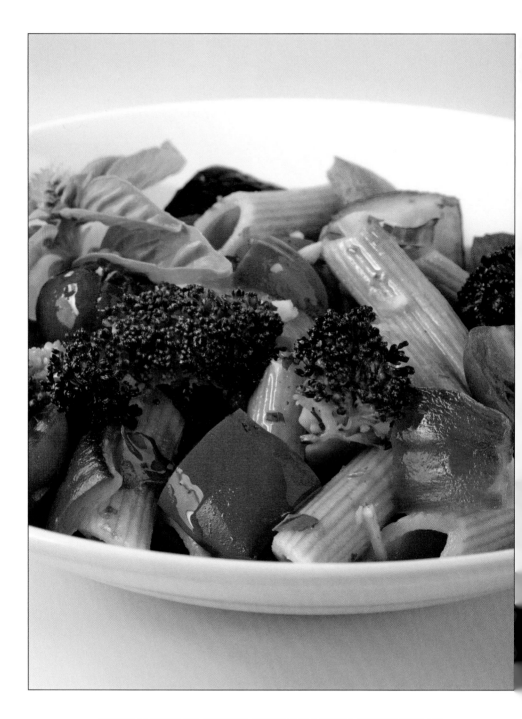

WHOLE WHEAT PENNE WITH ROASTED VEGETABLES

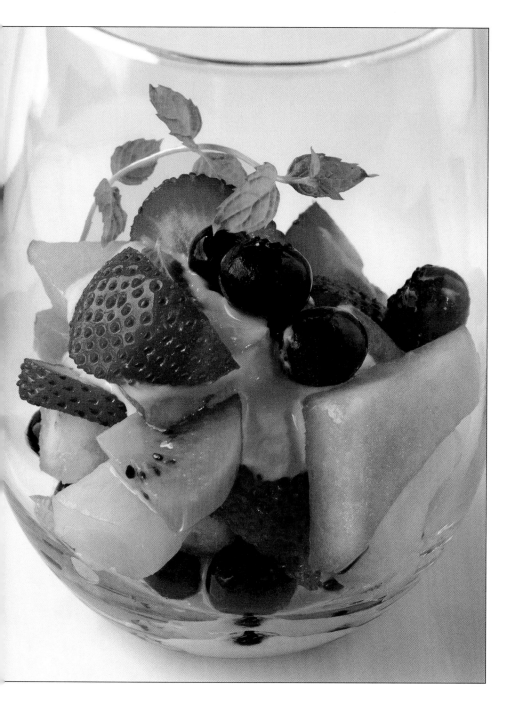

FAT-FREE YOGURT FRUIT TRIFLE

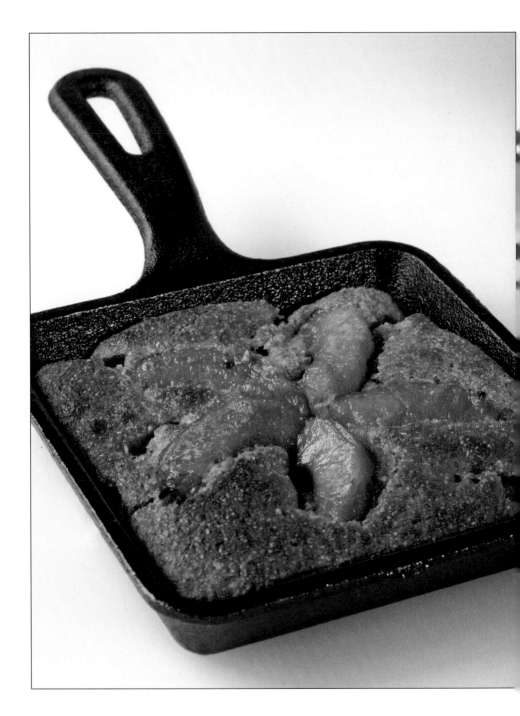

PEACH MULTIGRAIN GRIDDLE CAKE

- Avoid high-intensity resistance training, and be sure to not bear down or hold your breath when performing strength-training exercises.
- Circuit weight training is particularly effective in avoiding blood pressure fluctuations.
- Before doing activities at peak intensity, be sure to warm up—at least five minutes of low-level aerobic activity. After exercise, do an extended cool-down. Keep moving slowly for at least ten minutes to avoid large fluctuations in blood pressure.
- Do flexibility exercise five to seven days per week to decrease your stress.

Tips

- If your blood pressure is greater than 150/90, you should talk to your doctor before beginning your exercise program. You might need medication first, which you might be able to wean off of over time.

- Exercising while taking certain blood pressure medications—beta-blockers, diuretics, calcium channel blockers, alpha-blockers, and vasodilators—may cause side effects such as low blood sugar, overheating, and unusually low blood pressure (hypotension). Make sure you drink a lot of water, exercise in appropriate temperatures, and wear proper clothing to increase your ability to regulate your body temperature. Ask your doctor to monitor your blood sugar and potassium levels when you first begin an exercise program, and be sure to cool down slowly.

If your blood pressure is very elevated, don't exercise. Instead, try a stress-management regimen such as gentle yoga and meditation. If your blood pressure goes too high during exercise, stop and cool down slowly.

THE STRESS-MANAGEMENT SPECTRUM

In addition to its physiological benefits, exercise helps modulate the effects of stress on your blood pressure. For example, researchers at Duke University Medical Center found that regular exercise and weight loss significantly lowered blood pressure. "Our results show that exercise and weight loss helped to keep blood pressure lower even when individuals were under mental stress," said the study's lead investigator.

Many studies have shown that chronic emotional stress contributes to high blood pressure. Also, chronic anger and hostility as well as depression and hopelessness have a particularly strong effect on your blood pressure.

In one study, menopausal women who were put under mental stress (for example, by asking them to do mental arithmetic) had greater reactivity and showed greater increases in both systolic blood pressure and diastolic blood pressure than did men or premenopausal women. Thus, estrogen may help moderate some of the negative effects of stress.

In addition to your blood pressure at rest, how reactive your blood pressure becomes in response to stressful situations is another predictor of bad outcomes.

Meditation and other stress-management techniques may significantly lower your resting blood pressure within only a few weeks. In addition, these techniques may make your blood pressure less reactive.

As a patient once said to me after learning how to meditate, "I used to have a short fuse, and I'd explode easily. Now my fuse is longer. Things just don't bother me as much. Even if the situation hasn't changed, *I've* changed in how I react to it. So, I get more done and have more fun."

While meditation can make your fuse longer, caffeine often makes it shorter. Researchers studied medical students during exams. They gave half of the students grapefruit juice with hidden caffeine and the others juice without caffeine. Neither group knew who was receiving the caffeine.

On average, the students who drank the juice with caffeine had blood pressure readings 5 to 15 points higher than the others. For many people, this is the difference between needing to be on blood pressure medications for the rest of their lives or not at all. The caffeine also raised their level of chronic stress hormones such as cortisol. Students who already had high blood pressure, or who had a family history of high blood pressure, had the highest spikes in blood pressure after consuming the caffeine.

The researchers concluded, "Given the cumulative effects of stress and caffeine, it may be beneficial for individuals at high risk for hypertension to refrain from routine use of caffeinated beverages, particularly at times when work demands and attendant stressors are high."

A randomized controlled trial of African-American men and women showed that twenty minutes of meditation twice a day caused a significant decrease in both systolic blood pressure and diastolic blood pressure for at least one year and a reduced use of antihypertensive medications.

While meditation has a number of short-term benefits, it has long-term ones as well. In a study published in *The American Journal of Cardiology,* more than two hundred men and women who began meditating to treat their high blood pressure were followed for an average of 7.6 years. There was a 23 percent decrease in premature mortality from all causes, a 30 percent reduction in premature mortality due to cardiovascular diseases, and a 49 percent reduction in premature mortality from cancer.

Diet and stress may interact to increase your blood pressure. In a recent study, thirty healthy adults fasted the night before and then ate either a high-fat breakfast or a low-fat breakfast. Both meals contained about 800 calories, but the high-fat meal had 42 grams of fat and the low-fat meal only 1 gram of fat. A sodium supplement was added to the low-fat meal to even out the difference in sodium between the two meals.

Two hours later, the participants completed several stress-inducing tasks while researchers measured their cardiovascular response, including blood pressure, heart rate, and resistance within blood vessels. The tasks were designed to provoke mental and/or physical stress, such as completing a public speaking exercise about something emotionally provocative or holding a hand in ice water.

The results showed that regardless of the task, the blood pressure response was greater among those who ate the high-fat meal than among those who ate the low-fat one. Researchers say it's unclear how a single high-fat meal can sensitize the body to stress, but the results suggest a new way in which high-fat diets may contribute to heart disease.

Some of the mechanisms explaining why changes in nutrition, exercise, and stress management lower blood pressure are becoming clearer. The Nobel Prize in Medicine in 1998 went to Dr. Louis J. Ignarro for discovering the important role of nitric oxide (not to be confused with nitrous oxide, which is laughing gas).

Nitric oxide relaxes your arteries—in technical terms, it decreases vascular smooth muscle tone and inhibits your blood from clotting too quickly. When your arteries relax, your blood pressure decreases and more blood can flow where you want it to go. Drugs such as Viagra and Levitra improve nitric oxide production to your sexual organs, so increasing your body's production of nitric oxide is a good thing and has many benefits.

Moving toward the healthy end of the Spectrum increases your body's production of nitric oxide. For example, a study of people who went through the Pritikin program of diet and exercise for three weeks found that their systolic blood pressure and diastolic blood pressure showed significant decreases, their body's nitric oxide production increased, and their insulin levels decreased. Also, markers of oxidative stress showed improvement.

In addition, meditation and other stress-management techniques have been shown to increase nitric oxide production and to reduce oxidative stress.

An amino acid called L-arginine is converted into nitric oxide by your body. It's found in higher concentrations in soy protein and plant protein than in animal protein and may explain one of the mechanisms that makes eating more closely toward the healthy end of the Spectrum so beneficial.

A recent randomized controlled trial published in *The Journal of the American Medical Association* found that eating a small piece of dark chocolate (6 grams, or about ⅕ ounce) each day for eighteen weeks caused a significant reduction in systolic blood pressure (about 3 mm/Hg) and diastolic blood pressure (about 2 mm/Hg).

Why? Dark chocolate (but not white chocolate or milk chocolate) is high in protective substances called flavonols. Flavonols cause your arteries to produce more of a substance called "S-nitrosoglutathione," which is converted to nitric oxide. As noted earlier, nitric oxide relaxes your arteries and lowers your blood pressure.

An earlier study, also published in *The Journal of the American Medical Association,* found that a single dose of a cocoa drink rich in flavonols caused an increase in nitric oxide production and improvement in blood flow. Another study reported that chocolate may improve blood flow to your brain as measured by MRI scans.

Of course, chocolate is usually high in fat and sugar as well as flavonols, so the point here is to enjoy small amounts of chocolate. In chapter 3, I described how meditating on a single piece of rich, dark chocolate can be exquisitely satisfying.

In Woody Allen's 1973 movie *Sleeper,* twenty-second-century doctors marveled at how previous generations once avoided foods like hot fudge. "Those were thought to be unhealthy," a doctor said. "Precisely the opposite of what we now know to be true."

Won't be long . . .

PREVENTING AND REVERSING TYPE 2 DIABETES USING THE SPECTRUM

TESTIMONIAL:
Jeff Oliver, Monessen, Pennsylvania

I remember the conversation like it was yesterday.

Sitting around a table with a few of my friends, I listened as they complained about President's Bush's plans to revamp the Social Security system.

They ranted and raved that by the time they reached sixty-two, there would be little or nothing left for them.

Then one of them asked me what I thought.

Without blinking, I replied, "I don't care one way or the other because I won't be here then."

One of my friends took exception to what I said, retorting, "That isn't funny."

"Who's laughing?" I replied in an honest tone.

That was back in January, just a few months ago.

But that's how I felt. And I was okay with it.

Why would a 46-year-old man not think he would be living sixteen years from now? Well, for me, it was a matter of being realistic.

I weighed over 370 pounds, had high blood pressure, and was an out-of-control diabetic. Oh, did I add that I was taking medication for anxiety problems?

I had the energy of a sloth. And even less stamina.

I figured, "What the heck?"

And then my life changed.

In January, I received some information from my insurance provider, Highmark, about a nationally known program entitled

"Dr. Dean Ornish Program for Reversing Heart Disease." The program was being offered at the Monogahela Valley Hospital.

I don't have any heart problems (which, considering my condition, was truly amazing). However, since I was a type 2 diabetic, I qualified for the program.

"What do I have to lose?" I figured. So I signed up.

I had to overcome some early trepidation when I joined the Dr. Ornish program.

For example, I was told that while patients generally lose weight in the program, the main idea behind the Ornish experience was not a diet, per se, but a way of eating.

"Hmmm, no fun," I thought.

And, as part of the stress-management part of the program, I would have to do yoga.

I remember the first day I sat with the other members of our class. As I watched the slide show, while all the other members were seeing informative tidbits about the program, all I kept seeing was "Get out now!" on the screen.

But I did not. And I'm so glad that I didn't.

After the exercise was a forty-five-minute meal period in which Ornish-style healthy meals were prepared for the members by a hospital staff chef. The entire purpose behind this segment is to not only revamp our eating habits but to show us how many tasty foods there actually are in the program.

My new diet was to be made up mostly of whole grains, vegetables, legumes, and fruit.

Next up was a forty-five-minute group therapy session in which we met with a hospital case worker and discussed our feelings and everyday lives.

After that came stress-management yoga, under the auspices of one of the hospital's stress-management specialists. The deep breathing, meditating, and stretching techniques are aimed at improving each member's overall health.

In fact, we were told that of those who received substantial gains through the Ornish program, those who did the best were the ones who took full advantage of the group support and yoga, as well as the exercise and diet aspects.

Each week, we recorded everything we ate for that week and how much we exercised and did our yoga.

At first, I followed the program religiously . . . no meat, including chicken or fish. No oil or fried foods. No caffeine. I exercised as much as—and more than—was prescribed. I drink only fat-free milk, and I don't buy anything with more than 3 grams of fat in it or with much cholesterol in it.

I'm not quite so strict now, but I can probably count on one hand how many times I have eaten fried foods in the last year and a half. I eat fish and chicken sometimes and other low-fat meat on occasion. I have a cup of coffee most mornings.

And, yes, I do yoga.

In those first twelve weeks, I lost a whopping 47 pounds.

That translated into five inches off my chest, 2½ inches off my thighs, and another 1½ inches off my biceps.

Plus, I have found that I have energy to burn. I walk a minimum of two miles a day, sometimes doing as many as four.

To date, I've lost over 65 pounds and hope to keep that trend going. However, I should note that my large amount of weight loss is more the exception than the norm. The average weight loss for the first twelve weeks is anywhere from 12 to 25 pounds.

The thing to remember about this program is that it is not mainly a weight-loss program, but it is a road to better health through a change in lifestyle.

Before the program, I was averaging an intake of 3,800 calories per day, more than 40 percent fat, of which one third was saturated fat. I also had an average daily intake of more than 500 milligrams of cholesterol.

After twelve weeks, my food records showed that I was consuming 1,956 calories per day, less than 10 percent fat, and almost no saturated fat or cholesterol.

What also is impressive to me is that my cholesterol level dropped from a medication-aided level of 144 to 129 mg/dl without any medications and my triglycerides dropped from 203 to 129 mg/dl.

I don't need nearly as much sleep, and some of my coworkers have said that they have noticed a change for the better in my disposition. I no longer need to take medication for anxiety and depression.

My blood pressure, which once registered during a workout as high as 220/108, was whittled to an amazing 112/50 on one of my last exercise visits despite cutting my blood pressure medicines in half.

But the best news of all is my diabetes. My blood sugar was as high as 318 before I joined the program. Since then, I've had my medication cut four times by my family doctor, from a high of thirteen pills a day for diabetes to only two different ones now, and I have even had some bouts of low blood sugar. My goal is to someday soon go to no pills at all.

Of course, I put in a lot of hard work during my Ornish experience. Nothing ventured, nothing gained.

But make no mistake about it, I could never have found the success I have in this program without the constant support and care of the program's staff. I could go on and on about what each and every one of these loyal people has meant not only to me but also to anyone who has been in an Ornish program. I guess the best thing I can say is that I truly love these people and I give them as much credit for changing my life as I can give to myself.

After all, there is no value that can be put on an encouraging word, a compassionate pat on the back, or even an occasional kick in the butt.

It's funny, but only six months ago, I wasn't even worried about reaching Social Security age, and now I can't wait to play with my kids' children.

Of course, I'm not quite ready for grandchildren just yet. That would be another story.

Like the obesity pandemic, and in large part because of it, diabetes has become epidemic. It's the fastest-growing disease in the United States, and also in many other parts of the world. Diabetics have a shorter life expectancy than people without diabetes. One in ten adults in America has diabetes, and nearly twice as many are prediabetic and have abnormally high blood sugar. More than half are women. As with men, women with diabetes have a shorter life expectancy than women without diabetes, and they are at greater risk of blindness from diabetes than are men.

The prevalence of diabetes increased by 600 percent between 1950 and 1993 and has continued to increase since then. Clearly, our genes did not change during that time period, but our diet and lifestyle have changed considerably.

For example, Pima Indians who live in rural Mexico and follow their traditional lifestyle of a diet low in animal fat and high in unrefined carbohy-drates ("good carbs") have much lower rates of diabetes and obesity than Pima Indians living in the United States who consume a Western diet and are more sedentary. Their genes are comparable, but their diabetes rates are very different.

In the Harvard Nurses' Health Study, which followed 90,000 nurses over a sixteen-year period, investigators reported that 91 percent of the diabetes cases were attributed to lifestyle factors such as unhealthy diet and lack of exercise.

Your pancreas makes insulin, a hormone that binds to receptors on your body's cells and allows glucose (sugar) to enter these cells and be con-verted to energy.

Type 1 diabetes occurs when the pancreas doesn't make enough insulin, usually because antibodies have formed that attack the islet cells in the pancreas that make insulin. Type 1 diabetes, formerly called "juvenile-onset diabetes," accounts for only about 10 percent of diabetes.

Most diabetes—90 percent—is type 2 diabetes, formerly called "adult-onset diabetes." In this condition, the pancreas is actually making *more* insulin than in most people, not less.

Why does this occur? As I described in chapter 3, when you eat a lot of refined carbohydrates with a high glycemic index ("bad carbs"), your food is absorbed quickly, causing your blood sugar to spike. This stimulates your pancreas to make more insulin to bring your blood sugar back down to a normal range.

Over time, these repeated surges of insulin cause the receptors on your cells to become less sensitive to its effects—a little like the boy who cried wolf. This is called insulin resistance, and it often leads to type 2 diabetes. Too much insulin causes you to gain weight, and obesity causes insulin resistance in a vicious cycle.

Also, overconsumption of animal fat and "bad carbs," lack of exercise, and emotional stress play a role in the development of diabetes, which I discuss later in this chapter.

The consequences of diabetes are serious—eye damage that can lead to blindness, kidney damage that can lead to kidney failure, nerve damage that can lead to impotence, damage to arteries in the heart that can lead to coronary heart disease, and damage to arteries in the arms and legs that can lead to amputation.

As a result, diabetes care accounts for 12 percent of the $645 billion in federal health care spending each year, almost $80 billion more than for those without diabetes.

Even worse, because of the childhood obesity epidemic, diabetes is afflicting an increasing number of children and young adults—which is why type 2 diabetes is no longer called "adult-onset diabetes."

Diabetes in 30-year-olds has risen 70 percent in the past decade! Children exposed to diabetes in the womb have a greater likelihood of becoming obese during childhood and adolescence and of developing type 2 diabetes later in life than those who are not so exposed.

The good news is that diabetes is usually preventable or even reversible for those who are willing to go far enough toward the healthy end of the Spectrum, both adults and kids.

To prevent type 2 diabetes, move toward the healthy end of the nutrition, exercise, and stress-management spectrums. To reverse diabetes, you need to move even further.

A landmark study by the Diabetes Prevention Program Research Group, published in *The New England Journal of Medicine,* studied 3,234 men and women with prediabetes to determine whether lifestyle modification could prevent diabetes.

It did.

These patients were randomly assigned to one of three groups: one group received metformin, a commonly prescribed diabetes medication; one group made moderate changes in diet and lifestyle (asked to follow a step 1 diet of 30 percent fat and less red meat, to exercise, and to lose weight); and the third group was asked to make more-intensive changes in diet and lifestyle (to eat a diet lower in fat and calories, to lose at least 7 percent of their body weight, and to exercise at least 150 minutes per week).

Daily energy intake decreased by 250 calories in the group that made moderate lifestyle changes, by 300 calories in the medication group, and by 450 calories in the intensive lifestyle-modification group. Dietary fat intake decreased by less than 1 percent in the medication and the moderate lifestyle-changes groups and by 6.6 percent in the more-intensive lifestyle-changes group. Weight loss was .25 pound in the moderate lifestyle-change group, 4.6 pounds in the medication group, and 12.3 pounds in the intensive lifestyle-change group.

After three years, there was 58 percent less diabetes in the intensive lifestyle-change group than in the group that made moderate lifestyle changes and only a 31 percent reduction in diabetes due to the metformin medication.

The authors concluded, "The [intensive] lifestyle intervention was significantly more effective than metformin" in preventing diabetes.

The Finnish Diabetes Prevention Study was another large randomized controlled trial showing that comprehensive lifestyle changes can help prevent diabetes in those who are prediabetic. In this study, patients were randomly assigned to a usual-care control group or a group that consumed more whole grains, fiber, fruits, vegetables, low-fat dairy products, and low-fat meats, lost weight, and exercised more. After five years, the incidence of diabetes was reduced by 58 percent, the same as in the Diabetes Prevention Program study.

More recently, a study of more than 5,000 patients found that weight loss and exercise caused significant reductions in diabetes, high blood pressure, and the need for cholesterol-lowering drugs.

In our research, the Multicenter Lifestyle Demonstration Project, patients with heart disease and diabetes who followed our program for reversing heart disease (i.e., the healthiest end of the Spectrum) were able to show significant reductions in weight, body fat, and LDL cholesterol and substantial improvements in exercise capacity and quality of life. We found that 20 percent of these patients were able to discontinue or significantly reduce their diabetes medications. We also found some evidence for reduced insulin levels in men three months after following our lifestyle program. Interestingly, these men also showed evidence of improved C-reactive protein levels, indicating reduced inflammation.

The Diabetes Prevention Program Research Group study is a good example of the Spectrum in action. For some patients, moderate changes in lifestyle were enough to prevent diabetes, but not for most. Those who made bigger changes in diet and lifestyle showed even better results than those taking the drug, without the costs and side effects of a lifetime on the medication.

So if you want to prevent diabetes, start by asking your doctor to measure your blood sugar level, either with a fasting blood glucose test or with an oral glucose tolerance test. If it's normal, then whatever you're eating and doing is probably okay. If it's a little high, you can begin by moving a little in the healthy direction on the Spectrum and measuring your blood sugar again a month or two later. If moderate changes are enough to bring it down, great; if not, you can go further in the healthy direction on the Spectrum.

If you have diabetes, you may want to begin by going even further in the healthy direction on the Spectrum. Repeat your testing; if necessary, go even further.

THE NUTRITION SPECTRUM

While consumption of refined carbohydrates ("bad carbs") increases the risk of diabetes, studies have shown that consumption of unrefined, whole-food carbohydrates ("good carbs") actually lowers your risk of diabetes.

For example, the Harvard Physicians' Health Study of more than 40,000 health professionals found that higher intake of fruits, vegetables, whole grains, fish, and chicken was associated with a lower risk of diabetes, whereas a higher intake of refined grains, sweets, processed and red meat, and high-fat dairy products was associated with an increased risk of diabetes. A higher glycemic load also increased the risk of diabetes.

Similar findings were noted in a study of Native Canadians. Those who consumed more foods high in refined carbohydrates and fat and lower in fiber had a higher incidence of diabetes.

In the Harvard Nurses' Health Study, described earlier, consuming trans–fatty acids was found to increase the risk of diabetes. Consuming omega-3 fatty acids or fish may reduce the risk of diabetes.

Another example of the Spectrum approach was a study comparing the standard dietary recommendations of the American Diabetes Association (ADA) with a vegan diet (fruits, vegetables, whole grains, legumes, soy products) containing only 10 percent of calories from fats and low in refined carbohydrates. In the vegan diet, portion sizes and energy intake were unrestricted, whereas subjects on the ADA diet were asked to consume 500 to 1,000 fewer calories per day than usual.

After twenty-two weeks, blood glucose decreased two to three times as much in those on the vegan diet as in those on the ADA diet. Also, body weight decreased 14 pounds in those on the vegan diet but less than 7 pounds in those on the ADA diet since the vegan diet was very low in fat and high in fiber and thus low in energy density. LDL cholesterol decreased 21.2 percent in those on the vegan diet and 10.7 percent in those on the ADA diet.

The Weight of Evidence

A common thread in all of these studies is that weight loss has a markedly beneficial effect on preventing or reversing diabetes. As mentioned earlier, obesity promotes chronic low-grade inflammation, which in turn promotes insulin resistance as well as other chronic diseases such as coronary heart disease. Also, diets high in refined carbohydrates and high glycemic load increase inflammation, whereas many of the protective factors found in fruits and vegetables have been shown to reduce inflammation.

These changes in diet also improve insulin sensitivity. Both diets high in unrefined carbohydrates ("good carbs") and a Mediterranean diet have been shown to increase insulin sensitivity.

As described more fully in chapter 3, chronic inflammation is linked to a variety of chronic diseases besides diabetes. A recent study from the Karolinska Institute in Sweden showed that those with prediabetes as well as diabetes have a 70 percent higher risk of developing Alzheimer's disease and other forms of dementia later in life than those without prediabetes or diabetes.

The good news is that those with diabetes who kept their blood sugar in close control were able to reduce their risk significantly. The study, by researchers from the Karolinska Institute in Sweden and the Stockholm Gerontology Research Center, included 1,173 people 75 and older. But the higher risk occurred only in those who did not carry the gene apo E4, which is associated with some cases of Alzheimer's. Other studies have shown that compared with healthy people of the same age and sex, those with type 2 diabetes are twice as likely to develop Alzheimer's.

In another study, researchers at Kaiser Permanente in Oakland followed more than 22,000 patients with type 2 diabetes for eight years. None had dementia at the beginning of the study. Over the next eight years, they found a direct correlation between the subjects' blood sugar levels and their risk of dementia.

They measured hemoglobin A1C, which reflects average blood sugar levels during the past three months. A normal level is less than 7. The risk of dementia rose 13 percent in those with levels from 10 to 12, 24 percent in those with levels from 12 to 15. When the hemoglobin A1C was greater than 15, the risk of developing Alzheimer's disease was 83 percent higher!

The role of inflammation in Alzheimer's disease may be one of the reasons that the spice turmeric, which has powerful anti-inflammatory properties, decreases the risk of Alzheimer's disease, as I mentioned in chapter 3. Some research has found that too much insulin in the brain itself can contribute to amyloid buildup, which leads to Alzheimer's disease.

THE EXERCISE SPECTRUM

Exercise is important to help prevent or reverse type 2 diabetes and metabolic syndrome.

In a new study, investigators found that moderate to vigorous physical exercise reduced the risk of developing type 2 diabetes by affecting the expression of two genes involved in insulin secretion. There was a small number of patients with a rare genetic variant for whom exercise did not reduce the risk of diabetes. Thus, in the near future, genetic testing may make it possible to determine more precisely where you need to be on the Spectrum in order to tailor an exercise prescription just right for you.

Men who exercise less than one hour per week are 60 percent more likely to have metabolic syndrome than men who exercise for more than three hours per week.

In the HERITAGE study, after twenty weeks of endurance training, 30 percent of the people no longer met the criteria for metabolic syndrome. The Aerobics Center Longitudinal Study showed that aerobic fitness strongly protects against heart disease and mortality in people with metabolic syndrome.

Just one session of exercise can decrease blood sugar as much as 40 mg/dl. Studies (including ours) have shown that moderate exercise improves blood sugar levels by 10 to 20 percent. Again, consistency is important, since exercise-induced decreases in blood sugar disappear after about seventy-two hours.

In general, the more you exercise, the greater will be the impact on diabetes. Exercise more if you need to reverse diabetes than if just want to help prevent it. If you're taking diabetes medications, talk with your doctor before changing your amount of exercise (or diet or stress-management techniques), as these may reduce your need for medication. Otherwise, your blood sugar may get too low and you may become hypoglycemic.

People with diabetes-associated eye disease (retinopathy) need to avoid anaerobic exercise and activities that involve straining, jarring, or bearing down, as well as holding their breath.

People with kidney disease (nephropathy) should exercise at low to moderate intensity and avoid strenuous activity. Because they also tend to have difficulty regulating their body temperature, they should avoid exercising in the heat or cold and make sure that they drink plenty of water before and during exercise.

Resistance training should be adapted to include only low to moderate resistance. Light weights should be used and the number of repetitions increased.

Other safety tips:

• If you are a diabetic, monitor your blood sugar closely as you begin your Spectrum plan for diet and exercise. You may see big changes very quickly. The American Diabetes Association website has good information on blood sugar monitoring with exercise: www.diabetes.org/weightloss-and-exercise/exercise/getting-started.jsp.

• Good foot care is crucial. Diabetes impairs circulation to the feet. Practice blister prevention: make sure shoes fit well and don't chafe. Keep your feet dry with good socks. Monitor your feet regularly. If any blisters or wounds develop, see your doctor.

• Wear appropriate exercise clothes and drink water before, during, and after exercise.

THE STRESS-MANAGEMENT SPECTRUM

In our study of 869 patients described earlier, the amount of time people spent practicing stress-management techniques was directly correlated with their blood glucose level (as measured by hemoglobin A1C). In other words, the stress-management techniques helped reverse their diabetes. Other studies have confirmed this finding.

For example, a study at Duke University Medical Center reported that patients with type 2 diabetes who incorporated stress-management techniques into their routine care significantly reduced their average blood glucose levels. According to Richard Surwit, Ph.D., the lead author of the study and a medical psychologist at Duke, "The change is nearly as large as you would expect to see from some diabetes-control drugs."

Put another way, for some patients this may be the difference between needing to be on diabetes drugs for the rest of their lives or being off them altogether. According to Surwit, the effect cannot be explained by changes in body mass index, diet, or exercise because the two groups did not differ in these variables during the year they were followed. "Managing stress can significantly improve a patient's control of their diabetes," he said.

In another study, investigators studied 506 diabetic patients at the School of Medicine, University of California, San Francisco. They found that those who were depressed and stressed had higher hemoglobin A1C levels, lower exercise levels, and higher intakes of saturated fat and calories. This is consistent with what I described in chapter 2, the importance of addressing the deeper issues that underlie our behaviors. Also, chronically high levels of stress hormones may cause your blood sugar to rise.

Another study found that in women who were not diabetic at the beginning of the study, those who reported feeling depressed, had a lot of stressful life events, or frequently felt intensely angry, tense, or stressed were much more likely to develop diabetes and metabolic syndrome over the subsequent fifteen years—in some cases, more than double the risk.

Therefore, if you have no evidence of diabetes but have a strong family history of it, begin by moving a little further toward the healthy end of the Spectrum. Practice at least a few minutes of stress-management techniques each day, along with the changes in diet and exercise described earlier.

If you are prediabetic, go even further on the Nutrition Spectrum and spend more time each day on the stress-management techniques; after three months, ask your doctor to repeat your tests (including hemoglobin A1C, fasting blood glucose, and perhaps a glucose tolerance test). If you're no longer prediabetic and your tests are in a normal range, that may be as far on the Spectrum as you need to go. If not, go even further and recheck your tests again after three more months.

If you have diagnosed type 2 diabetes, you may want to go as far as you comfortably can in the healthy direction on the Nutrition Spectrum, exercise more, and practice the stress-management techniques even longer each day. Ask your doctor to recheck your tests after three months; if they're normal, great. If not, go even further in the healthy direction on the Nutrition Spectrum, exercise more, and practice more of the stress-management techniques. If necessary, your doctor may advise you to take medication, but you may be able to avoid it completely if you make sufficient changes in your diet and lifestyle.

PREVENTING AND REVERSING CARDIOVASCULAR DISEASE USING THE SPECTRUM

attack because two of the bypasses failed. It was just going on like that every year for me.

I couldn't even stand up long enough to wash the dishes. I just thought . . . I felt useless. I felt there was nothing . . . nobody could do anything for me and I couldn't do anything for myself, so why should I be around if I can't do anything for myself? I didn't want to be dependent on anybody.

I read an article about the Ornish program, so I called my doctor's office and she said, "Yes, that would be good for you." And when I got involved in the lifestyle-modification program, I thought, "Oh, my God, there is hope after all. Somebody can help me." And once I started the program, I really felt good. This is the best I've felt in a long time.

It was a complete change—a change of my eating habits, talking to people in group support, exercise, and stress management. And without this program, I wouldn't be here.

When I started doing the stress management, I wasn't able to get down on the floor and do it. But now I can get down on the floor and do it with the rest of the people. And it's just a beautiful thing to take time for meditation and just to relieve all that stress.

When I first started this program, I didn't know what group support was about. I thought we were going to talk about the diet and stuff, but I didn't think you were going to talk about yourself. I was kind of quiet at first, but now I talk a lot.

I was at our meeting last Thursday and I had just a little problem and I started to cry. The support you get from the other people in the group is so meaningful. When I came home, I felt like I had a lighter heart—just from being able to open up to somebody. And we're there for them whenever they need us. They can call on us anytime. Even if we don't have an answer, we can listen.

For much of my life there was lot of stuff I just kept to myself. I didn't want to tell anybody my problems or tell them how sick . . . well, some people know how sick I was. But I don't want to tell anybody, because I don't want anybody to feel sorry for me. I never let anybody know what was bothering me. But just by being able to talk to these people and telling them how I feel, it has changed my life. I never knew how good it is just to open up.

I learned to say "no." It came up for other people in the group, too. I have two daughters, and I'm always there for them. You drop anything . . . they want you to do something for them, and you're there. I have to learn how to say "no" to them because I have to take time to take care of myself or I won't be able to help anyone else and they'll have to take care of me. By taking care of myself, I can do more to help them as well.

I never thought I'd be able to exercise because I couldn't walk. Now I exercise twice a week for an hour. Also, I exercise on my bike for thirty minutes a day. My legs are always moving now. I have happy feet!

I wish this program had been around in 1997. Maybe I wouldn't have had to go through all this open-heart stuff. If it wasn't for this program, I wouldn't be here because this program has changed my life completely.

You can never underestimate the power to live. Whether you are lying in a hospital bed or at home, you have to take the first step on the path to living your life to the fullest. I feel like a new person who has a lot to live for. For the first time since 1993, I can do things I never dreamed I'd be able to do again. I recommend that everyone try this program because it really works. I am so glad that I am alive.

As I described in chapter 1, our program has been proven to reverse the progression of even severe coronary heart disease simply by changes in diet and lifestyle, without drugs or surgery. Even though heart disease still kills more people in this country and in much of the world than virtually all other causes of death combined, it is almost completely preventable for at least 90 to 95 percent of people by putting the Spectrum into practice.

Time out—take a moment and think about what that means. The number one cause of death in most of the world is almost completely preventable just by changing diet and lifestyle.

One of the basic premises of the Spectrum is that it usually takes more changes in diet and lifestyle to reverse disease than it does to prevent it. Several factors play important roles in your risk of heart disease. The more of these factors you have, the further you may need to go in a healthy direction on the Spectrum in order to prevent heart disease. These include:

- **Your genes.** If your mother, father, sister, or brother has heart disease, and especially if it occurred at a relatively young age, your risk is higher. But this is just a predisposition; it's not written in stone.

- **Your blood pressure.** Elevated systolic blood pressure or diastolic blood pressure may cause chronic damage to the lining of your arteries as the blood hits the arterial walls with too much force. Over time, as your body attempts to repair this damage, the arteries may become progressively more clogged. It's a little like putting a Band-Aid on a cut, then another on top of that, and so on.

- **Your blood sugar.** Even prediabetes significantly increases your risk of heart disease, whereas lowering your blood sugar substantially lowers your risk, as described in the previous chapter.

- **Your activity level.** As described in chapter 8, even moderate exercise such as walking for twenty to thirty minutes per day—and not even that fast or even all at once—may reduce your risk of premature death from heart disease by 50 percent or more compared to those who are sedentary.

- **Your stress levels.** Emotional stress increases your risk of coronary heart disease in several ways. First, as I described in chapter 2, many people smoke, overeat, drink too much, work too hard, and abuse substances when they're feeling stressed. It's their way of coping with stress and getting through the day. Also, emotional stress makes your arteries constrict and your blood clot faster, and these mechanisms may precipitate a heart attack or stroke. In addition, emotional stress makes atherosclerosis (plaque) build up faster in your arteries.

  As I describe later in this chapter, studies have shown that when monkeys who are genetically comparable and on the same diet are divided into two groups—one that's put under emotional stress and one that isn't—the stressed monkeys have 50 percent more plaque in their arteries than the unstressed monkeys even though their genes and diet are comparable in both groups.

- **Chronic anger, hostility, and depression.** It used to be thought that "type A" behavior—moving quickly, multitasking, not liking to stand in line, and so on—was a risk factor for heart disease. Fortunately (especially for type A people like me), only a few components of type A behavior were found to be harmful: chronic anger and hostility.

- **Your weight.** Being overweight increases your risk of developing coronary heart disease as well as many other illnesses.

- **Smoking.** The more you smoke, the higher your risk of a heart attack, but there isn't a safe level of smoking. People who smoke a pack of cigarettes a day have more than twice the risk of heart attack that non-smokers do. Women who smoke and also take birth control pills increase their risk of heart attack, stroke, and peripheral vascular disease several times. So, unlike just about everything else in this book, there is not a spectrum of smoking. Quitting is very good—only three years after quitting smoking, your risk of having a heart attack is almost as low as if you had never smoked before. Quitting smoking after a heart attack or cardiac surgery can decrease your risk of death by at least one-third.

- **Chronic inflammation.** A simple blood test can measure your C-reactive protein level, which is an index of chronic inflammation. As I described earlier, smoldering inflammation increases your risk of coronary heart disease and many other illnesses as well.

- **Your cholesterol level.** LDL cholesterol is the most strongly predictive factor for the risk of coronary heart disease of the various cholesterol fractions. The higher your LDL cholesterol, the greater your risk.

As I described in chapter 1, my colleagues and I at the nonprofit Preventive Medicine Research Institute demonstrated in a series of randomized controlled trial and demonstration projects over a thirty-year period that comprehensive lifestyle changes can reverse the progression of even severe coronary heart disease.

We found that the more people changed their diet and lifestyle, the more they improved—but to reverse heart disease, they needed to make bigger changes than most doctors had recommended. Our findings have been replicated by other investigators.

For example, a study by a group of German scientists found that a 20-percent-fat diet plus exercise caused regression (reversal) of heart disease in almost 40 percent of patients. In our research, we found that 82 percent of patients showed regression, but they made bigger changes in diet and also practiced stress-management techniques. This is yet another example of one of the major principles of this book: the more you change your diet and lifestyle, the more you are likely to improve.

Another important validation of the Spectrum was a study directed by Dr. Stefano Sdringola and his colleagues at the University of Texas Medical School. They also found that the more people controlled their risk factors, the more improvement they showed in blood flow to the heart, heart attacks, bypass surgery, angioplasty, and deaths from heart disease. They found that moderate changes were not enough to reverse heart disease in most people.

In summary, if you're trying to prevent coronary heart disease, see where you are with respect to each of the above risk factors.

If your cholesterol level is too high, please go to chapter 9. Begin by making moderate changes in your diet and lifestyle. If that's enough to bring it down to an LDL level less than 100 mg/dl, preferably below 70 mg/dl if you have heart disease, that may be sufficient. If not, move progressively further toward the healthy end of the Spectrum until you achieve these goals. If you're not interested in changing your diet and lifestyle to that degree, consider taking cholesterol-lowering drugs. The more changes you make in your diet and lifestyle, the less medication you are likely to need.

If you find that your triglycerides start to go up when you change your diet, it probably means that you're consuming too many refined carbohydrates ("bad carbs"). In that case, progressively reduce your intake of sugar, white flour, white rice, alcohol, high-fructose corn syrup, and other refined carbohydrates. Also, exercise lowers triglycerides, as does fish oil or other sources of omega-3 fatty acids.

If your blood pressure is too high, please go to chapter 11 and move progressively toward the healthy end of the Spectrum until your blood pressure comes down to where you want it to be.

If your blood sugar is too high, please go to chapter 12 and move progressively toward the healthy end of the Spectrum until your blood sugar comes down to a normal range.

If you weigh too much, please go to chapter 10 and move progressively toward the healthy end of the Spectrum until your weight is where you want it to be.

If you need to exercise more, please follow the guidelines in chapter 8.

If you're feeling stressed, please practice some of the stress-management techniques I described in chapter 7. Even a few minutes a day can make a powerful impact on how you feel. In our research, people practicing stress-management techniques also showed a substantial decrease in chronic anger and hostility as well as significant reductions in depression, so they received several benefits.

If you have a significant number of these risk factors, talk with your doctor about having a test to find out if you have early heart disease. Some of the newer screening tests, such as the ultrafast CT scan (sometimes called a heart scan), can reveal whether or not you have significant coronary calcifications in your arteries.

Even more definitive, although with a somewhat higher radiation dose, is the 64-slice CT scanner. This provides an extraordinary view of the plaque throughout your coronary arteries. Over time, I'm sure newer technologies for early diagnosis of heart disease will become more widely available, more accurate, and less expensive.

Other tests such as a treadmill test are more commonly used but are less sensitive and specific for diagnosing early heart disease. Invasive tests such as coronary angiography are usually reserved for people who have a high likelihood of coronary artery disease and are considering bypass surgery or angioplasty.

Finding out that you have early heart disease can be lifesaving. First, about 30 percent of people first learn that they have heart disease when they die from it, which is clearly not a good way to find out. If you find out that you have heart disease, then you can do something about it.

Second, it can be very motivating to find out that you have heart disease. It's one thing to know that you may have several risk factors for heart disease, but it's easy to discount the significance of this: "Oh, it's not going to happen to me." In my experience, the more terrifying the possibility (heart attack or death), the greater the denial. On the other hand, if you find out that you have early heart disease, that can break through the denial and be highly motivating, especially if you know that you can do something to reverse the progression of heart disease if you're willing to go far enough in the healthy direction on the Spectrum.

It may be worth mentioning again that the moderate changes in diet and lifestyle recommended by many physicians and health agencies may be sufficient to prevent heart disease for some people but are often not sufficient to make much of a difference in reducing cholesterol levels or preventing heart disease in others.

A study of more than 50,000 men followed for eight years and 67,000 women followed for twelve years found that adherence to these dietary guidelines caused only a modest reduction in the risk of developing coronary heart disease.

Similar findings were seen in the Women's Health Initiative Study, which followed nearly 49,000 middle-aged women for more than eight years, comparing those on a regular diet to those on a low-fat diet. The women in the dietary change group were asked to eat less fat and more fruits, vegetables, and whole grains each day to see if it could help prevent heart disease and cancer. The women in the comparison group were not asked to change their diets.

Headlines proclaimed, "Low-fat diets don't protect against heart disease (or stroke or breast cancer or colon cancer)." However, the study participants did not reduce their dietary fat very much—more than 29 percent of their diet was made up of fat, not the study's goal of less than 20 percent. Even this may be an overestimation, since it's very common for people to report that they're following a diet better than they really are. Also, they did not increase their consumption of fruits and vegetables very much. The comparison group reduced its consumption of fat almost as much and increased its consumption of fruits and vegetables, making it harder to show between-group differences. Neither group significantly changed its consumption of grains.

As a result, LDL cholesterol decreased only about 2 percent more in the low-fat-diet group than in the comparison group, hardly any difference at all. Blood pressure decreased hardly at all in either group—by only about 2 percent.

Here's the good news: in this study, the risk of a heart attack *was* reduced in the subgroup of patients who consumed the lowest amount of saturated fat and trans fats and the highest amount of fruits and vegetables.

A recent study in the *Journal of the American Medical Association* compared the risk of colon cancer recurrence in those consuming a typical Western diet (high intakes of meat, fat, refined grains, and dessert) with a diet closer to the healthy end of the Nutrition Spectrum (high intakes of fruits and vegetables, poultry, and fish).

After a median of 5.3 years, the more closely the subjects followed the high-fat, high-sugar Western diet, the more likely they were to have a recurrence. Those with colon cancer who had the highest intakes of meat, fat, refined grains, and dessert had more than a threefold higher risk of recurrence of colon cancer or death compared to those consuming a healthier diet.

These findings are consistent with the theme of this book—in other words, based on your genetic predisposition, moderate changes in diet may be sufficient for some people to prevent heart disease, but not for most. However, for those who don't respond to moderate changes, moving further toward the healthy end of the Spectrum may be highly effective in preventing heart disease.

THE GOOD, THE BAD, AND THE UGLY

There are a lot of misconceptions about HDL cholesterol and LDL cholesterol. Most people, including many physicians, believe that HDL is "good cholesterol," and the higher it is, the better. LDL is often called "bad cholesterol."

It's easier to lower LDL cholesterol than raise HDL cholesterol. I think there should be less emphasis on raising HDL and more on lowering LDL via diet and lifestyle or, as a second choice, with lipid-lowering drugs. If you reduce your LDL below 100 mg/dl or even lower—below 70 mg/dl if you have coronary heart disease—your risk of heart disease is very low and your HDL level will be much less important.

Not everything that raises HDL is good for you and not everything that lowers HDL is bad for you.

Your body makes HDL to remove excessive cholesterol from your blood and tissues, a process known as "reverse cholesterol transport." Think of HDL as the garbage trucks of your body. HDL transports cholesterol back to your liver, where it is metabolized and removed from your body. Your body's ability to make more garbage trucks (raise your HDL) is, in part, genetically determined. Some people can make more garbage trucks than others.

Most Americans eat a diet that's relatively high in saturated fat and cholesterol—i.e., a lot of "garbage." People who have a lot of garbage trucks—in other words, who have high HDL levels—are more efficient at getting rid of extra fat and cholesterol in their diet. As a result, they have a lower risk of a heart attack or stroke than those who eat a high-fat, high-cholesterol diet who have lower HDL levels. However, the relationship of HDL to the risk of heart disease and stroke assumes that people are not changing their diet.

Not everything that raises HDL is good for you. For example, if you increase the amount of fat and cholesterol in your diet (as in an Atkins diet), you may increase your HDL because your body is trying to get rid of the extra "garbage" (fat and cholesterol) by increasing the number of available garbage trucks (HDL) if you are genetically able to do so. Eating a stick of butter will raise HDL in those who are able to do so, but that does not mean that butter is good for your heart. It isn't.

After spending almost a billion dollars, Pfizer recently discontinued a study of its drug torcetrapib. It was designed to prevent heart attacks by raising HDL cholesterol. Midway through the study, researchers found that this new drug actually *increased* the risk of a heart attack, so they had to stop the study and take the drug off the market.

This drug raised HDL by interfering with reverse cholesterol transport, causing HDL to build up. It was like having a traffic jam of garbage trucks—more trucks, but they didn't work as well. It's possible that new drugs that raise HDL via different mechanisms may eventually be shown to be beneficial.

Not everything that lowers HDL is bad for you. If you change from a high-fat, high-cholesterol diet to a healthy low-fat, low-cholesterol diet, your HDL level may stay the same or even decrease because there is less need for it. When you have less garbage, you need fewer garbage trucks to remove it, so your body may make less HDL. Thus, a reduction in HDL on a low-fat diet is not harmful.

We know this is true because instead of just measuring risk factors like HDL, we measured what actually happens to the progression of coronary heart disease in people who went on diets that were very low in "garbage"—that is, very low in cholesterol, saturated fat, total fat, and refined carbohydrates and high in fruits, vegetables, whole grains, legumes, and soy products.

Their HDL levels came down by 9 percent after one year, but their LDL ("bad") cholesterol levels came down even more, by an average of 40 percent. None of the patients was taking cholesterol-lowering drugs.

Even though their HDL levels decreased, these patients showed reversal of their heart disease as measured by state-of-the-art techniques such as quantitative coronary arteriography, cardiac PET scans, thallium scans, and radionuclide ventriculography in randomized controlled trials published in the leading peer-reviewed journals. On average, they showed even more reversal of their heart disease after five years than after one year. Also, there were 2.5 times more cardiac events such as heart attacks, bypass surgery, and angioplasty in the comparison group than in these patients.

A low HDL level in the context of a healthy low-fat diet has a very different prognostic significance than a low HDL level in someone eating a high-fat, high-cholesterol diet. People living in countries such as Asia where a low-fat diet is prevalent have low HDL levels yet among the lowest rates of heart disease in the world.

Conversely, some people believe that high-fat diets like an Atkins diet are good for your heart because they raise HDL levels. However, studies of people who go on an Atkins diet have showed that their heart disease worsens.

In our larger demonstration projects, we found that people whose HDL levels decreased in the first few months saw an increase during the remainder of the year, when they were more mindful about decreasing their intake of refined carbohydrates ("bad carbs").

APO A-1 MILANO

What will the future bring? One of the more interesting areas of research involves a protein called apo A-1, which becomes part of the HDL cholesterol molecule.

About thirty years ago, researchers at the University of Milan discovered that one of the men who lived in the lakeside town of Limone sul Garda in northern Italy had a very low level of HDL cholesterol and high levels of triglycerides. Despite this, he had no evidence of cardiovascular disease, and his parents lived a long time.

When blood tests were done on all 1,000 inhabitants of Limone, about forty individuals had a similar cholesterol finding. Using birth records maintained in the local church going back several hundred years, it was found that these forty individuals were all traceable to common ancestors from the year 1780. This led to the discovery that these forty people had a genetic mutation in the gene that makes a protein called apo A-1, which becomes a part of the HDL cholesterol molecule.

It was speculated that this mutant form of apo A-1 (now called apo A-1 Milano) may be protecting its carriers from cardiovascular disease. In 1994, Dr. P. K. Shah and his colleagues at Cedars-Sinai Medical Center showed for the first time that intravenous injection of a genetically engineered form of apo A-1 Milano markedly reduced arterial plaque buildup in the arteries of rabbits that were fed a high-cholesterol diet. In subsequent studies, Dr. Shah's laboratory found that injecting mice with apo A-1 Milano halted the progression of plaque buildup in their arteries and induced reversal (regression) of preexisting plaque within only five weeks.

Based on these encouraging findings in animals, Dr. Steven Nissen and his colleagues at the Cleveland Clinic studied the effects of apo A-1 Milano in humans with coronary artery disease. They found that injecting this into patients once a week for five weeks caused significant regression in coronary artery disease as measured by intravascular ultrasound.

Larger-scale studies of this approach are now in progress. It remains to be determined whether injecting people with apo A-1 Milano will turn out to be an accepted beneficial intervention or whether larger-scale trials may find, as in the case of torcetrapib, that patients become worse.

What is clear is that scientists will become more precise about identifying genes and gene mutations that may significantly increase or decrease your risk of developing coronary heart disease. If you find that you're at higher risk, you may benefit from moving closer to the healthy end of the Spectrum; conversely, if you're at lower risk, you may be able to make fewer changes in your diet and lifestyle.

THE NUTRITION SPECTRUM

The relationship between nutrition and coronary heart disease has been known since the early 1900s. Since then, we have developed a much greater understanding of the mechanisms that influence how what you eat affects your heart, how dynamic these mechanisms are, and how quickly these changes may occur—for better or for worse.

It was first observed many years ago that increased intake of saturated fat and cholesterol was associated with a higher risk of heart disease. These substances raise blood levels of both total cholesterol and LDL cholesterol. For example, the Seven Countries Study by Ancel Keys studied more than 12,000 men and found that their intake of saturated fat and its effects on LDL cholesterol were strongly linked with the risk of coronary heart disease. Similar findings were seen in the Framingham Heart Study, which tracked half of the people living in Framingham, Massachusetts, over a period of several decades.

The China Study, directed by T. Colin Campbell, found that the intake of animal protein and fat was much lower and the intake of fiber was higher in rural China than in the United States. As a result, average total cholesterol levels were only 127 mg/dl in China compared with over 200 in the United States. Heart disease mortality was almost seventeen times higher in men and almost six times higher in women in the United States than in China.

It's not just the amount of LDL cholesterol in your blood that determines your level of risk of heart disease. Other factors include oxidative stress, inflammation, and the particle size of the LDL. When LDL is oxidized, it's more likely to end up in your arteries.

I want to emphasize that it's not just the amount of fat in your diet that determines how it affects your heart. If you eat a very-low-fat diet that's high in refined carbohydrates such as sugar and other concentrated sweeteners, white flour, white rice, pasta, and so on, this may actually worsen your risk of cardiovascular disease.

A lot of "low-fat, low-cholesterol" foods are very high in sugar and other refined carbohydrates. For example, one SnackWell cookie has only 3 grams of fat but 13 grams of sugar, which is a lot.

When you have a lot of small, dense LDL particles—sometimes referred to as "pattern B"—they are more likely to end up in your arteries. Studies have shown that low-fat diets that are high in *refined* carbohydrates increase the number of harmful small, dense LDL particles.

However, low-fat diets that are high in *unrefined* carbohydrates such as whole grains, fruits, vegetables, and legumes in their natural forms—in other words, the healthy end of the Spectrum—cause a reduction in the number of harmful small, dense LDL particles. In our research, we found that levels of apolipoprotein B, which carries the harmful LDL particles, decreased significantly.

In the Harvard Nurses' Health Study of more than 75,000 women, researchers found a strong inverse relationship between intake of whole grains and the risk of developing coronary heart disease. This provides another validation of the Spectrum approach—in other words, it's not all or nothing. The more whole grains you consume, the lower your risk of heart disease.

So if your triglycerides are high, or if they increase when you change your diet, chances are that you're consuming too many refined carbohydrates. Use this information to, well, refine your diet by being more mindful about reducing your intake of refined carbohydrates and increasing your consumption of whole foods.

Saturated fats increase your risk of heart disease, but trans–fatty acids may increase it even more. A study in *The Lancet* of almost seven hundred Dutch men followed for ten years found that just a 2 percent increase in trans–fatty acid intake caused a 25 percent jump in the risk of heart disease.

According to Dr. Meir Stampfer, "My colleagues and I from the Harvard School of Public Health estimate, from laboratory and epidemiological studies, that between 72,000 and 228,000 heart attacks could be prevented each year in America if industrially produced trans fats were eliminated from our diet."

What you eat plays an important role in your risk of heart disease independent of its effects on your fasting blood cholesterol level. Studies have shown that there is a surge in triglycerides and harmful cholesterol fractions after you eat a meal high in saturated fat and cholesterol, and it is not affected by cholesterol-lowering drugs. This surge has a genetic component, as it is abnormally high and prolonged in people with heart disease and their children.

In chapter 9, I mentioned that some physicians believe that their patients are not going to change their diet, and they have neither the time nor the training to counsel their patients about nutrition, so why not just prescribe cholesterol-lowering drugs like Lipitor? One reason (besides costs and side effects, both known and unknown) is that these drugs lower your fasting cholesterol levels but don't affect the surge in your blood cholesterol that occurs after eating a fatty meal. This may be one of the reasons why lowering your cholesterol level with comprehensive lifestyle changes causes even more improvement in your arteries than lowering your cholesterol level an equivalent amount with cholesterol-lowering drugs alone.

As I mentioned in chapter 3, what you *include* in your diet is as important as what you *exclude*. This is especially true for preventing and reversing coronary heart disease. Many studies have shown that a higher intake of fruits and vegetables helps prevent heart disease. Some of the mechanisms for this are becoming increasingly well understood.

One of these is inflammation. Fruits and vegetables help reduce inflammation, whereas saturated fat, trans–fatty acids, and refined carbohydrates help promote inflammation. Foods that are high in refined carbohydrates also increase inflammation. Although inflammation has been recognized since ancient times, its contribution to cardiovascular diseases and other illnesses has only recently been fully appreciated.

The classic signs of inflammation are redness, heat, swelling, and pain. When you cut your finger or skin your knee, inflammation results. It's part of your body's defense system and helps speed wound healing.

Unfortunately, like the fight-or-flight response, our body's healing mechanisms can help *cause* disease when they are chronically stimulated. When overactivated, the same mechanisms that protect us can harm us, even kill us.

How do you know if your body is in a state of chronic inflammation? A simple blood test, called C-reactive protein, has been strongly linked with an increased risk of heart attack, stroke, and peripheral vascular disease, as well as other illnesses. It may be an even better predictor of risk than LDL cholesterol.

You may want to ask your doctor for this test, called "high-sensitive C-reactive protein." If it's elevated, it may be useful in both motivating you to make changes in diet and lifestyle and tracking your progress over time.

A study in *The Journal of the American Medical Association* found that adding C-reactive protein to other risk factors improved the accuracy of assessing the risk of heart disease in women. You can calculate your risk (free) at www.reynoldsriskscore.org.

C-reactive protein allows LDL cholesterol to enter the lining of your arteries more easily. It accelerates the buildup of plaque in your arteries and increases the likelihood that these plaques may rupture. C-reactive protein also increases the risk of your arteries constricting and blood clots forming. All of these mechanisms increase the risk of a heart attack occurring.

As with other aspects of the Spectrum, you can begin by making moderate changes in your diet and lifestyle. Recheck your C-reactive protein after a month or two. If it's down to a normal range, great. If not, consider making bigger changes and then rechecking it again.

In our research, we found a dose-response correlation between the adherence to the diet and lifestyle changes I recommend in this book and the changes in C-reactive protein:

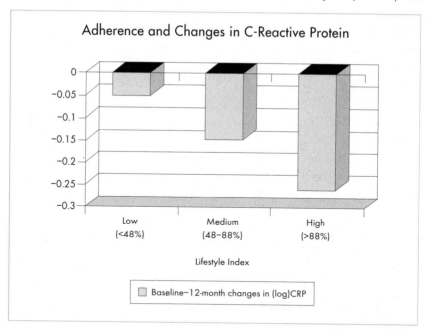

In other words, as we found in most of what we measured, the more people changed their diet and lifestyle, the more their C-reactive protein decreased, meaning the more their inflammation improved. This is yet another affirmation of the Spectrum approach.

In another study, patients who went through the Pritikin program showed a 45 percent decrease in C-reactive protein after only two weeks. Consuming fewer calories and losing weight also reduce C-reactive protein levels.

One of the reasons that cholesterol-lowering drugs called statins, such as Lipitor and Zocor, reduce the risk of a heart attack is that they reduce LDL cholesterol. Equally important may be the effect of statin drugs on reducing inflammation.

However, you don't have to take cholesterol-lowering drugs to decrease chronic inflammation. One study compared the effects of a low-fat diet high in soy, plant sterols, and fiber with the effects of a statin drug and found that both reduced C-reactive protein by about one third.

Another important factor in preventing heart disease is nitric oxide, as I described in chapter 11. An amino acid called L-arginine is converted by your body into nitric oxide. It's found in higher concentrations in soy protein and plant protein, and is one of the mechanisms by which eating more closely toward the healthy end of the Spectrum is so beneficial.

THE EXERCISE SPECTRUM

You already know that exercise is good for your heart. What you may not know is that you don't have to exercise very much to reduce your risk of heart disease.

The more you exercise, the more fit you become, but not necessarily the healthier. In an important study, Drs. Kenneth Cooper and Steven Blair studied more than 13,000 men and women over a period of more than eight years.

They expected to find that the more people exercised—in other words, the more fit they were—the lower their risk of premature death would be.

They didn't find what they expected. Instead, they found that the greatest reduction in premature death occurred when going from being a sedentary couch potato to exercising moderately—walking just twenty to thirty minutes per day, and not necessarily very fast or even all at one time. Those exercising more than this showed only slight, if any, additional reductions in premature death.

This is good news—a little goes a long way.

A randomized controlled trial comparing regular exercise with angioplasty in patients with heart disease found that people who chose exercise did much better than those undergoing angioplasty after one year. They had a higher event-free survival rate, fewer hospitalizations and surgical operations, and a significant improvement in exercise capacity—at half the cost of an angioplasty and without the costs, risks, and trauma.

Regular exercise also reduces inflammation. It may also lower your LDL cholesterol and triglyceride levels, increase HDL cholesterol, lower blood pressure, improve nitric oxide production, reduce oxidative stress, and help you lose weight. The benefits of exercise are described more fully in chapter 8.

If you have coronary heart disease, a treadmill test can be very helpful in tailoring an exercise prescription that's just right for you. Your doctor can monitor your EKG during exercise. If there are any indications that your heart is not receiving enough blood during the treadmill test, your doctor can show you how you can monitor your heart rate to keep it below the level at which abnormalities begin to occur.

THE STRESS-MANAGEMENT SPECTRUM

Emotional stress plays a major role in heart disease, both directly and indirectly.

There are direct connections between your brain and arteries throughout your body. Your brain communicates with your body in a number of ways, primarily via your nervous system and your hormones.

During times of stress, your brain stimulates your sympathetic nervous system, as I described in chapter 7. Your adrenal glands secrete stress hormones. Working together, these give you more energy to fight or to run, which helps you survive during times of danger.

Your heart beats faster. Also, the arteries in your arms and legs constrict and your blood clots more easily. This has survival value, so if you get wounded in battle or if a saber-toothed tiger bites you, you don't bleed as much.

However, when stresses become chronic, as many people experience, these same mechanisms that are supposed to protect you may cause a heart attack if the arteries in your heart constrict or if blood clots form there.

In the past, it was believed that plaque built up in arteries over a period of decades until they became so clogged that a heart attack ensued. We now know that these mechanisms are much more dynamic, with minute-to-minute changes in how dilated or constricted arteries are.

Surprisingly, arteries that are only 30 to 40 percent clogged may actually be more likely to cause a heart attack than those that are 90 to 95 percent blocked. Why? Because when there is a significant amount of plaque in your arteries, it's more likely to be calcified and stable.

Also, over time, new blood vessels called collaterals grow around blocked arteries—a type of "built-in bypass." So if an artery becomes completely obstructed, a heart attack may not necessarily ensue since there is another pathway for blood to flow around the blockage.

In contrast, an artery that is only 30 to 40 percent clogged has not had time to grow new collateral vessels. Also, it's not likely to be calcified and stable, so there is a greater risk of it constricting during times of emotional stress. When an artery in your heart constricts, it may cause rupture in plaques that are weakened, called vulnerable plaques.

When a plaque ruptures, the artery may go from 30 to 40 percent clogged to 100 percent blocked within seconds to minutes. This is called catastrophic progression (it's as bad as it sounds) and may lead to a heart attack, stroke, or sudden cardiac death. Plaque rupture can occur due to sudden physical or emotional stress.

This helps explain why the studies I mentioned in chapter 1 failed to show that angioplasty or bypass surgery prolongs life or prevents heart attacks in most patients. Most doctors are not going to put a stent or a bypass graft in an artery that's only 30 percent blocked, yet these are the ones that are most likely to cause a heart attack.

The more severely blocked arteries are more likely to cause angina (chest pain) due to the significant reduction in blood flow to the heart. However, most people don't need an angioplasty to reduce angina. Our studies show that you can reduce the frequency of angina by more than 90 percent in just a few weeks if you go far enough toward the healthy end of the Spectrum.

In addition to causing your arteries to constrict and your blood to clot more readily, chronic emotional stress may cause plaque to build up faster in your arteries. Studies of monkeys, which are genetically similar to humans, found that monkeys that were emotionally stressed by their social networks being disrupted had significantly more coronary artery blockages (atherosclerosis) than did another group of monkeys that wasn't put under stress, even though both groups of monkeys were on the same diet.

In another study by the same investigators, monkeys who were stressed showed constriction of their coronary arteries even when on a low-cholesterol diet.

In the INTERHEART study, emotional stress was found to be as potent a risk factor for heart disease as cholesterol, smoking, and lack of exercise. In one study, for example, public speaking about a topic that was personally relevant caused reduced blood flow to the heart and abnormal beats in the majority of patients. In another study, 75 percent of people with heart disease who were subjected to moderate mental stress showed abnormalities in the ability of the heart to pump blood.

Mental stress can trigger a lack of blood flow to the heart and increase the risk of death in people with coronary artery disease. Researchers asked heart patients to talk on an assigned topic for five minutes. The topic required role-playing in which a close relative was being mistreated in a nursing home. They found that heart patients who had reduced blood flow to their heart in response to mental stress had a threefold increase in the risk of death five years later compared to people without mental stress.

As I described in chapter 6, being in a stressful environment without much control over it is especially toxic to your heart. This is one of the reasons why people of lower socioeconomic status have higher rates of heart disease even when scientists adjust their findings for other known risk factors. Marital stress also increases the risk of a heart attack as well as increasing the rate of plaque buildup in coronary arteries.

As I mentioned earlier in this chapter, chronic anger and depression are strongly linked with an increased risk of developing coronary heart disease and sudden cardiac death. Studies show that the more depressed you feel, the greater your risk of developing coronary heart disease and having a heart attack. Depression increases C-reactive protein, interleukin-6, and other inflammatory proteins. Emotional stress also increases inflammation, which, in turn, raises the risk of coronary heart disease and other illnesses as well.

Emotional stress may also cause irregular heartbeats. In some cases, these can be lethal.

Stress may also cause strokes. For example, a study of more than 70,000 Japanese men and women who reported high levels of mental stress had double the risk of stroke-related and heart-related deaths than those reporting low stress levels. Similar findings came from a thirteen-year study of more than 12,000 people in Denmark. People who said they had high stress levels had almost double the risk of fatal stroke.

In some cases, emotional stress may damage your heart even if your coronary arteries remain normal. This syndrome, called "stress cardiomyopathy," sometimes referred to as "broken heart syndrome," is just that, and it is becoming increasingly recognized. The flood of stress-related hormones can temporarily stun or even disable your heart. In extreme cases, this can be fatal.

In a study published in the American Heart Association's major scientific journal, *Circulation,* investigators found that a three-month cardiac rehabilitation program that included both exercise and stress-management counseling significantly reduced feelings of distress in 150 men with heart disease. After nine years, the mortality rate was four times higher in a similar group of men who did not receive this intervention than in the patients who received it. Also, it was highest in men who reported more emotional distress.

A study by researchers at Duke University Medical Center followed ninety-four men with severe coronary heart disease. After five years, members of the stress-management group had 38 percent fewer cardiac events than did the group that received only the usual care. When medical costs over five years were calculated, the stress-management group averaged expenses of $9,251 each compared with $14,997 for the members of the control group.

Social support also plays an important role. In my book *Love and Survival,* I summarized hundreds of studies showing that people who feel lonely and isolated are many times more likely to die prematurely than are those who do not feel this way—not only from coronary heart disease but from virtually all causes.

So if you're feeling stressed, lonely, or chronically angry, you might consider spending more time each day on the stress-management techniques described in chapters 6 and 7 than you might otherwise. Part of the value of these research studies is to show us how important it is to address these psychosocial, emotional, and spiritual aspects of our lives.

As I mentioned earlier, awareness is the first step in healing. When we understand the effects of our choices, we can make different ones. For example, we sometimes view the time we spend relaxing, meditating, and hanging out with our friends and family as luxuries that we do only after the important stuff in our lives is done. These studies make it clear that this *is* the important stuff.

PREVENTING AND TREATING PROSTATE CANCER AND BREAST CANCER USING THE SPECTRUM

TESTIMONIAL:
Leonard Norwitz, San Francisco

I've been a participant in the research study directed by Dr. Ornish and his colleagues at the Preventive Medicine Research Institute to see if the progression of prostate cancer could be stopped or reversed by making comprehensive lifestyle changes. I've been in the program about eight years.

The program helped me a lot. It was more than just the diet. It was the entire program, including the support of the community, which was a major factor, especially since I live alone.

I felt better when I made these changes in my diet and lifestyle. Especially considering the anxiety I felt at the time about the diagnosis, I was surprised that I was able to slow down as much as I did. I had a fairly low threshold for anxiety, and I have been a lifelong hypochondriac. The nice thing about hypochondria is that it makes you very aware of what's going on in your body. So I just needed to turn that into a kind of vigilance that was productive instead of one that created more distress.

I never expected to live this long because of the history of cancer in my family. I'm sixty-five now; my mother died when she was sixty, and I have already outlived my father by forty years, so I never expected to do this well. I was kind of fatalistic about this.

After my prostate biopsy and ultrasound, my urologist thought that I needed a radical prostatectomy right away. He thought that delaying this surgery was irresponsible.

I got a second opinion from a different urologist, who said, "Why don't you take a little break and go see the people running the Ornish study and see what they can do for you?" I asked a third urologist, "Can I wait a year to do this surgery?" and after looking at the biopsy results, he said, "Sure." Because the disease was not that aggressive.

For the first bunch of years while I was vigorously doing the program, I felt so much better. I've always had an anxiety disorder, but I almost never felt anxious or stressed while I was doing the program on a regular basis, including the yoga and meditation. I don't remember being anxious at all during that time. That gave me confidence that the rest of the program had value as well.

I hadn't been doing the stress-management techniques as rigorously lately, and I was feeling more anxious again. My fuse got shorter. But I'm starting to do the stress-management techniques again, and I can already see that they're helping me. I still follow the diet pretty well.

Before I started the program, I felt fine. I felt even better once I began changing my diet and lifestyle on this program, but it was a subtle thing because I didn't feel there was anything wrong before I began, and I felt like I was in fine shape. I didn't feel that anything needed fixing. But when I started the program, I felt even better. I could climb stairs easier; I could do everything easier; everything worked better.

At the time I began, my PSA was 4.1 ng/ml, and over the next five years it rose to only 5.3. My other tests—the ultrasound, MRI, and MR spectroscopy—showed that the prostate cancer has been stable and has not advanced at all during the past eight years. That's a very good feeling.

Can the Spectrum approach to comprehensive lifestyle changes affect the progression of cancer?

My colleagues and I at the nonprofit Preventive Medicine Research Institute published the first randomized controlled trial showing that the progression of early-stage prostate cancer may be slowed, stopped, or perhaps even reversed by making changes in diet and lifestyle similar to the ones that we showed could reverse heart disease in our earlier studies.

As described in chapter 1, this may be the first randomized controlled trial showing that the progression of any type of cancer may be modified just by changing what we eat and how we live. What's true for prostate cancer may be true for breast cancer as well.

As described earlier, this study was done in collaboration with Peter Carroll, M.D. (chair, Department of Urology, School of Medicine, University of California, San Francisco), and William Fair, M.D. (chief of urologic surgery and chair of urologic oncology, Memorial Sloan-Kettering Cancer Center, now deceased).

In our prostate cancer research, we recruited ninety-three men with diagnosed prostate cancer who had decided, for reasons unrelated to our study, not to have conventional treatments. Now, you might wonder why someone with diagnosed prostate cancer might not rush to have the tumor surgically removed or irradiated before it spreads.

However, there is a surprising lack of rigorous evidence proving that men with prostate cancer—especially those who are older at the time of diagnosis, have a smaller tumor volume, a less-aggressive and less-invasive form of the tumor, and a PSA level that is not rapidly rising—benefit from or live longer after undergoing radical prostatectomy (surgical removal of the prostate) or radiation therapy in its various forms.

Unfortunately, these treatments leave many men impotent, incontinent, or both, so some men are not eager to have interventions that may not help them live longer but may affect their quality of life in major ways. Most men who live long enough are likely to eventually be diagnosed with prostate cancer, but they're more likely to die *with* prostate cancer than *from* prostate cancer.

There is a subgroup of men with prostate cancer who may benefit from conventional treatments, although the scientific evidence is not yet definitive. These tend to be men who are diagnosed with prostate cancer early in life, have rapidly rising PSA levels, have a Gleason score greater than 6, have a large tumor, have a PSA level that is rapidly rising, and so on. If you have prostate cancer, talk with your doctor to see if you're in a subgroup of patients whom surgery or radiation treatments may benefit—and ask to see evidence that this is true.

One of my patients was diagnosed with prostate cancer and decided to visit leading specialists around the country to find out the best course of treatment. In almost every case, each doctor recommended his own specialty area of therapy. In other words, the surgeons recommended surgery, the radiation oncologists recommended radiation treatments, and so on. In the absence of clear data showing safety and efficacy, people tend to default to their own methods of treatment. As Abraham Maslow once observed, "When the only tool you have is a hammer, you tend to view everything as a nail."

The decision to forgo conventional treatment in prostate cancer is sometimes called "watchful waiting," which was recently changed to "active surveillance." "Watchful waiting" implies that patients are sitting around under a sword of Damocles, waiting for the other shoe to drop, whereas "active surveillance" has a different connotation, of taking an active role in their treatment beginning with changes in nutrition and lifestyle.

In our research, we didn't recommend that our study patients should (or should not) have conventional treatments, as they had already made this decision for reasons unrelated to our study. The advantage of limiting enrollment in our study to patients who were not having conventional treatments was that it provided us with a unique opportunity to compare men who made comprehensive lifestyle changes with a similar group of men with prostate cancer who were not having conventional treatments.

Thus, we could see what the effects of changing diet and lifestyle alone were without being confounded by other surgical or medical treatments in the comparison group. This wouldn't have been possible in a study of breast cancer, since almost everyone receives conventional treatment shortly after diagnosis.

We randomly divided the men with prostate cancer into two groups. The experimental group was asked to make the comprehensive lifestyle changes described in this book—that is, making their nutrition and lifestyle decisions on the most healthful end of the Spectrum (that is, following the healthiest versions of Art Smith's recipes). The comparison group was not asked to make any specific changes in their diet or lifestyle but were free to do so.

PSA is the most commonly used marker for whether prostate cancer is progressing or improving. In our study, we drew the patients' blood samples at the beginning and again after one year.

PSA is an imperfect marker for prostate cancer, but it's the best one available for looking at interval changes in the disease's severity. If PSA increases, the disease is likely getting worse; if it decreases, it may be improving. There is considerable variability in quality and reproducibility among laboratories, so we overnight-couriered the blood samples from the patients in San Francisco to the laboratory at Memorial Sloan-Kettering Cancer Center, which is one of the most accurate and reliable anywhere.

After one year of intervention, we found that PSA levels decreased (improved) in the experimental group but increased (worsened) in the comparison group, who were making more moderate changes. These differences were not huge but were statistically significant. Prostate cancer tends not to spread if PSA is not rising, so these differences are clinically significant since PSA did not increase. This study was published in the *Journal of Urology*, the leading peer-reviewed urology journal.

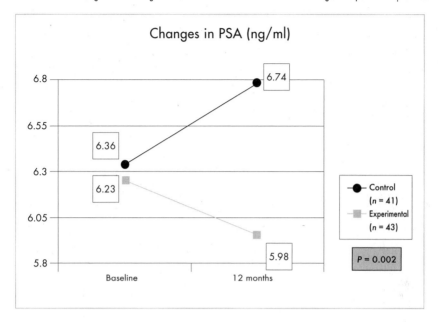

Also, there was a direct correlation between the degree of change in diet and lifestyle and the degree of change in PSA levels in both the experimental group and the comparison group. In other words, just as we found in the earlier cardiac studies, the more people changed their diet and lifestyle, the more improvement we measured.

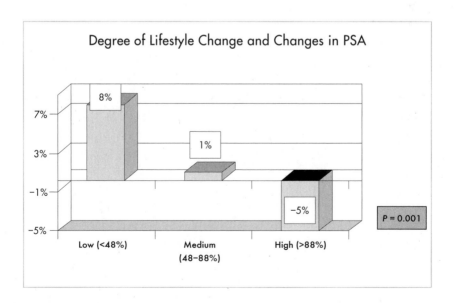

As you can see from the graph on page 223—which is a type of spectrum—a high degree of change in diet and lifestyle was required for PSA levels to go down rather than up. As we've been discussing throughout this book, moderate changes in diet and lifestyle are often enough to help prevent diseases such as prostate cancer, but bigger ones are often required to stop or reverse its progression.

This may be one of the reasons why no one had previously shown in a randomized controlled trial that the progression of prostate cancer (or, in our earlier studies, of coronary heart disease) could be stopped or reversed by changing diet and lifestyle alone—because they may not have gone far enough toward the healthy end of the Spectrum.

We also found that prostate tumor growth in vitro was inhibited 70 percent in the experimental group but only 9 percent in the comparison group. Not surprisingly, these large differences were also statistically significant.

To me, one of the most interesting findings in our research was the strong correlation between the degree of change in diet and lifestyle and the degree of inhibition of the prostate tumor growth in both the experimental group and the control group. Here again, the more people changed their diet and lifestyle—the closer they moved toward the healthy end of the Spectrum—the more the changes affected the growth of their prostate cancer tumors in vitro.

Patients in the lifestyle-change group also reported substantial improvements in their quality of life. These included better sexual functioning and reduced perceived stress, as well as less anxiety, fear, and feelings of vulnerability.

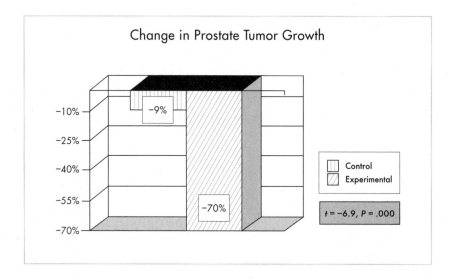

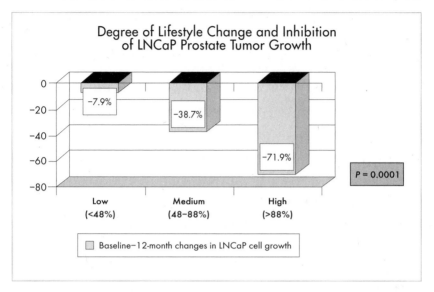

We found that six of the patients who were randomly assigned to the control group of this study needed conventional treatment such as surgery, radiation, or hormonal treatments during the first year of the study, whereas none of the patients in the experimental group (who were making more intensive changes in diet and lifestyle) needed conventional treatment. After four years, twenty-one of the control group patients needed conventional treatment compared with only six of the experimental group patients, and these differences were statistically significant.

Even if a person is diagnosed with prostate cancer that appears localized to the prostate and decides to have it surgically removed (called a radical prostatectomy) or has treatment with other modalities such as radiation, there is a surprisingly high rate of recurrence of 35 percent or more.

Why? Because the tumor may have spread microscopically in ways that were undetectable at the time of surgery. Therefore, if a person has prostate cancer, whether or not he decides to undergo conventional treatment, moving to the healthiest end of the Spectrum is wise and may help reduce the risk of recurrence.

Also, a year after our research was published, scientists at the University of California, San Diego, reported that a similar low-fat plant-based diet and stress-management techniques reduced the rise in PSA in men with recurrent prostate cancer.

Although our research focused on prostate cancer, our study may have implications for treating and helping to prevent breast cancer as well. There are many similarities between the two diseases.

THE NUTRITION SPECTRUM

The risk of both breast cancer and prostate cancer is increased by the intake of red meat, full-fat dairy products, and animal fats—i.e., the less healthy direction of the Spectrum—and decreased by consumption of fruits, vegetables, fiber, and soy products on the healthier end of the Spectrum. Frying or charbroiling red meat forms substances called aromatic hydrocarbons that are especially carcinogenic.

The healthiest end of the Spectrum is similar to a traditional Asian diet, which may be part of the reason why the incidence and age-adjusted mortality rate of both prostate cancer and breast cancer is more than ten times higher in the United States than in Asia. However, when Asians immigrate to the United States, their rates of both prostate cancer and breast cancer increase to levels seen in the U.S. population.

Unfortunately, as Asians begin to eat like us and live like us, they're starting to die like us. The incidence of both prostate cancer and breast cancer is rising rapidly in Asia, along with diabetes, heart disease, and other chronic diseases. Other countries are rapidly forgoing their own healthier diets and lifestyles and copying ours. As a result, a globalization of illness is occurring that is almost completely preventable.

In only one generation, cardiovascular disease, diabetes, obesity, and other chronic diseases have gone from being among the least common to the most frequent causes of premature death and disease in most of the developing world. Cardiovascular deaths now equal HIV/AIDS deaths in most African countries. It used to be uncommon to see an overweight person walking down the street in China or India, but not anymore. Because this is a recent phenomenon—the number of overweight people is on the steep rise of the exponential curve—intervention now can make a powerful difference.

A recent study showed that patients with prostate cancer who are overweight have a higher risk of recurrence than those with normal body weight. Thus, bringing weight into a normal range by moving further toward the healthy end of the Spectrum may reduce the risk of recurrence and lower the risk of ever getting prostate cancer.

Estrogen increases the risk of both prostate cancer and breast cancer. It stimulates cell growth and proliferation, which, if unchecked, may lead to cancer. Estrogen also promotes inflammation as well as oxidative damage to DNA. One reason why being overweight increases the risk of both prostate cancer and breast cancer is that fat cells convert precursors of estrogen into estrogen. In other words, the more fat you have, the more estrogen you are likely to have.

One reason why soy may help reduce the risk of both breast cancer and prostate cancer is that it reduces the harmful effects of estrogen. The phytoestrogens in soy have a structure similar enough to that of estrogen that they bind to estrogen receptors. They stimulate estrogen receptors only weakly but block the regular estrogen molecules from binding to these estrogen receptors.

It's a little like having a key that fits well enough to go into a lock but not accurately enough to open it—but it blocks any other keys from being able to open the lock. The net effect is to reduce the effects of estrogen.

As I mentioned in chapter 4, our genes have hardly changed during the past hundred years, but our diet and lifestyle have altered considerably. Dr. Donald Coffey is Professor of urology, oncology, pathology, and molecular biology and Director of research at the Brady Urological Institute at the Johns Hopkins Medical Institutions. In a major review article, Dr. Coffey wrote:

This major phase shift in food style occurred only about 10,000 years ago, when humans became farmers and domesticated both plants and animals. This technology quickly evolved into a tighter focusing of human diets from wild fresh vegetables and fruits to an eating pattern toward limited plants that could be domesticated and grown in great quantities and stored, like wheat, rice, barley, corn, potatoes, and other tubers.

This resulted in approximately 20 plant types rapidly replacing the high diversity of 3,000 plants and fruits that were earlier eaten fresh as they came into season and were gathered from the wild.

With large-scale domestication and breeding of cattle came a high meat intake, and this was combined with storage, curing, drying, and cooking as well as a propensity to use milk and cheese from dairy processing. Cooking, burning, and smoking produce high levels of heterocyclic molecules, many of which make adducts to DNA, and are carcinogens.

Since separating from the great apes and chimpanzees approximately 8 million years ago, humans evolved into *Homo sapiens sapiens* that are very similar to our present form in as little as 150,000 years. However, we dramatically changed to a Western-style diet only in the very recent past (i.e., 15,000 years)—at a pace much faster than we could biologically evolve. This Western diet consists of high meat and fat; dairy products; stored, processed, and cooked meats; and low fruit and fiber intake, along with a more sedentary lifestyle.

In summary, we were not biologically selected by the evolution process to eat the way we do today, and the damage is manifested in prostate and breast cancer.

Dr. Coffey summarized these changes in diet and exercise in this table:

Human Development and the Change of Diet

DIET	Time During Human Development (150,000 years)	
	FIRST 90% (135,000 YEARS)	LAST 10% (15,000 YEARS)
Fruit	High	Low
Fiber	High	Low
Plant diversity	High (3,000)	Low (20)
Red meat	Low	High
Animal fat	Low	High
Dairy products	Low	High
Food	Fresh/wild	Cooked/preserved
Movement	High	Sedentary

As I mentioned in chapter 13, the Women's Health Initiative Study followed nearly 49,000 middle-aged women for more than eight years. It was supposed to compare women consuming a typical American diet with those on a low-fat diet. The women in the dietary change group were asked to eat less fat and more fruits, vegetables, and whole grains each day to see whether this could help prevent heart disease and cancer. The women in the comparison group were not asked to change their diets.

Although the U.S. government spent almost a billion dollars on this study, it didn't show very much, and its results were widely misinterpreted when it was published in *The Journal of the American Medical Association.* The authors concluded, "A low-fat dietary pattern did not result in a statistically significant reduction in invasive breast cancer risk over an 8.1-year average follow-up period." Gina Kolata of *The New York Times* reported, "The largest study ever to ask whether a low-fat diet reduces the risk of getting cancer has found that the diet has no effect."

More balanced voices were found in places like the *Columbia Journalism Review,* which is considered one of the most credible and scholarly watchdog and friend of the press. They wrote:

The problem with the study, *The Wall Street Journal* went on to point out, was that it did not distinguish between so-called "good" fats, like omega-3 fatty acids found in fish, and "bad" fats, such as the saturated and trans fats found in fried and processed foods. Also, the *Journal* noted, the women on the low-fat diet didn't do a great job of sticking with it. As a result, the overall difference between the two diets ended up being fairly minimal. That the resulting health differences were also fairly minimal, therefore, was not exactly big news. Perhaps the best article of the bunch was penned by one of the skeptics quoted in Kolata's story. Writing on *Newsweek*'s Web site, in his debut health column, Dr. Dean Ornish provided a clear and nuanced take on the study. On this one, we recommend a little less Kolata in the diet, and a few more caveats.

As I wrote in chapter 13, the study participants did not reduce their dietary fat very much—29 percent of their diet was comprised of fat, not the study's goal of 20 percent. Also, they did not increase their consumption of fruits and vegetables very much. The comparison group also reduced its consumption of fat almost as much and increased its consumption of fruits and vegetables, making it harder to show between-group differences. Neither group significantly changed its consumption of grains.

As a result, LDL cholesterol decreased only about 2 percent more in the low-fat-diet group than in the comparison group, hardly any difference at all.

Seen from a different perspective, the Women's Health Initiative Study validates the concept of the Spectrum outlined in this book. In short, if you don't change much, you don't improve much.

As I mentioned in the last chapter, the risk of a heart attack *was* reduced in the subgroup of patients who consumed the lowest amount of saturated fat and trans fats, and the highest amount of fruits and vegetables. In the Women's Health Initiative, the incidence of breast cancer was 9 percent lower in the study group than in the comparison group, although not enough to be statistically significant.

Part of the problem may be the way the diets were measured. The relationship of dietary fat to breast cancer was not statistically significant when measured using what's called a "food frequency questionnaire," which asks a person to estimate the frequency of foods consumed on average during the past year. I can barely remember what I had for lunch yesterday, which is why this questionnaire is not considered as accurate as what's called a "food record," in which people write down everything they eat in a given day at the time they are consuming it.

In the Women's Health Initiative Study, there *was* a statistically significant relationship between total fat consumption and incidence of breast cancer in women when fat intake was measured using the food record but not when using the food frequency questionnaire.

Also, women who reported the highest levels of fat intake at baseline (i.e., those who consumed diets containing more than 37 percent of calories from fat), and therefore may have achieved the greatest reduction in fat intake (more room for improvement), also had a statistically significant decreased risk of breast cancer.

Similarly, a study by Dr. Rowan T. Chlebowski found that women who reduced their dietary fat intake to only 20 percent (about 33 grams of fat per day) reduced their risk of breast cancer recurrence by 42 percent after five years when compared with a randomized comparison group who consumed 51 grams of fat per day. However, this effect was only seen in estrogen-negative breast cancer.

These findings were supported by a study conducted by the National Institutes of Health (NIH) and the AARP, which examined women who made bigger reductions in dietary fat than did those in the Women's Health Initiative. In a study of almost 190,000 women with an average follow-up time of 4.4 years, the authors concluded, "In this large prospective cohort with a wide range of fat intake, dietary fat intake was directly associated with the risk of postmenopausal invasive breast cancer."

What made this study so important is that it examined a much larger range of fat intake than was seen in the Women's Health Initiative Study, in which only 2 percent of the women reported consuming a diet that was less than 20 percent fat. In contrast, 10 percent of the women in the NIH-AARP study reported consuming a diet that was less than 20 percent fat.

In the NIH-AARP study, the investigators found a direct relationship between consumption of *all* types of fat and the incidence of breast cancer in postmenopausal women. This contradicts those who say that mono-unsaturated and polyunsaturated fats have a neutral or protective effect on breast cancer.

This finding was also seen in a study of postmenopausal women in Sweden. The researchers found a direct association between the risk of breast cancer and the intake of total fat, saturated fat, monounsaturated fat, and polyunsaturated fat. They found that a high intake of omega-6 fatty acids increased the risk of breast cancer, which is why canola oil may be a better choice than olive oil, as I described in chapter 3, because it has fewer of the omega-6 fatty acids and more of the protective omega-3 fatty acids.

The NIH-AARP study also found a strong association between fat intake and risk of breast cancer in women who were on menopausal hormone therapy, suggesting that dietary fat intake may have more influence on breast cancer risk in those taking estrogen. This was also seen in the Women's Health Initiative Study, in which women who were assigned to the low-fat group and were taking estrogen showed a 17 percent reduction in breast cancer incidence compared to the control group, but this reduction was not seen in women who were not taking estrogen.

In the Harvard Nurses' Health Study II, mostly premenopausal women who consumed the highest amount of animal fat (but not vegetable fat) had a statistically significant increased risk of breast cancer.

Why does dietary fat increase the risk of breast cancer? Several mechanisms have been proposed. If the dietary fat is rich in omega-6 fatty acids, this may promote inflammation, which, in turn, may increase the risk of breast cancer. Dietary fat also stimulates your body to produce more estrogen, as previously discussed, and estrogen promotes breast cancer. Some studies have shown that reducing dietary fat intake reduces the amount of available estrogen in your body. Dietary fat also affects and regulates gene expression and modulates immune function.

The role of refined carbohydrates in the risk of both prostate cancer and breast cancer is less well established. In the Harvard Nurses' Health Study, no relationship was found among glycemic load, glycemic index, carbohydrate intake, and breast cancer, although other studies have shown some relationship.

Why? Because excessive insulin production increases the production of insulin-like growth factor (IGF), which, in turn, may promote cancer growth. Also, too much insulin reduces the amount of sex hormone binding globulin (SHBG), a protein that binds testosterone and estrogen. Reducing SHBG increases the amount of testosterone and estrogen in your blood, which, in turn, increases the risk of prostate cancer and breast cancer.

One of the themes of this book is that what you include in your diet is as important as what you exclude. Several studies have shown that diets high in fruits, vegetables, soy, fiber, lycopene, and omega-3 fatty acids reduce the risk of both breast cancer and prostate cancer. Diets high in whole grains, fruits, and vegetables contain high amounts of naturally occurring antioxidants that, combined with physical activity, have been shown to reduce oxidative stress. Vitamin D intake greater than 800 IU per day may also help prevent both prostate cancer and breast cancer.

One of the strongest examples showing the powerful effects of including fruits and vegetables in your diet was recently published in the *Journal of Clinical Oncology*. Investigators at the University of California, San Diego, followed almost 1,500 women who had early-stage breast cancer for several years. They found that walking at least thirty minutes six days per week, and consuming at least five servings of fruits or vegetables a day were associated with a 50 percent reduction in the risk of death from breast cancer. This substantial reduction in mortality was seen in both obese and nonobese women.

Unfortunately, a more recent publication from this group of investigators was very discouraging for many women. The researchers reported, "Among survivors of early stage breast cancer, adoption of a diet that was very high in vegetables, fruit, and fiber and low in fat did not reduce additional breast cancer events or mortality during a 7.3-year follow-up period."

However, as in the Women's Health Initiative Study, these women did not reduce their dietary fat very much by their own self-report, and they probably were not accurate in what they reported. They should have lost weight based on the number of calories they reported consuming, but both groups actually gained weight.

Also, both groups actually reported consuming *more* fat at the end of the study than at the beginning, so the hypothesis could not be tested.

In other words, if I want to find out whether eating less fat reduces the risk of breast cancer recurrence but the patients in the study report eating more fat, then it's hard to draw the conclusion that a low-fat diet doesn't reduce the risk of breast cancer recurrence.

The real message of the study was that it was not possible to test the hypothesis because the experimental group did not follow the recommended diet and the control group changed about the same amount.

Since a randomized controlled trial is based on differences between groups, if both groups are following essentially the same diet (regardless of what they were asked to follow), then you're not going to see a difference in outcomes such as breast cancer recurrence between the groups. This is very different from saying that it has now been proven that diets low in fat and high in fruits and vegetables have no effect on breast cancer recurrence, which is scientifically unjustified and terribly misleading.

As noted in the editorial that accompanied the publication of this study:

The intervention goal to reduce fat intake to 15 percent to 20 percent of total calories was not achieved. Indeed, at no time during follow-up was average self-reported fat intake less than 21 percent of total calories, and by year 4, fat intake was more than 27 percent of total caloric intake in both groups.

Moreover, at the 6-year follow-up, the average percentage of calories from fat reported by both intervention group and control group participants was *higher* than reported at baseline. Whether this lack of adherence to the intervention goal for fat reduction explains any of the null findings in this study is unclear.

Of further concern is that baseline mean total daily caloric intakes were 1719 kcal in the intervention group and 1717 kcal in the comparison group, but by year 6, the respective mean total daily caloric intakes were 1538 kcal and 1559 kcal, respectively. In the absence of changes in physical activity, it would be expected that an average decrease of nearly 180 kcal per day would result in a decrease in body weight during the study period. However, these women experienced small increases in body weight during the study period.

These results call into question the validity of some components of the self-reported dietary data.

THE EXERCISE SPECTRUM

Exercise also plays an important role in both prostate cancer and breast cancer. Several studies have shown that exercise diminishes the risk of breast cancer and prostate cancer both directly (for example, by reducing levels of estrogen and testosterone and tissue responsiveness to these hormones) and indirectly (by promoting weight loss).

A review of more than sixty studies suggests that both premenopausal and postmenopausal women who exercise regularly may reduce their incidence of breast cancer by 20 to 40 percent. Exercise appears to reduce the incidence of prostate cancer by about the same degree.

An expert panel of the International Agency for Research on Cancer of the World Health Organization estimated a 20 to 40 percent decrease in the risk of developing breast cancer among the most physically active women, regardless of menopausal status, or type or intensity of activity.

A study of almost 3,000 nurses with stage 1, 2, or 3 breast cancer, published in *The Journal of the American Medical Association,* reported that walking just three to five hours per week at an average pace significantly reduced the risk of death from breast cancer by 26 to 40 percent. Even women who walked only one hour per week had a better survival rate than those who were sedentary. Also, those who exercised more intensively than walking three to five hours per week showed no additional reduction in mortality from breast cancer.

THE STRESS-MANAGEMENT SPECTRUM

Chronic stress may increase the risk of breast cancer. A recent study that followed nearly 60,000 African-American women for six years, published in the *American Journal of Epidemiology,* found that women who reported feelings of racial discrimination were more likely than their peers to develop breast cancer.

In this study, women who reported on-the-job discrimination had a 32 percent higher risk of breast cancer than women who did not. Women who said they faced discrimination on the job, in housing, and by the police were 48 percent more likely to develop breast cancer than those who reported no incidents of major discrimination.

Chronic stress may also increase the risk of prostate cancer. In another study, men who experienced high levels of stress were more than three times as likely to have elevated PSA levels than were men who experienced low levels of stress. Also, those with low social support were nearly twice as likely to have high PSA levels as those with high social support.

In a study published in one of the leading international medical journals, *The Lancet,* women with breast cancer were followed for five years. There was a significantly increased risk of relapse or death in women who were depressed. On the other hand, a "fighting spirit" was not associated with improved survival.

Social support may help prolong life in women with metastatic breast cancer. In a well-known study, also published in *The Lancet,* Dr. David Spiegel at Stanford Medical School randomly assigned women with metastatic breast cancer to a support group or to a usual-care group.

Women in the support group met once per week for a year in a supportive, nurturing environment in which they were encouraged to talk about authentic feelings with other women who really understood what they were going through. These support groups were very similar to the ones that my colleagues and I used in our studies of heart disease and prostate cancer.

Survival from time of entry into the study was an average of 36.6 months in the group of women who attended the support group but only 18.9 months in the comparison group. In other words, attending the support group had almost doubled their survival time, even though there were no other significant differences in diet, exercise, conventional treatments, or other factors known to affect survival.

Some, but not all, studies by other investigators have confirmed these findings. In an editorial in *The New England Journal of Medicine,* Dr. Spiegel speculated that his study was conducted in the 1970s, when conventional breast cancer treatments were not as effective and when most women did not receive psychological counseling or participate in support groups, so the impact of the support group in his study would have been easier to detect.

In a more recent study, Dr. Spiegel examined the relationship between spirituality and immune function in 112 women with metastatic breast cancer. Spirituality was assessed by patients' reports of frequency of attendance at religious services and the importance of religious or spiritual expression.

Women who rated spirituality as important in their lives had a greater number of circulating white blood cells and improved immune function.

Genes also play a role in the risk of breast cancer, but they exert a major role in only a minority of women. The BReast CAncer, or BRCA, genes 1 and 2 increase the risk of breast cancer, but only about 5 percent of breast cancers are due to these genes.

Women who have BRCA1 or BRCA2 gene changes have a 36 to 85 percent chance of developing breast cancer and a 16 to 60 percent chance of developing ovarian cancer during their lifetimes. These numbers show a wide range of risk and depend on other personal and family history. In a small study, it showed that men with BRCA1 or BRCA2 gene changes have about a 6 percent chance of developing breast cancer by age 70 and a 16 percent chance of developing prostate cancer by age 70.

If you have a BRCA gene, discuss the advantages and disadvantages of different treatment options with your physician. Also, if you have a BRCA gene, it may be to your advantage to move further in the healthier direction on the Spectrum than you might otherwise have done—better diet, more exercise, more stress management, less alcohol, no smoking.

For example, one study showed that women with the BRCA gene who consumed more calories and had a higher body mass index had a higher rate of breast cancer. In other words, both genetic predisposition *and* lifestyle choices are important. Two well-known researchers have proposed that dietary modification may modulate the risk of hereditary breast cancer by decreasing DNA damage (possibly linked to estrogen exposure) or by enhancing DNA repair.

Even if you don't have the BRCA gene, you may still be at higher risk of breast cancer for other reasons—for example, if you have a strongly positive family history of early breast cancer. About 10 to 15 percent of all breast cancers have a genetic component, but only about 5 percent of breast and ovarian cancers are linked to the BRCA1 or BRCA2 gene change. Jews of eastern European descent have a higher risk of having one of the BRCA genes.

Genetic testing is also identifying other genes that may affect the treatment of breast cancer. For example, women with a genetic variant called CYP2D6 may metabolize the cancer drug tamoxifen effectively and so may benefit from knowing this information before deciding which type of chemotherapy to undergo.

In summary, if you have a genetic predisposition to prostate cancer or breast cancer—because of a strong family history, the presence of risk factors, or based on the results of your genetic testing—you may benefit considerably by going further in the healthy direction of the Spectrum.

PART II

WELCOME TO ART'S KITCHEN: AN ABUNDANT SPECTRUM OF FOODS TO ENJOY

A NOTE BY ART SMITH

Several years ago, I met Dr. Dean Ornish at a dinner party for the music legend Quincy Jones. Imagine how nervous I was when Quincy told me that America's foremost health and nutrition adviser was an invited guest. I practically made myself sick worrying about my menu. Was it healthy enough for Dr. Ornish? Would he be scrutinizing every calorie on his plate? But once I met Dr. Ornish that night, I was relieved. Because besides being genuinely concerned about our nation's health and well-being, he is also a dear man with a gentle spirit and a kind heart. I was thrilled that he loved the meal I had prepared for him.

A few years later, I called him to see what he thought about combining our passions in a single book: his medical research and lifestyle philosophy with my recipes and my never-ending crusade to get people to sit down and share meals with their families. So when Dr. Ornish asked me to create the recipes for the book, I was thrilled again! It's true that I did feel the same nervousness I had felt years before when Quincy Jones read me his guest list. After all, people know me for my twelve-layer cake and melt-in-your-mouth buttermilk biscuits! I knew that creating healthy recipes that would be up to Dr. Ornish's standards would be a challenge, but I was up for it.

Over and over we hear how diets simply do not work, how people on diets become bitter and frustrated. I have seen this process happen hundreds of times, and I have experienced it myself, which is why I was so interested in Dr. Ornish's philosophy. The Spectrum involves positive lifestyle changes, not just two or three dreadful weeks of abstinence from all of the foods that taste good.

I kept these recipes simple, relying on one of the most basic and important components of good cooking: fresh, seasonal ingredients. Growing up on a farm in northern Florida, I am no stranger to the rich delicacies of the South, but I also learned very early in life that few things compare to the juicy tang of a just-picked summer tomato or the earthy sweetness of so many hearty autumn vegetables. But don't take my word for it. Eat foods when they are at their peak, and you will find out for yourself.

Over my many years as a professional chef, I have cooked nutritious meals for some of the most famous, on-the-go people on the planet— people who cannot afford to be bogged down by unhealthy meals. With this book, everyone can enjoy these wonderful, revitalizing dishes without sacrificing taste or simplicity. Make a point of enjoying them with your family. Sit down and talk. Laugh. Savor the tastes of the season. And if every once in a while you simply cannot go on without a bite of twelve-layer cake, I doubt that Dr. Ornish will mind.

Here's to a healthier you—and to a healthy family gathered around your table.

RECIPES

BREAKFAST

Multigrain Bagels

Mango and Blueberry Muesli

1-2-3 Tasty Morning Scramble

Whole-Grain French Toast

Blueberry and Flaxseed Smoothie

Curried Mushroom Scramble

Multigrain Pancakes with Strawberry "Syrup"

California Eggs

Zucchini Frittata

Morning Quinoa

Breakfast Taco

LUNCH

Marinated Vegetable Salad

Sesame Noodles

Chilled Marinated Lentil Salad with Curry-Spiced Artichokes

Tomato Salad with Fresh Herbs and Tofu Cheese Crumble

Miso Tofu Noodle Soup

Vegetarian Chili

Jicama Salad

Asian-Style Cabbage Salad

Asian Noodle Salad

Marinated Italian White Bean and Celery Salad with Basil

Savory Herbed Quinoa

Three-Bean Salad with Creamy Dill Dressing

Sicilian Vegetable Soup

Roasted Tomato Soup

Sweet Corn, Black Beans, and Tomato Salad

Super Crunch Salad

Citrusy Carrot Slaw

Romaine Salad with Creamy Grain Mustard Dressing

Fennel and Arugula Salad with Fig Vinaigrette

Rice Noodle Salad with Spiced Ground Tofu

Japanese Vegetable Pot

Watermelon, Radish, and Arugula Salad

Quick Mediterranean Quinoa Salad

DINNER

Roasted Cauliflower Salad with Parsley and Grapes

Pear, Butter Lettuce, and Fresh Herbs with a Honey-Infused Vinaigrette

Summer Bean Salad with Basil

Balsamic Roasted Beet, Fennel, and Orange Salad

Savoy Cabbage and Bean Stew

Omelet with Tomato and Basil

Indian Kebabs

Japanese Buckwheat Soba Noodles with Dashi

Stuffed Zucchini Squash

Roasted Parsnip Soup

Cannellini Bean Soup

Red Bell Pepper Soup

Dal Soup

Spelt Noodles with Roasted Eggplant and Roasted Tomatoes

Barley Grain, Lentil, Greens, and Roasted Butternut Squash Gratin

Firm Tofu with Green Chili Sauce
Tandoori Tofu Skewers with Cilantro and Lime Chutney
Curried Vegetable Hot Pot
Brined Tofu with Gingery Rice
Mediterranean-Spiced Seitan
Roasted Tofu with Pineapple and Cilantro Salsa
Baked Tofu with Tomato, Basil, and Black Olives
Pumpkin and Sage Pilaf
Sautéed Wild Mushrooms with Polenta
Portobello Mushroom Napoleon with Balsamic Reduction
Stuffed Roasted Anaheim Peppers with Spicy Black Beans
Autumn Simmered Butternut Squash with Lentils and Savory Fruit
Zucchini and Basil Quinoa Pilaf
Black Japonica Rice with Porcinis and Peas
Brown Rice Risotto with Winter Vegetables and Sage
Szechuan Roasted Fall Vegetables
Whole Wheat Penne with Roasted Vegetables
Spelt Spaghettini with Tomatoes, Kalamata Olives, and Toasted Pine Nuts
Miso Vegetable Stir-Fry with Ginger Brown Rice

SIDES, SAUCES, AND SNACKS

Quick-Cooked Okra with Indian Spices
Stuffed Grape Leaves
Green Pea Guacamole
Fiesta Black Beans
Garlic-Mashed Cauliflower with Herbs
Thyme-Scented Brussels Sprouts
Spicy Roasted Corn

Brown Rice with Ginger and Edamame

Fava and Potato Mash with Herbs

Stir-Almost-Fried Chinese Cabbage

Black Bean Dip

Pureed Swiss Chard with Nonfat Cottage Cheese

Tomato Chutney

DESSERTS

Floating Island with Custard and Strawberry Sauce

Ginger Cookies

Old-fashioned Egg Custard with Fresh Raspberry Jam

Fat-Free Yogurt Fruit Trifle

Peach Multigrain Griddle Cake

Yogurt Soufflés

Chocolate Yogurt Soufflés

Flourless Hazelnut Chocolate Cake

Strawberry Pie in Almond Crust

Almond Peach Cake

■ ■ ■ ■ ■ ■ ■ ■ ■ ■

MULTIGRAIN BAGELS

This is a very easy breakfast bread to make and is perfect to serve in the morning. Make them in advance and put them in the freezer for convenience. They are wonderfully delicious toasted.

MAKES 12 BAGELS

1½ cups warm water
5 teaspoons sugar
1 package dry yeast
1 tablespoon beaten egg white or egg substitute
1 tablespoon malt powder or syrup
Salt to taste
2½ cups bread flour
1 cup whole wheat flour
1 cup amaranth flour
¼ cup honey

Preheat the oven to 425° F. Gently stir the warm water, sugar, yeast, egg white, and malt powder until the yeast is dissolved. Combine the flours. Add the salt and 1 cup of the flour mixture to the yeast mixture, and then fold in 3 cups of the flour mixture to make a soft dough.

Knead the dough for 10 to 12 minutes, incorporating the rest of the flour as needed until the dough is firm. Cover with a cloth and let the dough sit for 10 minutes.

Cut the dough into 12 pieces. Roll each piece into an 8-inch rope, and shape it gently into a circle, pressing to connect the ends. (If needed, use a little warm water to help the ends stay together.) Cover with a cloth and let the bagels proof for 30 minutes.

Meanwhile, add the honey to 6 quarts of water in a stockpot and bring to a boil. Boil the bagels for 1½ minutes on each side (3 minutes total).

Line a sheet pan with parchment. Remove the bagels to the sheet pan. Place in the oven for 20 minutes, turn once, and bake for another 15 minutes. Let the bagels rest for 5 minutes before cutting. Serve with fat-free cream cheese.

Group 2: Before baking, sprinkle with sunflower seeds, pumpkin seeds, or untoasted sesame seeds.

Group 3 choices: Serve the finished bagels with 1 ounce of smoked salmon per bagel, or make the recipe with 5 tablespoons of sugar instead of 5 teaspoons of sugar.

MANGO AND BLUEBERRY MUESLI

Blueberries add great flavor and antioxidants to a morning staple.

SERVES 2

2 cups rolled oats
1 cup unsweetened apple juice
Juice of 1 lemon
1 cup coarsely grated apple
½ cup fat-free plain yogurt
⅓ cup cut-up fresh mango or thawed frozen mango
¼ cup fresh or frozen blueberries

Put the oats, apple juice, and lemon in a bowl and soak for at least 1 hour or as long as overnight. Add the grated apple and yogurt and top with the mango and blueberries.

Group 2: Add honey or maple syrup to the oat mixture.

■■■■■■■■■■

1-2-3 TASTY MORNING SCRAMBLE

Adding a touch of garlic to your eggs gives them a burst of flavor with no extra effort.

SERVES 1

    1 handful baby spinach
    1 beaten egg white or ¼ cup egg substitute
    1 sprinkle granulated garlic
    Salt and freshly ground black pepper to taste
    ¼ cup chopped tomato

Spray a nonstick pan with nonstick cooking spray and heat over medium flame. Add the spinach. After the spinach begins to wilt, add the egg white, garlic, salt, and pepper. Continue stirring the egg until it is cooked. Top with the tomato.

> *Group 2:* Top with an avocado slice.
> *Group 3 choices:* Add 1 tablespoon of grated reduced-fat Pepper Jack or reduced-fat sharp Cheddar cheese while cooking the eggs.

■■■■■■■■■■

WHOLE-GRAIN FRENCH TOAST

Make sure you check the ingredients on your bread label. Be wary of high-fructose corn syrup or sugars added to the bread. Look for whole or sprouted grains.

SERVES 1

    2 egg whites or ½ cup egg substitute
    Splash orange juice
    Pinch cinnamon
    Dash vanilla extract
    1 slice whole-grain bread
    Fresh berries

Mix the egg whites, orange juice, cinnamon, and vanilla. Soak the bread in the mixture until it has absorbed most of the liquid.

Heat a nonstick pan lightly sprayed with nonstick cooking spray. Cook bread over medium heat approximately 3 minutes per side or until brown. Top with fresh berries.

Group 2: Top with warm maple syrup.

■ ■ ■ ■ ■ ■ ■ ■ ■ ■

BLUEBERRY AND FLAXSEED SMOOTHIE

Using frozen fruit creates a milkshakelike texture. Frozen organic berries are higher in vitamins and flavor than out-of-season fruits.

SERVES 1

1 cup organic fat-free kefir or fat-free plain yogurt
½ cup pomegranate juice or fresh seeds
½ cup frozen organic blueberries
½ frozen banana or ¼ cup frozen raspberries
1 tablespoon ground flaxseed

Place all items in a blender and puree. If the mixture is too thick, add water. Serve.

■ ■ ■ ■ ■ ■ ■ ■ ■ ■

CURRIED MUSHROOM SCRAMBLE

The curry powder gives great color and depth of flavor to this easy breakfast alternative.

SERVES 1

½ cup crumbled silken tofu
1 teaspoon onion powder
1 teaspoon granulated garlic
1 teaspoon curry powder
½ cup sliced cremini or button mushrooms
½ tablespoon low-sodium soy sauce or Bragg's liquid aminos

Mix the tofu with the spices. Heat a nonstick skillet sprayed with nonstick cooking spray over medium-high heat. Add the mushrooms and soy sauce. When the moisture starts to cook out of the mushrooms, add the tofu and spice mixture. Cook, stirring constantly, until heated through, about 2 minutes. Serve.

Group 2: Turn this into a breakfast burrito by wrapping it in a reduced-fat whole-grain tortilla.

Group 3: Add 1 tablespoon reduced-fat cheese to the scramble.

MULTIGRAIN PANCAKES WITH STRAWBERRY "SYRUP"

SERVES 4–6

1 cup unsweetened apple juice
½ cup unsweetened applesauce
2 egg whites or ½ cup egg substitute
2 cups multigrain flour
1 teaspoon baking powder
¼ cup oats
½ teaspoon cinnamon
2 teaspoons baking powder
¼ teaspoon salt

Whisk the apple juice, applesauce, and egg whites together in a bowl. In a separate bowl, stir the dry ingredients together. Fold in the wet ingredients. Add a splash more juice if it's too dry.

Heat a nonstick skillet sprayed with nonstick cooking spray and pour in batter 1 heaping tablespoon at a time.

Serve with strawberry syrup.

Strawberry Syrup
1 cup fresh or frozen strawberries
1 teaspoon Splenda

Heat the strawberries in a pot over medium heat and cook until soft, about 5 minutes. Remove three-quarters of the berries and puree in a blender with the Splenda. Add the remaining berries to the puree and serve warm with the pancakes.

■■■■■■■■■■

CALIFORNIA EGGS

SERVES 1

2 egg whites or ½ cup egg substitute
Salt and freshly ground black pepper to taste
1 slice whole-grain toast or half of a whole-grain English muffin
1 tomato slice
2 fresh basil leaves

Spray a nonstick pan with nonstick cooking spray and heat over medium heat. Add the eggs, salt, and pepper and scramble until done.
Toast the bread. Layer the tomato, eggs, and basil on the toast.

Group 2 choices: Add 1 tablespoon of reduced-fat Pepper Jack cheese or a slice of avocado to the toast.

■■■■■■■■■■

ZUCCHINI FRITTATA

Frittatas are enjoyable at any meal. Serve with a side salad for lunch or dinner.

SERVES 4–6

1½ cups shredded zucchini
½ medium yellow onion, minced
½ red bell pepper, cut into ¼-inch strips
2 garlic cloves, minced
10 egg whites
2 tablespoons nonfat milk

Salt and freshly ground black pepper to taste
2 tablespoons chopped flat-leaf parsley or basil

Coat a large ovenproof skillet with nonstick cooking spray and warm over medium-high heat. Preheat the broiler.

Add the zucchini, onion, bell pepper, and garlic to the skillet and sauté until the vegetables are tender, about 5 minutes. Drain off any moisture from the vegetables.

In a bowl combine the egg whites, milk, salt, pepper, and half of the herbs. Pour the mixture over the vegetables in the skillet. Allow to cook undisturbed until the eggs begin to set and the edges appear done, then place under the broiler. Cook until the top is lightly browned and the eggs are set. Sprinkle with the remaining herbs. Cut into wedges and serve.

Group 2: Cook the vegetables in 1 tablespoon of extra-virgin olive oil.

Group 3: Sprinkle the frittata with your favorite reduced-fat cheese before putting it under the broiler.

MORNING QUINOA

This is a great way to start your day. You will be satisfied and ener-gized throughout the morning. This quinoa can be reheated.

SERVES 4

½ cup unsweetened apple juice
1½ cups water
1 teaspoon cinnamon
Pinch salt
1 cup rolled oats
1 cup quinoa, rinsed
½ cup dried fruit (raisins, apricots, cranberries, etc.)

Bring the juice, water, cinnamon, and salt to a boil. Add the oats and quinoa and reduce to a simmer. Cook for 15 minutes. Stir in the dried fruit and serve immediately.

Group 2 choices: Top with honey or maple syrup, or with toasted walnuts or pecans.

■■■■■■■■■■

BREAKFAST TACO

This is a satisfying way to start your morning and is very simple to make.

SERVES 1

> 2 egg whites or ½ cup egg substitute
> Pinch garlic
> Dash hot sauce
> 1 fat-free whole-grain tortilla
> 1 tablespoon fat-free salsa
> Few leaves cilantro
> Salt and freshly ground black pepper to taste

Spray a nonstick skillet with nonstick cooking spray and heat over medium heat. Add the egg whites, garlic, and hot sauce. Stir constantly until the eggs are cooked.

Heat the tortilla in the microwave for 15 seconds. Layer the eggs, salsa, cilantro, salt, and pepper on the tortilla.

Group 2: Serve with a slice of avocado.

Group 3: Add 1 tablespoon of your favorite reduced-fat cheese to the eggs.

■■■■■■■■■■

MARINATED VEGETABLE SALAD

Ideally, make this delicious lunch salad according to what is in season.

SERVES 2

Dressing
  ½ cup chopped flat-leaf parsley
  ¼ cup red wine vinegar
  ¼ cup lemon juice
  Pinch sea salt
  1 teaspoon freshly ground black pepper
  3 medium garlic cloves, minced

Vegetables
  1 cup cherry tomatoes, cut in half
  1 small zucchini, cut lengthwise
  1 small yellow squash, cut lengthwise
  ¼ pound mushrooms, cleaned and sliced
  1 red bell pepper, cut into strips
  1 cup arugula

Combine the dressing ingredients in a sealed container and shake to blend.
Place all the vegetables except the arugula in a bowl. Pour the dressing
over the vegetables, cover, and allow to marinate for at least 2 hours. When
ready to serve, spoon the mixture over the arugula.

Group 2: Add ¼ cup of extra-virgin olive oil to the dressing.

■■■■■■■■■■

SESAME NOODLES

I adore these noodles. They make a great lunch, side dish, or after-noon snack. Here is a simple recipe that everyone will love.

SERVES 4

¼ cup light soy sauce
½ cup oyster sauce
½ cup red wine vinegar
Dash chili sauce
1 packet Splenda
1 pound buckwheat soba noodles, cooked
1 cup shredded Chinese cabbage
1 cup shredded carrots
1 medium red bell pepper, thinly sliced
1 tablespoon rice wine vinegar

In a bowl, combine the soy sauce, oyster sauce, red wine vinegar, chili sauce, and Splenda. Whisk well. Add the noodles and toss to combine. Add the vegetables and rice wine vinegar. Toss gently until all the ingredients are blended.

Group 3 choices: Add 2 teaspoons of honey or brown sugar to the dressing.
Group 4: Add 1 cup of shredded cooked skinless chicken breast.

■■■■■■■■■■

CHILLED MARINATED LENTIL SALAD
WITH CURRY-SPICED ARTICHOKES

The small French du Puy lentils have a wonderful flavor and are packed with protein and other healthy nutrients. This is great as a lunch entrée or a dinner side dish.

SERVES 4

4 bay leaves
2 tablespoons minced shallot or onion
1 cup dried green or black lentils, rinsed

2 tablespoons apple cider vinegar
2 garlic cloves, minced
¼ cup roughly chopped cilantro leaves
Pinch dried red pepper flakes
1 teaspoon ground coriander
½ cup chopped roasted red bell pepper
One 14-ounce can artichoke hearts, quartered and drained
1 tablespoon lemon juice
2 teaspoons curry powder

Add 4 cups of water, the bay leaves, and the shallot or onion to a pot and bring to a boil. Add the lentils and return to a boil. Reduce the heat to medium-low and simmer for approximately 20 minutes, until the lentils are just tender. Drain the lentils in a colander and remove the bay leaves.

In a serving bowl, whisk together the vinegar, garlic, cilantro, red pepper flakes, and coriander. Mix the roasted bell pepper and the lentils into the dressing. In a separate bowl, toss the artichokes with the lemon juice and curry powder, then fold this into the lentil mixture in a serving bowl. Serve at room temperature or chilled.

> *Group 2:* Add 1 tablespoon of extra-virgin olive oil to the dressing while whisking.
> *Group 3 choices:* Serve with a piece of grilled salmon as a dinner entrée, or add salt to taste.

TOMATO SALAD WITH FRESH HERBS AND TOFU CHEESE CRUMBLE

I love tomatoes, especially when they are in season. Often you can even get amazing tomatoes out of season. Some fresh chopped herbs and a little vinegar can really give them a lot of flavor.

SERVES 4

4 medium tomatoes, sliced
1 cup thinly sliced red onion
2 tablespoons chopped fresh herbs (basil, tarragon, and flat-leaf parsley)
¼ cup red wine vinegar
Sea salt and freshly ground black pepper to taste
¼ cup crumbled tofu herb cheese

Place the sliced tomatoes on a serving platter. Arrange the red onion and the herbs on top. Drizzle with the red wine vinegar, and season with the salt and pepper. Sprinkle with the tofu cheese and serve.

> Group 2: Drizzle 1 tablespoon of extra-virgin olive oil over the tomatoes.
> Group 3 choices: Serve with a piece of grilled salmon as a dinner entrée, or replace the tofu herb cheese with 2 tablespoons of blue cheese.

MISO TOFU NOODLE SOUP

There are those days when we feel under the weather and a simple soup can hit the spot.

SERVES 4

Broth
    1 shallot, chopped
    1 garlic clove, chopped
    ½-inch slice ginger
    2 tablespoons rice or soybean miso

In a large saucepan, add all the ingredients to 2¼ quarts of cold water. Bring to a boil and simmer for 1 hour. Strain and cool. Keep refrigerated until ready to use.

    1 cup sliced shiitake mushrooms
    1 cup sliced canned bamboo shoots
    12 to 16 ounces cooked tofu noodles
    4 scallions, thinly sliced
    1 tablespoon light soy sauce
    1 tablespoon mirin
    1 tablespoon sake

In a Dutch oven, add the broth and bring to a simmer. Add the shiitake mushrooms, bamboo shoots, tofu noodles, scallions, and remaining seasonings. Serve this immediately or remove it from the heat and allow it to cool before putting it in the refrigerator.

> Group 3: Serve with 3 steamed or grilled shrimp per person.

VEGETARIAN CHILI

This vegetarian version of chili is always appreciated. The bulgur wheat adds a nice texture along with the vegetables.

SERVES 8

2 cups diced red onion
1 cup diced red bell pepper
1 jalapeño, minced
1 cup diced carrots
4 garlic cloves, finely minced
2 tablespoons chili powder
2 teaspoons ground cumin
1 teaspoon ground coriander
1 teaspoon ground cinnamon
¼ teaspoon cayenne pepper
Salt and freshly ground black pepper to taste
One 28-ounce can crushed Italian plum tomatoes
1 cup vegetable broth
½ cup bulgur wheat
½ cup lentils, cooked
1 can kidney beans
1 can lima beans

Spray a Dutch oven with nonstick cooking spray, add the vegetables and garlic, and sauté over medium heat. Add the chili powder, cumin, coriander, cinnamon, and cayenne pepper. Cook the vegetables in the spices, about 5 minutes. Season with salt and pepper. Add the tomatoes, broth, bulgur wheat, lentils, kidney beans, and lima beans. Bring to a simmer and cook until the bulgur is tender, about 10 minutes. Test to see if it's done then serve, or let it cool down and freeze it.

JICAMA SALAD

I love the crunchiness of jicama, and combining it with citrus juices and orange segments makes for a wonderfully cool summer salad.

SERVES 4

> 2 medium jicamas (approximately 1½ pounds)
> ¾ cup orange juice
> 2 tablespoons lime juice
> 1 teaspoon sea salt
> 1 garlic clove, minced
> 1 tablespoon chopped cilantro
> 2 large navel oranges, peeled and segmented

Peel the jicamas and slice them into strips. In a bowl, combine the orange juice, lime juice, salt, garlic, cilantro, orange sections, and jicama. Toss together and chill.

> *Group 2:* Add 2 tablespoons of extra-virgin olive oil.
> *Group 3:* Add 3 chilled poached shrimp per person.

ASIAN-STYLE CABBAGE SALAD

SERVES 4

> 4 cups finely shredded green cabbage or 1 bag coleslaw mix
> 1 medium carrot, shredded
> 1 bunch scallions, cut thin (just the white part)
> 1 medium carrot, minced
> 1 medium red bell pepper, cut into long strips
> 2 teaspoons honey
> 2 tablespoons light soy sauce
> ½ cup minced cilantro
> 1 small cucumber, peeled and cut into small pieces

Toss all the ingredients together in a large bowl. Chill. (This dish will keep for up to 24 hours without getting too soft.)

> *Group 2:* Add 2 tablespoons of sesame seeds and 1 teaspoon of sesame oil.
> *Group 3:* Add 3 ounces grilled shrimp per person.
> *Group 4:* Add 3 ounces grilled, skinless chicken breast per person.

■ ■ ■ ■ ■ ■ ■ ■ ■ ■ ■

ASIAN NOODLE SALAD

This is a great dinner-to-lunch meal. If I have leftovers I am set for lunch the next day. You can make this with shrimp or chicken as well.

SERVES 4

One 14-ounce package rice noodles or buckwheat soba noodles
½ medium red onion, cut into thin half-moon slices
1 medium red bell pepper, cut into long, thin strips
1 medium carrot, cut into small pieces or strips
2 tablespoons rice wine vinegar
1 handful cilantro, minced
1 tablespoon black or white sesame seeds
1 lime, cut into wedges
Salt and freshly ground black pepper to taste

Bring a pot of water to a boil, then remove it from the heat. Place the rice noodles in it until softened (about 7 minutes), then drain.

In a large bowl, toss the noodles with the vegetables, vinegar, and half of the cilantro. If noodles are dry, add a drop more vinegar.

Place the noodles in a serving bowl or on a platter and top with the remaining cilantro, sesame seeds, and lime wedges, and season with salt and pepper.

> *Group 2:* Add 1 tablespoon of toasted sesame seed oil.
> *Group 3:* Add 3 ounces grilled shrimp per person.
> *Group 4:* Add grilled, skinless chicken breast.

■ ■ ■ ■ ■ ■ ■ ■ ■ ■

MARINATED ITALIAN WHITE BEAN AND CELERY SALAD WITH BASIL

SERVES 4–6

Two 14-ounce cans Italian white beans (cannellini or butter beans), drained
1½ cups thinly sliced celery
1 cup minced flat-leaf parsley
1 medium red or green pepper, finely chopped
½ cup balsamic vinegar
1 teaspoon granulated garlic
¼ cup fresh basil leaves, chopped
Salt and freshly ground black pepper to taste

Toss all the ingredients together and season with salt and pepper. Serve at room temperature or chilled.

Group 4: Add 3 ounces skinless chicken breast per person (recipe below).

Chicken
1 package chicken tenders or breasts cut into strips
Balsamic vinegar for drizzling
Granulated garlic for sprinkling
Salt and freshly ground black pepper to taste
1 handful basil leaves, chopped

Preheat the broiler. Drizzle the chicken with the vinegar, and sprinkle with the garlic, salt, and pepper. Place under the broiler for 5 to 7 minutes. Remove and toss with the basil.

■ ■ ■ ■ ■ ■ ■ ■ ■ ■

SAVORY HERBED QUINOA

Quinoa has a texture between rice and couscous. It is one of the most nutrient-dense grains and is simple to prepare.

SERVES 4–6

> 2 cups quinoa
> 1 medium yellow onion, chopped
> 2 garlic cloves, minced
> 4 cups low-sodium vegetable broth
> ¼ cup sun-dried tomatoes (not in oil)
> Salt and freshly ground black pepper
> ¼ cup chopped fresh herbs (parsley, oregano, basil, thyme, or a mixture)

Dry-toast the quinoa in a pan, then rinse it.

Sweat the onions and garlic in ¼ cup of the broth in a medium-size pot. Add the sun-dried tomatoes, quinoa, a pinch of salt and pepper, and the remaining broth. Bring to a boil, cover, and reduce the heat to low. After 15 minutes, remove the lid and stir in the herbs. Place the lid back on for 2 minutes with the heat off.

Group 2 choices: Stir in ½ cup of Parmesan cheese at the end, and/or add onions and garlic sautéed in 1 teaspoon of extra-virgin olive oil.

THREE-BEAN SALAD WITH CREAMY DILL DRESSING

SERVES 4–6

> ⅓ cup fat-free sour cream
> ⅓ cup fat-free plain yogurt
> 1 tablespoon dried dill or 2 tablespoons chopped fresh dill
> 2 teaspoons granulated garlic
> 1 tablespoon white wine vinegar
> One 14-ounce can kidney beans
> One 14-ounce can chickpeas (garbanzo beans)
> 2 cups fresh green beans, cut into 1-inch pieces and blanched

Place the sour cream and yogurt in a medium-size bowl, then whisk in all the other ingredients except the beans. Stir until well blended. Toss the dressing with the beans a few tablespoons at a time. Keep extra dressing for up to a week in the refrigerator.

Group 3: Add 1 teaspoon salt.

■■■■■■■■■

SICILIAN VEGETABLE SOUP

SERVES 6

2 garlic cloves, minced
1 teaspoon dried red pepper flakes
64 ounces low-sodium vegetable broth (or 8 cups water)
One 8-ounce can Italian plum tomatoes
1 medium Yukon Gold potato, diced
1 cup red lentils, rinsed
One 14-ounce can Italian white beans
One 14-ounce can kidney beans
2 large carrots, diced small
2 ribs celery, diced small
1 bunch red chard, cut into 1-inch pieces, tough ribs removed
Juice of 1 lemon
2 tablespoons flat-leaf parsley, minced
Freshly ground black pepper

In a large pot sauté the garlic and red pepper flakes in 2 tablespoons of the broth. Add the remaining broth and the tomatoes. After about 5 minutes add the potato and lentils. Cook at a gentle boil for about 15 minutes. Add the beans, carrots, celery, chard, and lemon juice. Simmer for a few more minutes. Ladle into bowls and finish with the parsley and pepper.

> *Group 2:* Sauté the garlic and red pepper flakes in 1 tablespoon of extra-virgin olive oil and finish with ¼ cup of Parmesan cheese.
> *Group 4:* Add 2 half chicken skinless breasts or 1 full boneless, skinless breast cut into pieces. Add to the soup when it is boiling and cook for 15 more minutes.

■■■■■■■■■

ROASTED TOMATO SOUP

Tomatoes roasted in the oven with onions, garlic, and herbs make a simple and superb soup.

SERVES 6

4 cups halved plum tomatoes
1 onion, cut into wedges
1 garlic head, halved
1 red bell pepper, halved
3 cups vegetable broth
2 tablespoons chopped fresh herbs (basil, thyme, or tarragon)
Salt and freshly ground black pepper to taste

Preheat the oven to 400° F. Place the vegetables on a baking sheet. Spray with nonstick cooking spray and roast for 10 to 12 minutes until the vegetables are caramelized. Remove from the oven. In small batches, puree the vegetables in a blender with the broth until they have all been pureed. Add the chopped herbs, salt, and pepper.

Group 2: Drizzle with 2 tablespoons of extra-virgin olive oil.
Group 3: Add 3 grilled shrimp per person.

■■■■■■■■■■

SWEET CORN, BLACK BEANS, AND TOMATO SALAD

This can be eaten on its own, or makes a great side dish for grilled chicken or fish.

SERVES 4

One 14-ounce can black beans, drained
1 cup sweet corn (either frozen or scraped from 2 cooked fresh ears)
2 large ripe tomatoes, cubed; or 1 pint cherry tomatoes, halved
2 teaspoons ground cumin
1 jalapeño, seeded and minced
1 teaspoon minced garlic
¼ cup finely chopped red onion
Juice of 3 limes
Zest of 1 lime

Mix all the ingredients together and serve at room temperature or chilled.

Group 2: Add 2 tablespoons of extra-virgin olive oil to the beans.
Group 4: Serve with 3 ounces grilled, skinless chicken breast per person.

■■■■■■■■■■

SUPER CRUNCH SALAD

The combination of endive, celery, and radish gives this salad a wonderful crunchy texture. It is enjoyable year-round and very easy to throw together.

SERVES 4

> 6 bulbs endive, cut into ¼-inch circles
> 3 ribs celery, very thinly sliced on an angle
> 1 bunch radishes, sliced into thin matchsticks or thin circles or coarsely grated
> 1 tablespoon dried dill or ¼ cup fresh dill torn into small pieces
> ¼ cup chopped fresh herbs (basil, mint, and/or parsley)
> Juice and zest of 2 lemons
> Salt and freshly ground black pepper to taste

Place all the vegetables in a salad bowl with the herbs. Add the lemon juice and zest and season with the salt and pepper.

> *Group 2 choices:* Top with pine nuts, and/or add 2 tablespoons of extra-virgin olive oil to the salad.
> *Group 3:* Add ¼ cup reduced-fat crumbled feta cheese.

■■■■■■■■■■

CITRUSY CARROT SLAW

SERVES 4–6

> 1 pound carrots, grated
> 1 medium apple, grated
> 1 teaspoon ground cumin
> ¼ cup lemon or lime juice or a combination of the two
> ½ cup coarsely chopped cilantro leaves
> Salt and freshly ground black pepper to taste

Toss all the ingredients together and refrigerate for 1 to 24 hours.

> *Group 2:* Add 3 tablespoons of extra-virgin olive oil.

ROMAINE SALAD WITH CREAMY GRAIN MUSTARD DRESSING

This is similar to a Caesar salad, but the grain mustard adds a tasty new dimension without adding fat.

SERVES 4

2 tablespoons grain mustard or Dijon mustard
¼ cup water
Juice of 1 lemon
1 tablespoon fat-free mayonnaise
1 garlic clove, minced
1 bag romaine lettuce hearts
1 tablespoon capers

Whisk together the mustard, water, lemon juice, mayo, and garlic in a bowl. Toss with the romaine hearts and finish with the capers.

Group 2: Add 1 tablespoon of Parmesan cheese at the end.
Group 4: Add 3 ounces grilled, skinless chicken breast per person.

FENNEL AND ARUGULA SALAD WITH FIG VINAIGRETTE

The peppery flavor of the arugula combined with the sweet, jammy flavor of the figs is refreshing.

SERVES 4

1 cup chopped dried figs
½ cup water
½ cup unsweetened apple juice
1½ tablespoons minced shallots
¼ cup sherry vinegar
1 medium fennel bulb, thinly sliced vertically
3 cups baby arugula or a mixture of arugula and baby spinach

Boil half of the figs in the water.

Place the figs and water in a blender or food processor. Add the apple juice, shallots, and vinegar. Blend until smooth. Arrange the fennel, arugula, and remaining figs on a plate and drizzle with the dressing.

> *Group 3:* Serve with 3 ounces grilled salmon per person.
>
> *Group 4:* Serve with 3 ounces grilled, skinless chicken breast per person.

RICE NOODLE SALAD WITH SPICED GROUND TOFU

SERVES 4

Dressing
3 tablespoons lemon juice
3 tablespoons rice wine vinegar
1 tablespoon light soy sauce
1 tablespoon chopped scallion
1 tablespoon chopped cilantro

Noodles
4 ounces rice noodles, cooked
1 can straw mushrooms, drained and halved
1 cup julienned carrots
½ cup chopped red bell pepper
1 cup shredded Napa cabbage
1 cup crumbled low-fat silken tofu
¼ cup chopped raw peanuts
Pinch dried red pepper flakes

Combine all the dressing ingredients in a sealed container or jar. Shake well and reserve for the salad.

In a serving bowl, combine the rice noodles, vegetables, tofu, peanuts, and red pepper flakes. Pour the dressing over the salad and toss well. Serve immediately or chill.

> *Group 2:* Add 1 packet Splenda.
>
> *Group 3 choices:* Add salt to taste, and/or add 6 ounces of chilled, poached, or grilled shrimp.
>
> *Group 4:* Add 6 ounces of chilled, poached, or grilled, skinless chicken breast.

■■■■■■■■■

JAPANESE VEGETABLE POT

Add your favorite vegetables to this traditional Japanese dish. It can be served vegetarian or with grilled chicken or fish.

SERVES 4–6

Broth
1 cup vegetable broth
1 tablespoon light soy sauce
1 teaspoon chili paste
Salt and freshly ground black pepper to taste
4 tablespoons chopped scallions

Vegetables
3 cups julienned carrots
1 cup julienned leeks
2 cups sliced mushrooms
1 cup sliced zucchini
4 bok choy, halved
2 cups thinly sliced Napa cabbage
2 cups broccoli florets
1 medium tomato, quartered

Place all the broth ingredients except the scallions in a saucepan and bring to a simmer. Reduce the heat.

In a large pot, bring lightly salted water to a boil. Place the vegetables in the boiling water and blanch for 2 minutes, then remove them and shock them in cold water.

Arrange the vegetables in a deep serving dish. Pour the hot broth over the vegetables. Garnish with the chopped scallions.

WATERMELON, RADISH, AND ARUGULA SALAD

If you have never tried watermelon in a savory salad you are in for a treat! The peppery flavor of the arugula combined with the sweetness of the watermelon gives this dish a distinct taste.

SERVES 4

4 cups bite-size watermelon chunks, seeded
1 bunch radishes, thinly sliced
1 cup thinly sliced red onion (cut onion in half and make half-moon shapes)
2 cups baby arugula
1 small bunch mint leaves, torn into pieces
2 tablespoons balsamic vinegar
Salt and freshly ground black pepper to taste

In a large bowl, toss the watermelon with the radishes, onion, arugula, mint, and vinegar. Sprinkle with the salt and pepper.

> *Group 2:* Drizzle with 1 tablespoon extra-virgin olive oil.
> *Group 3:* Add ¼ cup crumbled low-fat feta cheese to the salad.

QUICK MEDITERRANEAN QUINOA SALAD

Quinoa is a superfood, with all eight amino acids. It is also the highest-protein grain.

SERVES 4–6

2 cups quinoa
4 cups water or low-sodium vegetable broth
½ tablespoon granulated garlic
Salt
¼ cup sun-dried tomatoes (not in oil)
⅓ cup lemon juice
2 tablespoons capers

1 cup shredded or minced zucchini
1 celery stalk, minced
1 cup minced flat-leaf parsley
Freshly ground black pepper to taste

Dry-toast the quinoa in a pan, then rinse it.

Bring the water to a boil with the garlic, a pinch of salt, and the sun-dried tomatoes. Add the quinoa and simmer for 15 minutes. Remove from the heat and fold in the lemon juice, capers, zucchini, celery, and parsley. Season with the pepper. Serve at room temperature or chilled.

Group 2: Add 2 tablespoons of extra-virgin olive oil.

■■■■■■■■■■

ROASTED CAULIFLOWER SALAD
WITH PARSLEY AND GRAPES

The earthiness of the cauliflower combined with the sweetness of the grapes is a surprising and delicious way to get in a few of your fruit and vegetable servings for the day.

SERVES 4

1 medium head cauliflower, cut into bite-size florets
Juice of 1 lemon
Salt and freshly ground black pepper to taste
1 cup flat-leaf parsley leaves
2 cups green or purple seedless grapes, halved

Heat oven to 300° F. Spray a baking dish with nonstick cooking spray. Toss the cauliflower with half of the lemon juice, and the salt and pepper. Roast for approximately 20 minutes. Remove and cool for 5 minutes. Toss with the parsley, grapes, and the rest of the lemon juice.

Group 2: Toss the cauliflower with 2 tablespoons of extra-virgin olive oil before roasting, then drizzle it with 1 tablespoon of olive oil before serving.

■ ■ ■ ■ ■ ■ ■ ■ ■ ■

PEAR, BUTTER LETTUCE, AND FRESH HERBS WITH A HONEY-INFUSED VINAIGRETTE

This is a wonderful salad for the fall season. Use your favorite apple if pears are not available.

SERVES 6

   1 small shallot, chopped
   2 tablespoons honey
   1 cup fresh herbs (basil, mint, flat-leaf parsley, and dill are good choices)
   2 tablespoons water
   ¼ cup champagne vinegar or white wine vinegar
   3 tablespoons extra-virgin olive oil
   Salt and freshly ground black pepper to taste
   1 medium Bosc or Bartlett pear, cut into thin slices
   2 small heads butter lettuce, separated, rinsed, and dried
   Edible flowers (optional)

In a blender, mix the shallot with the honey, half of the herbs, the water, and the vinegar, then slowly add the oil, salt, and pepper. Toss the mixture with the pear, greens, and the rest of the herbs. Serve with edible flowers sprinkled on top.

> *Group 2:* Serve with 3 ounces salmon per person.
> *Group 4:* Serve with 3 ounces grilled, skinless chicken breast per person.

■ ■ ■ ■ ■ ■ ■ ■ ■ ■

SUMMER BEAN SALAD WITH BASIL

SERVES 4–6

   1½ pounds mixed summer beans (yellow wax, green, Romano, etc.)
   Juice of 1 to 2 lemons
   1 piece shallot, minced
   1 tablespoon grain mustard
   1 tablespoon fat-free sour cream

Pinch salt
¼ cup torn flat-leaf parsley
¼ cup fresh basil, rough chopped

Bring a pot of salted water to a boil. Add the beans and cook them until crisp but tender. Remove the beans, plunge them into ice water, then drain them.

In a glass jar, add the lemon juice, shallot, mustard, sour cream, and salt. Shake vigorously.

Toss the beans, dressing, and herbs together.

Group 2 choices: Add ¼ cup of toasted pine nuts, and/or add 1 tablespoon of extra-virgin olive oil to the dressing.
Group 3: Serve with 3 grilled shrimp per person.

BALSAMIC ROASTED BEET, FENNEL, AND ORANGE SALAD

SERVES 6

1 pound beets, washed, peeled, and cut into quarters
1 to 2 fennel bulbs, cut into eighths (cut in quarters lengthwise, then in half again lengthwise)
¼ cup balsamic vinegar, plus a little extra for drizzling
Salt and freshly ground black pepper to taste
2 oranges, skin removed, cut into ½-inch circles

Preheat the oven to 375° F. Spray a baking dish with nonstick cooking spray. Add the beets and fennel to the baking dish, toss with ¼ cup of the vinegar, and sprinkle with the salt and pepper. Roast for 25 to 30 minutes. Remove the vegetables and let them cool for at least 10 minutes.

Spread the orange sections on a platter, top with the beets and fennel, and drizzle with a bit more balsamic vinegar.

Group 2: Toss the beets and fennel with 2 tablespoons of extra-virgin olive oil.
Group 3: Crumble ¼ cup goat cheese on top of the finished salad.

■■■■■■■■■■

SAVOY CABBAGE AND BEAN STEW

This is a hearty winter stew that makes for a wonderful supper on a cold evening.

SERVES 4

2 garlic cloves, chopped
1 teaspoon dried red pepper flakes
2 small heads Savoy cabbage, sliced
½ cup vegetable stock
One 28-ounce can crushed plum tomatoes
Two 19-ounce cans Great Northern beans, rinsed and drained
Salt and freshly ground black pepper to taste

Spray a Dutch oven with nonstick cooking spray and set it over medium heat. Add the garlic and red pepper flakes and cook until soft. Add the cabbage and cook until wilted. Add the vegetable stock, tomatoes, and beans. Season with the salt and pepper. Cook until the flavors of the mixture have married.

> *Group 3:* Add a smoked turkey leg cut into pieces (approximately 1 cup).

■■■■■■■■■■

OMELET WITH TOMATO AND BASIL

I enjoy omelets more often for supper than for breakfast. They are very simple and pure. Here is my favorite combination.

SERVES 1

3 large egg whites or ¾ cup egg substitute
Salt and freshly ground black pepper to taste
1 plum tomato, chopped
1 tablespoon chopped fresh basil
2 tablespoons Cheddar-flavored tofu cheese, grated

Spray a nonstick omelet pan with nonstick cooking spray, then set it over high heat. Beat the egg whites together with the salt and pepper. Pour the egg mixture into the pan once it's hot. Stir it around well in the pan, pulling the eggs from the sides into the middle, until it is completely done. Sprinkle the tomato, basil, and tofu cheese on the eggs. Fold the omelet over and serve.

■ ■ ■ ■ ■ ■ ■ ■ ■ ■

INDIAN KEBABS

I love ground turkey or soy made into meatballs. They are wonderful served by themselves or with a nice green salad. You can grill them outside or broil them in your oven.

SERVES 4

2 pounds ground soy burger
1 tablespoon chopped ginger
1 egg white or ¼ cup egg substitute
2 shallots, chopped
2 garlic cloves, chopped
3 tablespoons tandoori spice
¼ cup chopped cilantro leaves
Salt and freshly ground black pepper to taste
1 small zucchini, cut into 1-inch pieces
2 medium tomatoes, cut into wedges
1 dozen sugarcane skewers (usually available in Latin markets), or
  bamboo skewers, soaked for 5 minutes in water

Salad
1 cup fat-free plain yogurt
½ cup peeled and chopped cucumbers, all the water removed
¼ teaspoon chili paste, or to taste
Salt and freshly ground black pepper to taste

Mix the soy burger, ginger, egg white, shallots, garlic, and tandoori spice. Knead well. Add the cilantro and season with the salt and pepper. (This can be made ahead of time and kept in the refrigerator.)

Form ¼ cup of the soy mixture into a ball, insert a skewer through the ball, and repeat, alternating these balls with the zucchini and tomato. If grilling outside, spray the balls with nonstick cooking spray and place the kebabs on a medium-hot grill until thoroughly cooked.

Combine all the salad ingredients in a serving bowl and serve with the kebabs.

> **Group 4:** Replace the soy burger with 2 pounds of ground chicken or turkey breast.

JAPANESE BUCKWHEAT SOBA NOODLES WITH DASHI

Japanese buckwheat soba noodles are a healthy alternative to pasta. Serve these simple noodles with a Japanese fish broth or add steamed vegetables to create a more substantial meal.

SERVES 4

Dashi Broth
  1 piece kelp, approximately 2 inches long
  4 tablespoons bonito flakes

Add the kelp to a saucepan with approximately 4 cups of water. Bring to the beginning of a boil. Remove the kelp immediately and bring the water to a full boil. Add ½ cup cold water and the bonito flakes. Bring the water back to a boil, then remove it from the heat. Allow the broth to sit for 30 minutes to absorb the flavor. Strain the mixture and reserve it for the soup. The broth may be saved for up to 1 week.

Toppings for the Soup
  1 cup spinach leaves, cleaned and torn into pieces
  ½ cup sliced mushrooms
  ¼ cup shaved carrot
  ½ cup minced scallion
  ½ tablespoon light soy sauce
  12 to 16 ounces Japanese buckwheat soba noodles, cooked
  Chili paste to taste (optional)
  ½ cup cubed tofu

In a Dutch oven, heat the dashi broth to a simmer. Add the toppings (be sure to add the tofu cubes last), being careful not to overstir and break the tofu. Chili paste may be added for a spicy flavor.

■ ■ ■ ■ ■ ■ ■ ■ ■

STUFFED ZUCCHINI SQUASH

Here is a vegetable dish that kids will enjoy.

SERVES 6

7 small zucchinis, halved lengthwise to form "boats," with inside
flesh removed
½ pound ground soy burger
1 large onion, finely chopped
½ teaspoon ground cinnamon
2½ pounds tomatoes, chopped
2 garlic cloves, minced
2 tablespoons chopped fresh mint
2 tablespoons pistachio nuts, toasted
Salt and freshly ground black pepper to taste

Preheat the oven to 350° F.

Blanch the zucchini "boats" in boiling water for 3 minutes, then shock
them in cold water.

Spray a large skillet with nonstick cooking spray. Add the soy burger to
the skillet and brown it over medium heat. Add the onions, cinnamon,
tomatoes, and garlic. Allow the tomato juice to cook and reduce in the soy
mixture. Remove the pan from the heat and allow the mixture to cool. Add
the mint and pistachios. Season with the salt and pepper.

Fill the blanched zucchini boats with the soy mixture. Place them in a
casserole dish sprayed with nonstick cooking spray and bake until they're
thoroughly heated, about 30 minutes.

Group 2: Sprinkle the top of each zucchini boat with 1 teaspoon of Parmesan
cheese.
Group 3: Sprinkle the top of each zucchini boat with 1 teaspoon of reduced-fat
feta cheese.
Group 4: Replace the soy burger with ½ pound ground turkey breast.

████████▌▌

ROASTED PARSNIP SOUP

Parsnips are great vegetables for the colder months. Delicious cooking starts with seasonal ingredients.

SERVES 4–6

1 large onion, sliced
2 large parsnips, peeled and diced (about 3 to 4 cups)
5 cups hot vegetable stock
3 medium Jonagold apples (a Jonagold is a cross between a Jonathan and a Golden Delicious), peeled and sliced
1 tablespoon Dijon mustard
Salt and freshly ground black pepper to taste

Spray a Dutch oven with nonstick cooking spray and set it over medium heat. Add the onion and allow it to sizzle. Add 1 cup of water. Sweat the onion until it's soft, then add the parsnips and the hot stock. Cook until the parsnips are soft, then add the apples, and cook until they're tender.

Puree the mixture in a food processor, adding the mustard, salt, and pepper. Serve with a green salad.

> *Group 2:* Add 1 tablespoon of Parmesan cheese.

████████▌▌

CANNELLINI BEAN SOUP

These small Italian white beans are packed with protein and flavor.

SERVES 4–6

1 small eggplant
1 cup canned tomatoes
1 small Yukon Gold potato, peeled and diced
1 medium carrot, peeled and diced
One 15-ounce can cannellini beans, drained and rinsed
4 cups vegetable stock
1 teaspoon dried herbes de Provence

1 ounce dried mushrooms, rehydrated and rinsed
3 ounces basil pesto

Place all the ingredients in a Dutch oven and bring to a simmer. Cook until the vegetables are just tender, about 30 minutes.

RED BELL PEPPER SOUP

Bell peppers are loaded with vitamin C. This wonderful soup, with its Mediterranean flavor, showcases them with tomatoes, jalapeño pepper, and basil. It is a perfect summer soup to make while these vegetables are in season. I like to freeze it, so I can enjoy the flavor of summer in the middle of winter. This soup can be served hot or cold.

SERVES 4

8 ounces red bell peppers, seeded and sliced
1 small Vidalia onion, sliced
2 garlic cloves, minced
1 jalapeño, seeded and minced
1½ cups strained canned tomatoes
2½ cups vegetable broth
2 tablespoons chopped basil
1 tablespoon chopped rosemary or oregano

Place the red bell peppers, onions, garlic, jalapeño, and tomatoes in a saucepan with the vegetable broth, and bring to a boil over medium heat. When the vegetables are tender, puree the mixture in a blender a little at a time. Cool the soup and add the fresh herbs.

Group 4: Serve with 4 ounces of grilled, skinless chicken breast and 2 cups of salad greens per person.

■■■■■■■■■

DAL SOUP

This soup is based on the wonderful Indian dish made with lentils. It is a great main dish for dinner accompanied by a crisp green salad.

SERVES 4–6

½ teaspoon garam masala
¼ teaspoon cumin
1 teaspoon turmeric
5 cups vegetable broth
1 large onion, finely chopped
1 large leek, finely chopped
1 large carrot, grated
1 to 2 garlic cloves, finely chopped
½ teaspoon chili paste
9 ounces split red lentils, rinsed
Salt and freshly ground black pepper to taste

Set a Dutch oven over medium heat. Toast the spices in the Dutch oven, and when they become aromatic, add the vegetable broth. Bring to a simmer, then add the vegetables, chili paste, lentils, and salt and pepper and cook, covered, until tender. Carefully puree the soup in a blender a little at a time until it's smooth. Serve immediately or freeze.

> *Group 3:* Add 3 grilled shrimp per person to the soup (see preparation below).

Grilled Shrimp
12 medium shrimp, peeled
1 tablespoon Asian rub

Place the shrimp in a bowl, add the rub, and mix well. Grill approximately 2 minutes per side.

■■■■■■■■■

SPELT NOODLES WITH ROASTED EGGPLANT AND ROASTED TOMATOES

Spelt is one of the oldest grains still consumed. The Romans used it in everyday cooking. It is very healthy and a wonderful substitute for pasta, especially for those who are allergic to wheat.

SERVES 4

1 medium eggplant, cut in half, placed cut-side down on baking sheet
6 medium tomatoes, cut in half, placed cut-side down on baking sheet
Salt and freshly ground black pepper to taste
2 garlic cloves, minced
½ cup chopped basil
16 ounces spelt noodles
¼ cup white wine vinegar

Preheat the oven to 400° F. Coat two separate baking sheets with nonstick cooking spray. Place the eggplant and tomatoes on separate baking sheets. Roast the eggplant until it is soft, approximately 20 minutes. The tomatoes are ready once they begin to caramelize. Remove both baking sheets from the oven and cool the eggplant and tomatoes.

Peel the skin off the eggplant and tomatoes and cut them into 1-inch pieces. Season with the salt and pepper, then sprinkle with the minced garlic. Once the vegetables are completely cooled, sprinkle on the basil. Place all the vegetables in a large bowl. Set aside.

Cook the spelt noodles according to the package directions and drain, leaving half of the water in the pot. Add the vinegar to the noodles.

Pour the pasta into the roasted vegetable bowl. If the mixture is dry, add a bit of the reserved water, ¼ cup at a time, and toss well. Serve immediately, or cool and serve as a pasta salad.

■■■■■■■■■■

BARLEY GRAIN, LENTIL, GREENS, AND ROASTED BUTTERNUT SQUASH GRATIN

This recipe makes for a perfect lunch the next day if it doesn't get eaten up for dinner. You could add fish to it, too.

SERVES 4

1 cup unhulled barley
¼ cup sofrito (see page 326)
1¼ cup vegetable broth
Salt
1 small butternut squash, cut in half and seeds removed
¼ cup canned organic tomatoes
One 14-ounce can lentils, washed
4 cups greens (spinach, Swiss chard, collard, or mustard greens), blanched
¼ cup chopped flat-leaf parsley
Freshly ground black pepper to taste
½ cup grated tofu Pepper Jack cheese

Soak the barley overnight or for at least 1 hour to decrease cooking time.

Preheat the oven to 350° F. Place the barley, sofrito, and 1 cup of the broth in a saucepan and bring to a boil. Season with the salt and cover the saucepan. Cook about 20 minutes, until the grains are tender and plump, and all the liquid has evaporated.

While the barley is cooking, place the butternut squash halves cut side down on a baking sheet and roast them in the oven until a fork can pierce the flesh, approximately 40 minutes. Cool the squash, peel it, and cut it into chunks. Reserve for assembling.

Add the tomatoes and lentils to the saucepan and stir well. Allow to heat thoroughly.

In a second saucepan filled with water, blanch the greens until they're tender.

In a casserole dish, layer the barley mixture and the roasted squash, sprinkle with the parsley and the black pepper, add the greens, and sprinkle with the cheese. Drizzle with ¼ cup of the vegetable broth. Place in the preheated oven and bake for 20 minutes.

This can be prepared ahead of time (even up to two days).

■ ■ ■ ■ ■ ■ ■ ■ ■

FIRM TOFU WITH GREEN CHILI SAUCE

This is a wonderful main dish that my chef, Rey Villalobos, taught me.

SERVES 4

Sauce
 1 cup vegetable broth
 1 cup tomatillos
 1 jalapeño, seeded
 2 garlic cloves, chopped
 Pinch salt

 4 cups cubed firm tofu

Place the broth in a saucepan and bring it to a simmer. Add the tomatillos, jalapeño, garlic, and salt. Cook until the vegetables are tender. Remove from the heat and puree the mixture thoroughly in a blender. Add the tofu to the sauce and heat through, about 3 minutes.

Group 4: Add 4 poached, skinless chicken breasts, shredded.

■ ■ ■ ■ ■ ■ ■ ■ ■

TANDOORI TOFU SKEWERS WITH CILANTRO AND LIME CHUTNEY

SERVES 4

Chutney
 1½ cups cilantro (stems removed), and some for garnish (stems on)
 ½ cup mint, stems removed
 1 tablespoon lime zest
 1 green chile, minced
 ¼ teaspoon minced garlic
 1½ cups fat-free plain yogurt
 ¼ teaspoon ground cumin
 1½ tablespoons lime juice

Skewers
 1 pound firm tofu, cut into large cubes
 4 small zucchinis, cubed
 4 small yellow squashes, cubed
 4 medium red bell peppers, cubed
 1 medium yellow bell pepper, cubed
 1 medium green bell pepper, cubed

For the chutney, combine the cilantro, mint, lime zest, chile, and garlic in a blender, adding one tablespoon of water at a time until all the ingredients begin to blend into a paste. In a nonreactive bowl, combine the yogurt, cumin, and lime juice. Mix well.

Place the tofu, the vegetables, and about ¼ cup of the chutney in another bowl, and let it marinate for 30 minutes in the refrigerator. Save the remaining chutney for later use. Preheat the grill while the vegetables marinate. Remove the vegetables and tofu from the refrigerator and arrange them on metal skewers.

Place the skewers on the grill and cook on each side for 1 minute. This will allow the vegetables to cook evenly without drying out the tofu. (Also, remember that the metal skewer will heat up as well and cook the ingredients from the inside.) Serve with the chutney.

Group 2: Add 1 pound of salmon fillet, cubed (squeeze fresh lime juice over the fish and garnish it with cilantro).

CURRIED VEGETABLE HOT POT

Hot pots are very popular in Southeast Asia, where you can add any type of meat or vegetable. We like to add any white fish, shrimp, or scallops. It's great with lobster, too.

SERVES 6

Broth
 3 cups vegetable broth
 3 tablespoons yellow curry paste
 1 teaspoon chopped ginger

Noodles and Vegetables
>12 ounces whole wheat angel hair pasta
>2 medium Yukon Gold potatoes, diced (medium)
>2 small zucchinis, cubed
>2 large carrots, peeled and diced (medium)
>1 cup snow pea pods, blanched

Place all the broth ingredients in a saucepan and bring to a boil, then add the pasta and the potatoes. Cook for about 5 minutes. Add the zucchini and carrots. Cook until the vegetables are tender, approximately 8 minutes. Add the snow pea pods. Garnish with cilantro and chopped chiles, if desired.

Group 3 choices: Add 1 cup of medium peeled and deveined shrimp, 1 cup of cleaned scallops, or 1 cup of white fish.

Group 4: Add one 15-ounce can of light coconut milk and reduce the vegetable broth to 2 cups.

■■■■■■■■■■

BRINED TOFU WITH GINGERY RICE

SERVES 4

>1½ cups water
>3 tablespoons low-sodium tamari or soy sauce
>1 tablespoon rice wine vinegar
>1 package reduced-fat firm tofu
>1 medium red bell pepper, cut into ½-inch strips
>2 tablespoons sesame seeds
>2 satsuma oranges or 1 navel orange, diced
>Handful cilantro, chopped

Combine 1½ cups water with the tamari and vinegar in a large sealable plastic bag or a shallow glass dish. Add the tofu and bell pepper to the brine and let it marinate for 15 minutes or as long as overnight.

Turn the broiler on high. Remove the tofu and bell pepper from the brine. Place them on a baking sheet sprayed with nonstick cooking spray and coat them with the sesame seeds. Broil for approximately 7 min-

utes. Remove and finish with the diced oranges and sprinkl
cilantro.

> *Group 2:* Add a splash of toasted sesame oil to the oranges.

Rice
  3½ cups water
  2 cups short-grain brown rice or sushi rice
  2 tablespoons minced fresh ginger
  1 cup shelled edamame
  Handful cilantro, chopped
  1 teaspoon tamari

If you have a rice cooker, place all the ingredients in it except the
edamame. If not using a rice cooker, bring the water, rice, and ginger to a
boil. Turn the heat down to low and cover with a tight lid. Add the
edamame when the rice is almost cooked. Cover and let stand. Garnish
with the cilantro and a drizzle of tamari.

■ ■ ■ ■ ■ ■ ■ ■ ■ ■

MEDITERRANEAN-SPICED SEITAN

Seitan is made from wheat gluten. It has a texture similar to meat and,
like tofu, lends itself well to different flavors.

SERVES 4

  2 cups flat-leaf parsley, coarsely chopped
  ¼ cup fresh mint
  ¼ teaspoon turmeric
  ½ tablespoon ground cumin
  Salt and freshly ground black pepper to taste
  ¼ cup freshly squeezed lemon juice (use a Meyer lemon if available)
  1 box chicken-style seitan

50° F. Combine the herbs, spices, and lemon juice
seitan, then transfer it all to a baking dish. Bake

tra-virgin olive oil to the herb-and-spice mix.

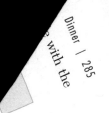

ROASTED TOFU WITH PINEAPPLE AND CILANTRO SALSA

*Tofu lends itself to almost any flavor. When you freeze it, then thaw it,
it has a meaty texture. The Latin flavors in this dish are great for the
summer months.*

SERVES 4

2 tablespoons ground cumin
1 teaspoon ground turmeric
2 teaspoons ground coriander
Salt
1 box extra-firm low-fat tofu, frozen, then thawed, drained, and cut
into ½-inch slices

Preheat the oven to 450° F. Mix the dry spices and salt, then rub the
mixture onto the tofu. Place the tofu on a foil-lined baking sheet. Roast for
approximately 5 minutes.

Salsa

1½ cup chopped pineapple (you may substitute mango or mix the
two)
1 fresh pepper, such as jalapeño or serrano, minced (without seeds
for less spicy, with for spicier)
1 shallot, minced
Handful cilantro, roughly chopped
Juice of 1 to 2 limes
1 teaspoon ground cumin
Salt

Chop the pineapple into small pieces and toss it with the pepper, shallot, cilantro, lime juice, and cumin. Season with the salt and serve the salsa
over the tofu or on the side.

Group 2 choices: Add half of a cubed avocado to the salsa, or add 1 tablespoon of extra-virgin olive oil to the salsa and drizzle more on the tofu before cooking. *Group 3:* Replace the tofu with 1½ pounds of red snapper and cook for an additional 5 minutes.

BAKED TOFU WITH TOMATO, BASIL, AND BLACK OLIVES

This dish will take minutes but seem like it took hours.

SERVES 4

1½ pints cherry tomatoes, halved
2 to 3 garlic cloves, minced
Handful fresh basil, chopped
1 teaspoon dried red pepper flakes
⅔ cup dry white wine
Handful cured black olives
Salt
1 package extra-firm low-fat tofu, drained and sliced into 1-inch
  rectangles

Preheat the oven to 475° F. Mix the tomatoes with the garlic, basil, red pepper flakes, wine, olives, and salt. Make an "envelope" out of foil or parchment. Place half of the tomato mixture on the bottom. Lay the tofu on top. Top with more of the tomato mixture. Seal the envelope and bake for approximately 20 minutes. Remove from the oven and allow to stand for a few minutes before serving.

Group 2: Drizzle the tofu and tomatoes with extra-virgin olive oil before cooking.
Group 3: Substitute 1 pound of tilapia for the tofu.

■■■■■■■■■■

PUMPKIN AND SAGE PILAF

This simple dish is full of fall flavors.

SERVES 4-6

One 14-ounce can pureed pumpkin
4 cups low-sodium vegetable or chicken broth
¼ cup minced yellow onion (about ½ small onion)
1 tablespoon minced fresh sage, or 2 teaspoons dried sage
2 cups brown rice
½ cup dry white wine
Salt
¼ cup pumpkin seeds, shelled

Stir the pumpkin and broth together and heat in a small pan over medium heat. Coat the bottom of a stockpot that has a tight-fitting lid with nonstick cooking spray and sauté the onion and sage over low heat. When the onion starts to get soft, add the rice. Stir the rice, then add the wine. When the wine is almost completely absorbed, add the pumpkin and broth mixture. Add a pinch of salt and bring to a boil. Place the lid on the pot and turn down to low. Cook until the rice is tender, about 40 minutes. Finish with the pumpkin seeds.

> *Group 2 choices:* Add ¼ cup of grated Parmesan cheese to the finished rice, or sauté the onion in 1 tablespoon of canola oil.

■■■■■■■■■■

SAUTÉED WILD MUSHROOMS WITH POLENTA

SERVES 4-6

1 package cooked polenta (comes in a log shape)
Salt
2 tablespoons low-sodium vegetable broth
1 teaspoon dried red pepper flakes
1 tablespoon chopped fresh thyme
2 tablespoons minced garlic

3½ cups coarsely chopped mixed mushrooms (Some stores sell a
   mixture of mushrooms prepacked. If you cannot find these, make a
   mixture of your own, including cremini, shiitake, oyster, and
   chanterelle, if available.)
1 cup dry white wine
Freshly ground black pepper to taste
¼ cup chopped flat-leaf parsley

Preheat the oven to 350° F. Cut the polenta into ½-inch disks. Spray a
baking sheet with nonstick cooking spray and line the pan with the polenta
disks. Sprinkle with salt and place the sheet in the oven.

Place the broth, red pepper flakes, thyme, and garlic in a large sauté
pan. Cook on medium heat for 2 minutes. Add the mushrooms. Sauté until
the liquid from the mushrooms has started to cook down. Add the wine.
Cook until the liquid has reduced by half. Season with the pepper.

Remove the polenta from the oven. Using a flat spatula, place 2 disks on
each plate. Top with the mushrooms, and generously sprinkle with the
chopped parsley.

Group 2 choices: Sauté the garlic in extra-virgin olive oil, and/or stir in 2 tablespoons of butter to the mushrooms when they are three-quarters of the way
cooked, or ¼ cup fat-free mozzarella.

PORTOBELLO MUSHROOM NAPOLEON
WITH BALSAMIC REDUCTION

4 to 6 large portobello mushrooms
½ cup balsamic vinegar
2 medium red bell peppers
¼ cup low-sodium vegetable broth
2 tablespoons chopped fresh garlic
10 ounces baby spinach
Salt and freshly ground black pepper to taste
2 tablespoons minced parsley or basil

Preheat the oven to 350° F. Remove the stems from the portobellos and
wipe them clean with a paper towel. Place the mushrooms on a plate and
brush both sides with balsamic vinegar.

Cut the bell peppers into quarters and spray them with nonstick cooking spray. Place the pepper quarters on a cookie sheet and roast them in the oven for 30 minutes.

Combine the vegetable broth and garlic in a sauté pan. Cook until the garlic is soft but not browned. Add the baby spinach and cook it until it is wilted. Season with salt.

Place the portobellos on a baking sheet, sprinkle them with the pepper, and roast them in the oven for 10 minutes.

While the mushrooms are cooking, place the remaining balsamic vinegar in a small saucepan or sauté pan. Reduce the liquid over medium heat until the mushrooms are done.

Layer the spinach and then a piece of bell pepper on top of each mushroom, and place them back in the oven for 5 minutes.

Remove the mushroom napoleons from the oven. Place them on plates with a spatula, drizzle each one with the balsamic reduction, and sprinkle with the fresh herbs.

> Group 2: Sauté the garlic and spinach in extra-virgin olive oil and drizzle the peppers with extra-virgin olive oil before roasting them.
>
> Group 3: Add ¼ cup goat cheese to the mushrooms before you place them back in the oven the second time.

■ ■ ■ ■ ■ ■ ■ ■ ■ ■

STUFFED ROASTED ANAHEIM PEPPERS WITH SPICY BLACK BEANS

SERVES 4–6

Peppers
6 small Anaheim peppers or 3 to 4 medium red bell peppers
4 cups orange juice
1 cup instant polenta
1½ cups fresh corn (off the cob, 2 ears) or frozen sweet corn
¼ cup coarsely chopped cilantro

Preheat the oven to 350° F. Roast the peppers over an open low flame on a gas stove (roast them in the oven at 350° F for 30 minutes if you do not have a gas stove), turning them to blacken them evenly on all sides.

Place them in a paper bag for 10 minutes to soften the skin. Remove the peppers from the bag, peel off the skin, and discard it. Make an incision lengthwise on the peppers and remove the seeds and membranes. Set the peppers aside.

Bring the orange juice to a boil and add the polenta in a steady stream. Stir constantly with a whisk to avoid clumps (approximately 2 to 3 minutes). Remove from the heat and stir in the corn and cilantro.

Fill the peppers with the polenta mix and hold them closed with toothpicks or wooden skewers. Place them on a baking sheet and roast them in the oven for 15 minutes. Remove the peppers from the oven, take out the toothpicks, and serve them open side down over the spicy black beans.

Beans

  2 tablespoons vegetable or chicken broth
  ½ medium yellow onion, diced
  1 tablespoon minced garlic
  1 small jalapeño, diced
  Two 12-ounce cans black beans, drained and rinsed
  2 tablespoons ground cumin
  1 tablespoon fresh lime juice
  Salt

Heat the broth and the onion in a sauté pan over medium-high heat. Cook the onion until it's translucent, then add the garlic and jalapeño and cook for 2 to 3 minutes. Add the black beans and cumin, and cook on low heat for 5 minutes. Stir in the lime juice. Season with the salt.

Group 3: Add reduced-fat cheese of your choice.

Group 4 choices: Add 1 cup of grated Vermont or sharp white Cheddar to the polenta when you stir in the cilantro, and/or add grilled or rotisserie skinless chicken breast, chopped, to the polenta before you place it in the oven.

■■■■■■■■■ ▪

AUTUMN SIMMERED BUTTERNUT SQUASH WITH LENTILS AND SAVORY FRUIT

This one-dish wonder is a fall favorite. Use whichever seasonal apples you love.

SERVES 4

> 1 large butternut squash (or 3 8-ounce bags frozen)
> ½ medium yellow onion, cut into thin slices
> 1½ tablespoons ground cumin
> 2½ cups low-sodium vegetable broth or water
> ½ cup red lentils, rinsed
> Handful fresh thyme, chopped
> 1 medium apple, cut into ½-inch slices

Peel the squash and cut it into 1-inch chunks. Spray the bottom of a heavy-bottomed pan with nonstick cooking spray and heat on high. When the pan is very hot, add the squash, onion, and half of the cumin. Let the squash get a bit stuck on the bottom of the pan, then stir and scrape it with a wooden spoon. Add ¼ cup of the broth and place the lid on the pot for 5 minutes. Add the lentils, thyme, apples, and the remaining broth. Replace the lid and simmer for 15 minutes. Turn off the heat and let the pan stand for a few minutes. Serve with rice or chicken or both.

> *Group 2:* Sauté the onions and squash in 3 tablespoons of extra-virgin olive oil.
> *Group 4:* Use 3 ounces turkey breast tenderloin instead of butternut squash.

■■■■■■■■ ▪ ▪

ZUCCHINI AND BASIL QUINOA PILAF

Toasting quinoa in a dry pan and then rinsing it gives more depth of flavor.

SERVES 4–6

> 2 cups quinoa
> 1 medium yellow onion, chopped
> 3 garlic cloves, minced

4 cups low-sodium vegetable broth
Salt and freshly ground black pepper to taste
2 small zucchinis, cut into pea-size pieces
Juice of 2 lemons
½ cup slivered raw almonds
1 cup basil leaves, torn up

Dry-toast the quinoa in a pan, then rinse it.

Sweat the onion and garlic in ¼ cup of the broth in a medium pot. Add the quinoa, a pinch of salt and pepper, and the remaining broth. Bring to a boil, cover, and reduce the heat to low. After 15 minutes, remove the lid and stir in the zucchini, lemon juice, almonds, and three-quarters of the basil. Place the lid back on for 2 minutes with the heat off. Finish with the remaining basil and season with salt and pepper.

> *Group 2 choices:* Sauté the onion and garlic in extra-virgin olive oil, and/or stir in ½ cup of Parmesan cheese at the end.

BLACK JAPONICA RICE WITH PORCINIS AND PEAS

SERVES 6–8

3 ounces dried porcini mushrooms
½ medium onion, minced
6 cups low-sodium vegetable broth (can be water, stock, or a
  combination of both)
1 garlic clove, minced
Pinch dried red pepper flakes
3½ cups Black Japonica rice or other short-grain brown rice
Porcini water
1½ cups frozen or fresh peas
½ cup chopped flat-leaf parsley
1 tablespoon minced thyme

Soak the porcinis in 1½ cups boiling water. When they are hydrated, drain them through a paper coffee filter and save the strained liquid (porcini water). Chop the mushrooms.

In a heavy-bottomed pot, sauté the onion in a bit of vegetable broth. When the onion begins to soften, add the garlic and red pepper flakes, then add the rice and stir. Add the rest of the broth and the porcini water. Replace the lid and cook at a low simmer until the rice is done (read the cooking instructions on the rice package). Remove the lid and add the peas and herbs. Replace the lid for a few minutes, then stir the rice and serve.

> *Group 2 choices:* Sauté the onion and garlic in 1 tablespoon extra-virgin olive oil or add 1 tablespoon grated Parmesan cheese.
> *Group 4:* Add 3 ounces grilled, skinless chicken breast to the finished rice.

BROWN RICE RISOTTO WITH WINTER VEGETABLES AND SAGE

This is a very earthy dish. It is extremely satisfying in the cold winter months and is wonderful for kids.

SERVES 4–6

- 7 cups low-sodium vegetable broth
- 1 shallot or ½ medium onion, minced
- 2 garlic cloves, minced
- 2 tablespoons minced fresh sage leaves
- 2 cups short-grain brown rice
- 1 cup dry red wine
- 1 medium carrot, diced
- 1 medium turnip or rutabaga, diced
- 1 small bunch red chard, cut into 1-inch strips, tough ribs removed

Heat the broth in a saucepan and keep it next to a risotto pot on the stove. Sauté the shallot, garlic, and half of the sage in ¼ cup of vegetable broth. Add the rice and stir constantly for a few minutes. When the rice starts to appear translucent, add the wine. When the wine is almost completely absorbed, start adding the hot broth one ladleful at a time.

When the broth is halfway incorporated, add the carrot, turnip, and the rest of the sage. Continue adding broth and stirring. When the rice is creamy and tender, fold in the chard and serve immediately.

> *Group 2 choices:* Sauté the garlic and shallot in 1 tablespoon of extra-virgin olive oil, and/or finish with ¼ cup grated Parmesan cheese.

■■■■■■■■■■

SZECHUAN ROASTED FALL VEGETABLES

SERVES 4–6

1 cup 1-inch butternut squash cubes
1 small sweet potato or garnet yam, cut into 1-inch wedges
1 cup carrots, peeled and cut into 1-inch pieces
1 medium red or yellow onion, cut into eighths
1 small parsnip or turnip, cut into 1-inch rounds
1 tablespoon five-spice powder (see page 325)
2 tablespoons low-sodium soy sauce
Freshly ground black pepper to taste

Preheat the oven to 375° F. Put all the vegetables in a large bowl and coat them with the five-spice powder, soy sauce, and pepper. Spread them on a baking sheet sprayed with nonstick cooking spray and roast for 20 minutes. Turn the vegetables and roast them for another 10 to 15 minutes, until golden brown.

■■■■■■■■■■

WHOLE WHEAT PENNE WITH ROASTED VEGETABLES

SERVES 4–6

2 cups coarsely chopped roasted vegetables (zucchini, red bell
  pepper, broccoli, and tomatoes)
1 pound whole wheat penne pasta
½ cup vegetable broth
2 tablespoons minced garlic
1 teaspoon red pepper flakes (optional)
2 tablespoons chopped parsley
2 tablespoons chopped fresh basil, mint, or oregano
Salt and freshly ground black pepper to taste

Preheat the oven to 400° F. Place the vegetables on a baking sheet sprayed with nonstick cooking spray and roast them for 20 minutes.

Salt a large pot of water (1 tablespoon salt) and bring it to a boil. Add the pasta and cook it until it is al dente.

Place the broth, garlic, and red pepper flakes, if using, in a large sauté pan. Cook over medium heat for a few minutes. Do not let the garlic get brown. Add the roasted vegetables and turn the heat down to low.

Drain the pasta (reserving ½ cup of the pasta water) after it is cooked, then place it back in the pot with the reserved water. Add the vegetable mixture and the herbs. Season with the salt and pepper. Serve in one large bowl or individual bowls.

> *Group 2 choices:* Drizzle extra-virgin olive oil on the vegetables before roasting them and sauté the garlic in 1 tablespoon of extra-virgin olive oil instead of broth, and/or pour the pasta tossed with the sauce into an ovenproof baking dish, top with ¼ cup fat-free mozzarella cheese, and place under the broiler for 5 minutes.

SPELT SPAGHETTINI WITH TOMATOES, KALAMATA OLIVES, AND TOASTED PINE NUTS

SERVES 4–6

1 pound spelt or whole wheat spaghettini
1½ tablespoons minced garlic
½ teaspoon red pepper flakes
¼ cup low-sodium vegetable broth
One 14-ounce can crushed tomatoes
1 cup pitted kalamata olives, coarsely chopped
Salt and freshly ground black pepper to taste
2 tablespoons chopped flat-leaf parsley
2 tablespoons chopped fresh basil
¼ cup toasted pine nuts

Add the pasta to a large pot of salted, rapidly boiling water. Drain the pasta when it is al dente.

In a large pan over medium heat, cook the garlic and red pepper flakes in the broth. Do not let the garlic brown. When the garlic starts to become soft, add the tomatoes. Cook over medium heat until the pasta is ready (approximately 10 to 15 minutes).

Add the olives to the tomato sauce. Season with the salt and pepper. Add the pasta to the sauce, sprinkle with the herbs and pine nuts, and toss. Serve immediately in a warm serving bowl or in individual bowls.

> *Group 2:* Finish with Parmesan cheese.
> *Group 4:* Add grilled or rotisserie skinless chicken breast to the pasta.

■■■■■■■■■

MISO VEGETABLE STIR-FRY WITH GINGER BROWN RICE

SERVES 4

1½ cups uncooked brown basmati rice
2 tablespoons grated fresh ginger
Pinch salt
2 tablespoons light-colored miso
2 tablespoons low-sodium vegetable broth
1 medium yellow onion, diced
2 cups sliced mushrooms
½ pound snow peas
1 celery rib, chopped
1 small head broccoli
1 carrot, cut into thin strips
1 tablespoon low-sodium soy sauce
¼ cup lemon juice
6 ounces low-fat tofu, cut into cubes

Bring 3 cups of water to a boil, then add the rice, half of the ginger, and a pinch of salt. Return the pot to a boil and cover it. Reduce and cook on low for 25 to 30 minutes. Fluff the rice with a fork before serving.

Blend the miso with 2 tablespoons of water until smooth, and set it aside. In a wok, heat the vegetable broth, and add the onion and the rest of the ginger. Sauté for about 3 minutes. Add the mushrooms and cook until the moisture comes out (about 3 minutes), then add the snow peas, celery, broccoli, and carrot. Stir for a few minutes. Add the soy sauce, miso mixture, and lemon juice, stirring frequently. Add the tofu and cook until warmed through. Serve with the rice.

> *Group 3:* Replace the tofu with 1 pound of boneless skinless chicken breast cut into 1-inch pieces.

SIDES, SAUCES, AND SNACKS

■■■■■■■■■

QUICK-COOKED OKRA WITH INDIAN SPICES

High in vitamin C and low in calories, okra is a great side dish and cooks in minutes.

SERVES 4–6

2 tablespoons minced onion
2 tablespoons curry powder
1 teaspoon mustard seeds
1 tablespoon extra-virgin olive oil
1 pound okra, cut into ½-inch pieces
Salt and freshly ground black pepper to taste

Sauté the onion and spices in the oil in a skillet until the onion is soft. Add the okra and cook for 2 minutes. The okra will be warm but still firm. Season with the salt and pepper and serve.

■■■■■■■■■

STUFFED GRAPE LEAVES

This is a Mediterranean favorite from Greece to Syria. I love them because they are fun to eat, they are healthy, and they taste great.

SERVES 12 (MAKES 24 ROLLS)

One 16-ounce jar grape leaves
2 large onions, minced
2 bunches flat-leaf parsley, minced

¼ cup chopped fresh mint
1 pound ground chicken breast
Juice of 1½ lemons
1½ cups cooked brown rice
3 small tomatoes, peeled, seeded, and finely diced
1 teaspoon sea salt
¼ teaspoon allspice
¼ teaspoon nutmeg
3 cups vegetable broth
1 lemon, cut into wedges

Cover the grape leaves with cold water and soak them for 20 minutes, then wash and dry them well.

In a bowl, mix the onions, parsley, mint, ground chicken breast, lemon juice, cooked brown rice, and tomatoes. Season with the sea salt, allspice, and nutmeg. Chill well.

Place the grape leaves on a cutting board 6 at a time. Use a tablespoon to make balls out of the chilled meat mixture. Place one ball into each grape leaf and roll up eggroll-style: First fold in the sides, left and right, then roll them away from you tightly. Make 24 rolls and set them aside.

Place a circle of parchment paper on the inside bottom of a stainless-steel pot. Arrange extra unrolled leaves on the parchment paper. Stack the stuffed rolls in the pot. Pour the vegetable broth over the rolls and place a ceramic plate directly on top of the rolls in the pot to weigh them down. Cover the pot. Bring it to a simmer and cook the rolls for 45 to 60 minutes. Add more broth if it cooks away. Remove the pot from the heat. Let it cool and then remove the stuffed grape leaves from the pot. Serve garnished with the lemon wedges.

Group 2: Drizzle 2 tablespoons of extra-virgin olive oil over the stuffed grape-leaf rolls.

GREEN PEA GUACAMOLE

MAKES 2 CUPS

1 cup defrosted green peas, drained
1 pecked and destoned avocado
Juice of 1 lime

2 tablespoons minced red onion
1 teaspoon minced serrano chile
1 small tomato, chopped
½ cup chopped cilantro leaves
Salt and freshly ground black pepper to taste

In a food processor, pulse the peas until smooth. Spoon them into a mixing bowl. Add the avocado, lime juice, red onion, chile, tomato, and cilantro. Season with the salt and pepper. Carefully mix everything. Serve immediately with vegetables.

Group 2: Add 1 extra avocado, peeled and pitted, cut into small pieces.
Group 3: Add salt to taste.

FIESTA BLACK BEANS

Black beans are high in protein and fiber. Adding ground cumin gives them a nice Latin flavor.

SERVES 2–4

½ medium onion, finely chopped
1 tablespoon vegetable broth
3 to 5 garlic cloves, minced
½ tablespoon ground cumin
1 teaspoon dried red pepper flakes or ½ fresh jalapeño, minced
One 14-ounce can black beans, drained and rinsed
Salt

Spray a pan with nonstick cooking spray, and place over medium heat. Add the onion. Sauté for a few minutes, then add the broth and cook until the onion begins to soften, about 5 minutes. Add the garlic, cumin, and red pepper flakes. Sauté for a few more minutes. Add the beans and cook for about 5 minutes. Season with the salt. Serve in tacos or with a piece of grilled chicken or fish.

Group 2 choices: Cook the onion in 1 tablespoon of extra-virgin olive oil, and/or top with shredded reduced-fat Pepper Jack cheese.
Group 4: Add 1 cup of ground turkey to the onion while it is cooking.

■■■■■■■■■■

GARLIC-MASHED CAULIFLOWER WITH HERBS

This is a tasty alternative to mashed potatoes and takes only about 10 minutes to make!

SERVES 4

> 1 large head cauliflower
> 7 garlic cloves, peeled and cut in half lengthwise (use more if you
>   want it extra garlicky)
> ¼ cup fresh herbs (dill, flat-leaf parsley, thyme, and basil are all great)
> Salt and freshly ground black pepper to taste

Remove the greenery and core from the cauliflower, and chop it into roughly 1-inch chunks. Bring the cauliflower and garlic to a boil in a pot of salted water. When the cauliflower is soft, drain it and place it in a food processor or blender with the herbs, salt, and pepper. Blend until chunky, or mash the whole mixture by hand.

> *Group 2 choices:* Add 2 tablespoons of extra-virgin olive oil to the cauliflower mixture in the food processor, and/or sprinkle with Parmesan cheese when it is finished.

■■■■■■■■■■

THYME-SCENTED BRUSSELS SPROUTS

SERVES 4

> 1 pound brussels sprouts
> ¼ cup low-sodium vegetable broth
> ½ small yellow onion, minced
> 1 teaspoon dried red pepper flakes
> 2 tablespoons chopped fresh thyme
> Salt

Remove the tough bottoms of the sprouts, then cut them in half lengthwise (remove outer leaves if they are damaged). Add the broth and onion to a large skillet over medium-high heat. Add the red pepper flakes, and sauté until the onion is soft, about 5 minutes. Add the brussels sprouts and thyme and cook about 5 more minutes, turning occasionally. Season with the salt. If the sprouts seem to be getting a bit dry and sticking to the pan, you can add more broth to loosen them up.

> *Group 2:* Substitute 2 tablespoons of extra-virgin olive oil for the broth when sautéing the onion.

SPICY ROASTED CORN

SERVES 4

> One 16-ounce package frozen organic corn (or 4 fresh ears, corn cut from the cob)
> 1 jalapeño, seeds removed, minced (or ¼ teaspoon chili powder)
> 1½ tablespoons ground cumin
> Salt
> Handful cilantro, minced

Preheat the oven to 400° F. Toss the corn with the jalapeño and cumin. Spread the corn on a sheet pan sprayed with nonstick cooking spray and sprinkle with the salt. Roast for 15 minutes (or longer if you want them to be a bit crispy). Finish with the cilantro.

> *Group 2:* Add 2 tablespoons of extra-virgin olive oil to the corn before roasting it.

BROWN RICE WITH GINGER AND EDAMAME

SERVES 4

> 4 cups low-sodium vegetable broth or water
> 1-inch piece of ginger, peeled and grated
> Salt and freshly ground black pepper to taste
> 2 cups brown or wild rice
> 1 cup frozen edamame (substitute peas if edamame is unavailable)

Place all the ingredients except the edamame in a rice cooker. When the rice is finished, add the edamame and place the lid back on for 5 minutes. If you are not using a rice cooker, bring the broth, ginger, salt, and pepper to a boil. Add the rice, place a tightly fitting lid on the pot, and reduce the heat to low. Remove the lid and add the edamame 5 minutes before the rice is finished. Replace the lid, then fluff the rice before serving. Serve with fish, chicken, or stir-fry.

■ ■ ■ ■ ■ ■ ■ ■ ■ ■

FAVA AND POTATO MASH WITH HERBS

SERVES 4–6

4 large Yukon Gold potatoes, peeled and cut into cubes
1 tablespoon granulated garlic
1 cup frozen fava, lima, or broad beans
2 tablespoons chopped fresh herbs (parsley, basil, or thyme)
Salt and freshly ground black pepper to taste

Place the potatoes and garlic in a pot of salted water. Bring to a boil and cook until the potatoes are soft. Add the beans and cook for 1 minute. Remove the potatoes and beans with a slotted spoon and place them in a food processor or blender, or a large bowl (to mash by hand). Reserve the cooking liquid. Puree (or mash), adding some of the cooking liquid if it's too dry. Fold in the herbs, salt, and pepper, and serve immediately.

> *Group 2:* Fold in ¼ cup grated Parmesan cheese.

■ ■ ■ ■ ■ ■ ■ ■ ■ ■

STIR-ALMOST-FRIED CHINESE CABBAGE

Every time I travel to Chicago's Chinatown near my home, I find the most interesting and amazing new green vegetables. If you are bored with spinach, why not try a different kind of green? It will change your "vegetable life."

SERVES 4

3 pounds baby bok choy
2 sliced ginger, peeled and chopped (2 tablespoons)
1 garlic clove, chopped

1 tablespoon water
1 tablespoon rice wine vinegar
Salt
1 teaspoon toasted sesame seeds

Trim the baby bok choy and set it aside. Spray a wok with nonstick cooking spray and place it over high heat. Add the ginger and garlic. Begin to stir-fry. Add the baby bok choy, water, vinegar, salt, and toasted sesame seeds. Toss well and serve immediately.

> *Group 2:* Add 3 peeled, deveined shrimp per person after the ginger and garlic.

■ ■ ■ ■ ■ ■ ■ ■ ■ ■

BLACK BEAN DIP

Dip is a great source of quick protein. If you eat it with some raw vegetables, it makes a delicious lunch or a wonderful afternoon snack. You can use any of your favorite beans.

MAKES 2 CUPS

2 cups canned black beans, drained and rinsed
3 garlic cloves, smashed
¼ cup tahini
1 teaspoon lemon juice
1 teaspoon lemon salt
½ cup water
Salt and freshly ground black pepper to taste
Fresh vegetables for dipping

Place the black beans, garlic, tahini, lemon juice, lemon salt, and water in a food processor and puree. Season with the salt and pepper.

Chill for several hours and bring to room temperature before serving. Serve with the fresh vegetables.

> *Group 2:* Add ¼ cup of extra-virgin olive oil.

■■■■■■■■■

PUREED SWISS CHARD WITH NONFAT COTTAGE CHEESE

This dish is great served either hot or cold.

SERVES 6

> 1 large onion, chopped
> 1 garlic clove, minced
> ½ teaspoon dried red pepper flakes
> 2 pounds Swiss chard, torn into coarse pieces (discard the stems)
> 1 cup nonfat cottage cheese, drained
> Juice of 1 lemon

Spray a pan with nonstick cooking spray and heat over medium heat. Add the onion, garlic, and red pepper flakes, and cook until the onion is soft. Add the Swiss chard and cook until it is wilted. Remove from the heat and cool slightly. Stir in the cottage cheese and season with the lemon juice.

■■■■■■■■■

TOMATO CHUTNEY

When serving grilled tofu, chicken, or fish, tomato chutney is a great sauce to have on the table. This chutney is best made in season, but you can store it in a canning jar and have a taste of summer all year long.

MAKES 2 CUPS

> 4 medium apples, peeled, cored, and sliced
> 6 large ripe tomatoes
> 1 cup golden raisins
> Salt
> 1 tablespoon peeled and coarsely chopped fresh ginger
> 1 teaspoon cayenne pepper
> ½ cup finely chopped sweet onion
> 2 teaspoons Splenda
> ½ cup apple cider vinegar

Place the apples, tomatoes, raisins, salt, ginger, cayenne pepper, and onion in a heavy stainless-steel pot. Cook over low heat until thickened, approximately 1 hour. Add the Splenda and apple cider vinegar. Remove from the heat and allow to cool slightly. Serve or place in sterilized jars and process according to the jar manufacturer's suggestions.

DESSERTS

■ ■ ■ ■ ■ ■ ■ ■ ■ ■

FLOATING ISLAND WITH CUSTARD AND STRAWBERRY SAUCE

SERVES 4

6 egg whites
Pinch cream of tartar
8 packages Splenda
4 cups nonfat milk
One 16-ounce container egg substitute
1 cup pureed strawberries

Using a countertop electric mixer, beat the egg whites with the cream of tartar until stiff. Gradually add 4 packets of Splenda until it is all blended into a meringue.

Heat the milk in a saucepan over medium heat until hot but not boiling (or milk will curdle). Using spoons dipped in hot water, make egg-size shapes of meringue and place a few at a time in the hot milk. Cook meringue "eggs" for 4 to 5 minutes. Remove them and cool them on clean dishtowels. Set the milk mixture aside.

In a separate bowl, beat the egg substitute with the remaining 4 Splenda packets and add this mixture to the milk. Cook until it coats the back of a wooden spoon. Remove it from the heat and cool. When ready to serve, pour the custard into a serving dish and place the meringue eggs on top. Serve with the pureed strawberries on the side.

Group 4: Prepare with 2 percent reduced-fat milk instead of nonfat milk.

■■■■■■■■■

GINGER COOKIES

Although these cookies are delicious when they're just made, they taste even better as they age.

MAKES 2 DOZEN SMALL COOKIES

¾ cup organic cane sugar
¼ cup unsalted butter
2 egg whites or ½ cup egg substitute
¼ cup natural molasses
1¾ cups multigrain flour, sifted
1 teaspoon baking soda
1½ teaspoons pumpkin pie spice
¼ teaspoon salt

Using a countertop electric mixer, beat the sugar and butter until fluffy. Add the egg whites into the mixing bowl one at a time until well incorporated. Add the molasses. In a separate bowl, combine the sifted flour, baking soda, and pumpkin pie spice. Mix well. Gradually stir the flour mixture into the dough. Add the salt. Stir well. Refrigerate the dough until firm.

Preheat the oven to 350° F. Place oiled parchment paper on a sheet pan. Remove the dough from the refrigerator and roll it into ¾-inch balls. Place them on the parchment-lined pan 2 to 3 inches apart. Bake for 10 minutes, until the cookies are set. Remove them from the oven and allow them to cool. Serve or store in airtight containers.

Group 2: Prepare with ½ cup of chopped walnuts.

■■■■■■■■■

OLD-FASHIONED EGG CUSTARD
WITH FRESH RASPBERRY JAM

SERVES 6

2 egg whites, beaten, or ½ cup egg substitute
¼ cup Splenda
1 teaspoon vanilla extract
Salt

2½ cups nonfat milk, warmed
6 tablespoons sugar-free raspberry jam
Freshly ground nutmeg
Handful fresh raspberries

Preheat the oven to 350° F. In a bowl, mix the egg whites, Splenda, vanilla, and salt. Gradually pour the warm milk into the bowl and blend.

Place 1 tablespoon of the jam in each of six 6-ounce glass custard containers. Carefully pour the custard into each container and sprinkle with the nutmeg.

Place the containers in an ovenproof dish at least two inches deep. Pour warm water into the pan until it is a quarter filled to ensure that the custards bake evenly. Bake 45 minutes or until a knife comes out clean.

Remove the custards from the oven and the water bath, and place them on a kitchen towel. Allow them to cool. Serve them warm or place them in the refrigerator and chill. Serve with the fresh raspberries.

Group 3 choices: Add a pinch of salt, and/or prepare with 2 percent milk.

FAT-FREE YOGURT FRUIT TRIFLE

SERVES 4

Two 6-ounce containers plain yogurt
2 tablespoons unsweetened cranberry juice
2 cups fresh pineapple chunks
1 cup blueberries
1 cup strawberries, cut into ½-inch slices
1 kiwi, peeled and cut into pieces
2 cups cubed cantaloupe

In a bowl, mix the yogurt and juice. In a clear serving bowl, layer the fruit and yogurt. This can be made in advance and refrigerated.

Group 3: Add 1 tablespoon of honey to the yogurt.
Group 4: Sprinkle ¼ cup of unsweetened coconut, shredded and toasted, on top.

■ ■ ■ ■ ■ ■ ■ ■ ■ ■

PEACH MULTIGRAIN GRIDDLE CAKE

SERVES 8

> One 14-ounce can peaches, drained
> 2 tablespoons brown sugar
> 2 cups multigrain flour
> ½ tablespoon baking powder
> 1 teaspoon ground cinnamon
> Pinch salt
> 2 egg whites
> ¾ cup fat-free milk or soy milk
> 1 cup fat-free plain yogurt

Preheat the oven to 350° F. Spray a nonstick ovenproof skillet with nonstick cooking spray. Over medium heat, add the drained peaches and brown them lightly on one side. Sprinkle with the brown sugar and remove from the heat.

Mix the flour, baking powder, cinnamon, and salt with a whisk. In a separate bowl, beat the egg whites and milk. Do not overmix. Pour the liquid mixture into the flour mixture and blend until it becomes a batter. Pour the batter into the skillet over the peaches.

Place the skillet in the oven and bake approximately 12 minutes, until the cake is firm. Cut into 8 wedges and serve with the yogurt.

■ ■ ■ ■ ■ ■ ■ ■ ■ ■

YOGURT SOUFFLÉS

MAKES 4 SOUFFLÉS

> 1 tablespoon unsalted butter
> 3 tablespoons organic cane sugar
> 3 egg whites or ¾ cup egg substitute
> Pinch cream of tartar
> 1 small container fat-free fruit yogurt with raspberries or
>   strawberries
> 4 tablespoons pureed raspberries or strawberries

Preheat the oven to 350° F. Lightly butter 4 small soufflé cups and dust them with 1 tablespoon of the sugar. Set them aside.

With an electric mixer, beat the egg whites and cream of tartar until they form soft peaks. Gradually add the remaining 2 tablespoons of sugar, and beat until stiff peaks form.

In another bowl, mix the yogurt and fruit puree together. Fold the egg-white mixture into the yogurt-fruit mixture until just blended. Spoon the new mixture into the soufflé cups and gently tap them against the countertop. Place the cups in a baking dish. Pour warm water into the baking dish until it is a quarter filled to ensure even baking.

Bake the soufflés for 12 minutes, until they are puffed and lightly browned. Remove them from the oven, and serve with an additional fruit puree.

CHOCOLATE YOGURT SOUFFLÉS

MAKES 4 SOUFFLÉS

1 tablespoon unsalted butter
3 tablespoons organic cane sugar
1 small container fat-free vanilla yogurt, warmed
¾ cup bittersweet chocolate, melted
3 egg whites or ¾ cup egg substitute
Pinch cream of tartar
Cocoa powder for dusting

Preheat the oven to 350° F. Lightly butter 4 small soufflé cups and dust them with 1 tablespoon of the sugar. Set them aside.

In one bowl, mix the yogurt and melted chocolate.

In another bowl, with an electric mixer, beat the egg whites and cream of tartar until they form soft peaks. Sprinkle in the remaining 2 tablespoons of sugar. Beat until stiff peaks form. Fold the yogurt-chocolate mixture into the egg-white mixture. Carefully spoon the new mixture into the sugared cups. Pour warm water into a baking dish until it is a quarter filled to ensure even baking. Set the sugared cups containing the soufflés into the baking dish.

Bake the soufflés for 12 minutes, until they are puffed and lightly browned. Remove them from the oven and dust them with cocoa powder. Serve immediately.

FLOURLESS HAZELNUT CHOCOLATE CAKE

SERVES 6

2 tablespoons unsalted butter
1 tablespoon rice flour or semolina
2 tablespoons cocoa powder
¼ cup hazelnuts
2 tablespoons plus ¾ cup organic sugar
3 ounces bittersweet chocolate
4 tablespoons unsalted butter
4 ounces fat-free sour cream
2 egg yolks
1 teaspoon vanilla extract
5 egg whites
½ teaspoon salt
Fresh fruit

Preheat the oven to 350° F. Grease a 9-inch springform pan with the 2 tablespoons of butter, dust it with the flour and cocoa powder, and set it aside.

In a food processor or blender, combine the hazelnuts and 2 tablespoons of the sugar, then process until fine.

In a double boiler, melt the chocolate and the 4 tablespoons of butter. Remove from the heat and beat in the sour cream and egg yolks. Once incorporated, add the vanilla.

In a bowl, beat the egg whites with the salt and the remaining sugar. Carefully fold the chocolate mixture into the egg-white mixture, then mix gently until well incorporated. Sprinkle the hazelnut mixture in bottom of the springform pan, then spoon the chocolate mixture into pan and bake for 30 minutes. Check it with a toothpick. The cake should still be moist in the center or it will be dry when you serve it.

Allow the cake to cool in the pan. Loosen the cake around the edges and carefully remove it from the pan. Serve with the fresh fruit.

■ ■ ■ ■ ■ ■ ■ ■ ■ ■

STRAWBERRY PIE IN ALMOND CRUST

8 SERVINGS

Crust
3 tablespoons unsalted butter
1½ cups almond flour
2 tablespoons liquid Splenda

Preheat the oven to 350° F. Melt the butter in a microwave or in a saucepan over low heat. Mix the butter, almond flour, and Splenda until they form a dough. Pat the dough into a 9-inch glass pie dish. Bake the crust for 12 minutes and allow it to cool.

Filling
¾ cup orange juice
4 tablespoons tapioca powder, dissolved in a little water to make a paste
4 cups hulled strawberries, cut in half
3 tablespoons liquid Splenda
1 tablespoon unsalted butter

Optional
1 cup fat-free plain yogurt
1 tablespoon chopped mint

In a saucepan, whisk together the orange juice and tapioca paste over medium heat. Bring this to a simmer and allow it to thicken. Add the strawberries, Splenda, and butter. Mix the ingredients well. Pour the mixture into the prebaked pie shell. Place in the refrigerator and chill. Serve with fat-free yogurt on the side. Also, try adding a little chopped fresh mint to the yogurt.

ALMOND PEACH CAKE

8 SERVINGS

1 stick soy butter
½ cup pureed peaches
4 tablespoons Splenda
¼ teaspoon ground ginger
¼ teaspoon ground cinnamon
1 teaspoon vanilla extract
Pinch salt
5 egg whites
1 teaspoon cream of tartar
2 cups almond flour mixed with 2 teaspoons baking powder
Optional peach slices for garnish

Preheat the oven to 350° F. Grease and flour a 9-inch springform pan. With an electric mixer, blend the butter, peaches, Splenda, spices, vanilla, and salt until nice and light.

In another clean bowl, beat the egg whites with the cream of tartar until stiff.

Fold the egg-white mixture and the almond flour into the peach batter, alternating ingredients, until well incorporated. Spoon into the springform pan and gently tap the bottom.

Place the pan in the oven and bake the cake approximately 25 to 30 minutes, until it is puffed. A toothpick in the center of the cake should come out clean to show that it is cooked. Allow the cake to cool in the pan for approximately 10 minutes. Expect the cake to deflate slightly. Remove the cake from the pan carefully and serve it with the extra peaches.

ESSENTIAL KITCHEN TOOLS
FOR LOW-FAT COOKING

■ ■ ■ ■ ■ ■ ■ ■ ■

You will find specialty utensils and pans in some of these recipes, but to cook healthy low-fat meals in your kitchen you will need at least these essential tools—the tools you will find yourself using most.

Two knives. For the home chef, two good knives are essential, three are ideal, and four start to lean toward excessive. Every kitchen needs a knife that can slice, dice, chop, and do whatever mass-quantity cutting is necessary. That knife is called a chef's knife or French knife. A proper kitchen also needs a good paring knife for jobs that are too small and delicate for the mighty chef's knife. You might also consider investing in a serrated bread knife, but you could certainly get by without one (although they do move through soft, malleable baked goods more efficiently than do nonserrated blades). Because you will not be portioning a great deal of meat (including fowl and fish), you do not need a slicing knife. Considering your low-fat menu, you will be well equipped with a chef's knife and a paring knife. And you will have less to wash.

CHOOSING A CHEF'S KNIFE

This is the knife you will use the most, by far. To find a knife that best suits you, consider three factors: weight, balance, and length. Six-inch knives are gaining popularity, but the most common lengths are 8 and 10 inches, and neither is better for any reason other than what feels good in your hand. Same with weight and balance. Some knives are so light you forget you are even holding them, while others are hefty enough to let you know that you have a serious piece of equipment in your possession. To test the balance of a knife, rock it forward and back from the tip to the rear edge. This is how chef's knives are designed—to rock back and forth, never leaving the cutting board. If you try a few knives and get no sense of balance—

either good or bad—don't worry about it. Base your decision on weight and length alone. Can you control the knife? Could you chop efficiently and comfortably with it? If so, you have found your knife. Many specialty stores will let you try knives out before you buy them—at least let you rock them back and forth on a cutting board—and if you splurge a little and spend anywhere from $75 to $150 on a knife you may never have to buy another one as long as you keep it sharpened (at a few bucks per sharpening, once or twice a year). Carbon-steel blades get very sharp but do not hold the sharpness as long as other blades do. They can also become discolored, and they require the most care. Ceramic blades are intensely sharp and light and hold their sharpness well. But they are delicate and can chip or break if they are dropped. Stainless-steel blades stay clean, hold a sufficiently sharp edge, and last the longest. They are also the least expensive of the three. No matter which knife you choose, make sure it has a full tang, meaning that the blade is one piece, extending all the way through the handle. This makes a knife stronger and extends its lifetime.

One vegetable peeler. You are about to eat a lot of vegetables. A good vegetable peeler will save you a lot of time. They are easy to use and easy to clean. Peel with a peeler, and use your knives for the big stuff.

Two baking sheets. For roasting vegetables and baking. Do not skimp on these. Make sure your baking sheets are not thin, flimsy, or shallow. Get some nice sturdy ones with high sides. They will last a long time, and they will perform better than cheap ones.

Two 10-inch nonstick frying pans. Here is where you can save a little money. At some point, inevitably, the nonstick surface on your frying pan will get scratched. Then it will get scratched again. And then you will have to throw it away because it is not good for you to be cooking on a scratched nonstick surface. You can get a decent nonstick pan for $25 at a department store or a large discount store. Make sure to get two—you will use them both at once sometimes. And make sure they are not too thin. When they start to break down after five years or so, pitch them and get new ones. If you cannot bear throwing them away every five years, make sure you are extra careful when washing them. And be vigilant about using wooden or plastic tools; no scraping the pans with steel utensils.

One pair of tongs. Think of them as an extension of your fingers. Tongs are not just for the grill. Professional chefs use them in their kitchens all the time.

One electric blender or food processor. Both can be used to puree, and a food processor can also be used to chop. With your new knife skills, though, who needs a machine to do the chopping? Then again, it is a time-saver.

One Dutch oven. This cast-iron pot can be on the expensive side, but just like those good-quality knives and baking sheets, it will be with you for-ever.

One stockpot. For soups and stews. Make sure the bottom is thick to prevent easy burning.

One 2-quart saucepan. Basically a little pot with a long handle, this thing is a workhorse. Use it for making sauces; boiling water and cooking grains; blanching, simmering, or poaching vegetables; simmering stock—you name it.

One roasting pan. Roasting is one of the fundamental low-fat cooking methods, and you will soon be a pro at it.

Two ovenproof, flameproof casseroles (1.5 and 2.5 quarts). It's the old "bake" or "roast" question: Is a casserole baked or roasted? Either way, these dishes are what you need to get that job done.

One grater. The box grater is classic (they've been used for decades), efficient (the grated ingredients fall down in the middle of them), and versatile (many have at least four different grating options). But if you do not have room for one, go with a modern microplaner instead. Some of them are the size and shape of a large shoehorn; you can easily find room in a drawer for one or two of them.

One set of dry measuring cups. Until you can measure by sight, you need these cups. Some chefs swear by them even after they've been cooking for years. Get a set that is held together at the handles, like a set of keys. That way, you'll never have to wonder, "Now, where did I leave that ⅓ cup?"

One liquid measuring cup and one set of measuring spoons. Get a glass measuring cup with a handle, and make sure you do not forget to buy a set of measuring spoons because they are much easier and more accurate to use than flatware teaspoons and tablespoons. The designers of those spoons are more concerned with aesthetics and ease of use.

Measuring spoons are all about the amounts, so they are guaranteed to be precise.

Two mixing bowls. Buy two different sizes (one large enough to hold a dinner party salad and one a little smaller), and make sure they are nonreactive (see page 324). Stainless steel, glass, glazed ceramic, enamel, and plastic are all nonreactive.

One wire whisk. Why? That's a fair question. The answer is that while a fork or wooden spoon can easily mix ingredients, they cannot introduce air into the mix the way a whisk can. You see many specialty tools hanging from kitchen shelves or standing in open-top canisters on the counter, and you may wonder how many of them are actually used. In baking and in low-fat cooking, the whisk is a key player.

Two rubber spatulas. These are used not only to scrape the last remnants from a jar but also to fold ingredients, which is a delicate job that requires proper tools.

One flat spatula. This is the thing you use to flip pancakes. To distinguish it from a rubber spatula, it is also called a "turner."

One citrus reamer. You will use this almost as much as your whisk. It looks like a giant drill bit, and it is used to extract juice from a citrus fruit once it has been sliced in half. Unless you are the type of person who can rip a telephone book in two, you cannot rely on your hand strength to get all of the juice out of a lemon. If you have the counter space and budget for an electric juicer, more power to you. Otherwise, get in there with a reamer and give it a twist. The juice will flow.

COOKING LESSONS

■ ■ ■ ■ ■ ■ ■ ■ ■ ■

The information below will help you better understand some select cooking techniques and ingredients included in the recipes in this book.

The most important lesson comes first: There is no tool in any kitchen that is more dangerous than a dull knife. Anyone who has ever used a dull knife knows that it can cut through a firm surface more easily than a more delicate surface. You might not have much trouble slicing a zucchini with a dull knife, but if that same knife has trouble with a tomato and slips off the side, it will have no problem cutting your finger. Even a dull knife is sharp enough to hurt you when it is moving fast with a lot of force behind it (and this will always be the case when you are struggling to cut something). Find a sharpening service where you live and get your knives sharpened (both of them or all three of them) at least once or twice a year. It's cheap (a few bucks per knife), and it will keep your knives useable and safe for decades. Most important, you will never have to mix cooking with bandages.

If you want to sharpen your knives yourself, fine. It is not that dangerous or complicated. But you need to buy a sharpening steel—a diamond sharpening steel—because a honing steel does not sharpen. It hones. Thus the name. Both sharpening steels and honing steels are metal rods with handles at one end. But they are not interchangeable, so make sure you get the one you need. You could actually use both. The easiest way to sharpen a knife with a sharpening steel is to hold the steel out in front of you with the handle in your hand and the other end of the steel resting on a countertop. Place the back edge of the knife blade near the top end of the steel, so that the handle of the steel and the handle of the knife are close together. Position the side of the blade at a 45-degree angle against the steel, and slowly pull the knife toward you and down, as if you were attempting to make an angle cut through the rod. When you finish the movement, the tip of the knife should be close to the far end of the steel, down by the counter. Do this six or eight times and then repeat the movement on the other side of the blade. You could also hold the steel upright, the way chefs do. They are usually honing their blades, though, when you see this; it's something they do constantly. Honing puts a fine edge on a blade only after it has been sharpened. Honing a dull blade is like putting tomato sauce on uncooked pasta. Incidentally, the speed with which professional chefs sharpen and hone their blades has nothing to do with how well they are doing it. They do it well, and they do it fast. But a slow, precise movement will do the trick just as well. Go at your own pace; you will speed up naturally as you become more comfortable with the movement. Using a sharpening stone is more complicated and is best left to a professional knife sharpener. Keep your knives sharp; it cannot be said enough.

Now for something a little lighter: getting garlic smell off of your fingers. Three words: salt, lemon, steel. One way to remove the odor is to rub salt on your fingers. The salt will absorb the odor, and then you can rinse the salt away with hot soapy water. Another way is to rub lemon juice on your hands, and a third way is to rub your garlicky digits on anything made of stainless steel. Give your faucet a little good-luck rub and see it if does the trick. To be safe, do all three. These tricks work for onions, too.

Okay, back to the serious stuff. Put a moist towel underneath your cutting board to keep it from slipping. A moving cutting board is the first cousin of the dull knife in terms of danger. Both dull and sharp knives are dangerous when they are used on a moving surface. The safest—and most efficient—combination is: sharp knife, stable surface. The key word here is "precision."

Furthering that point, always make sure the ingredient you are cutting has a flat or otherwise stable bottom. If it does not have one naturally, the way a brick of tofu does, create one with a single careful slice of your knife. An orange, for instance: you don't have to cut it in half and put the flat side down, but you should cut off enough so that the orange does not wobble when you start to slice. Do this with everything you are about to cut into pieces.

One more serious thing and that's it, promise. To save the fingers of your non–knife hand from errantly sneaking out in front of a blade as you are cutting, curl those fingers under and dig your fingernails into the food you are cutting. It might be awkward at first, but if you do it enough it will become second nature.

To keep eggshell fragments out of egg white, crack the egg on a flat surface such as the counter instead of on the rim of a bowl. It works. If you somehow still manage to get a shell fragment in with the egg, scoop the little piece out with one of the halves of the shell. The thin, curved shell is a natural shell-fragment retriever—much better than your finger or a spoon. You will never make a crunchy muffin or omelet again—unless, of course, you plan it that way.

There are two ways to separate egg whites from their yolks. After you have cracked open the shell, you can use the two halves as cups and pass the yolk back and forth between them over a bowl. After about five passes the whites will have dropped into the bowl below and one half of the egg shell will contain a lonely yolk. Another way to do it is in your hand. Simply hold the yolk, and the whites will drip through your fingers into the bowl. The yolk will be firm enough to hold its shape as long as you don't squeeze it. Be gentle. Imagine that you are handling . . . an egg yolk.

Chopping a bell pepper can become the most efficient, most satisfying thing that you do in your kitchen if you follow these simple steps. You must first promise that from this day forward you will never again cut a circle around the stem of a bell pepper. Instead you will turn the pepper on its side and chop off the thinnest layer from the bottom to create a flat surface. (If the bottom is very even, with four equal humps, you can skip that step.) Next, you will hold the pepper upright, stem on top, and slice straight down on each of the sides, one side at a time. In the end you will have four mostly flat pieces of pepper in front of you—four cuts, four beautiful pieces—and minimal waste. You will then be able to throw away the stem and the core. If you want to dice the four pieces, simply cut them into equal squares. You will not believe how easy this is until you do it. Then you will find yourself seeking out recipes with bell peppers in them.

Chopping a mango is not as easy as chopping a bell pepper, but it just might be more interesting. The pit inside a mango is oddly shaped, about the size of a thin oval bar of soap from a hotel. To extract it, skin the mango first. A sturdy vegetable peeler may do the trick, but mango skin can be thick and might require a knife. If this is the case, turn the mango upright, so that it is taller than it is wide, make a very shallow cut at the top, and follow that line down to the bottom. (Remember to first create a flat surface on the bottom of the mango.) Imagine that you are shaving off the thinnest layer of skin, cutting as shallowly as you can manage; you can always take more of the skin off if you do not get it the first time. Once the skin is off, slice from top to bottom about one fifth of the way in from the edge of the fruit. If you run into resistance, you have found the pit. Make another cut closer to the edge. If you run into resistance again, turn the fruit one quarter and go back to your original cut; the pit is much wider than it is thick; therefore, you will get two good chunks of fruit and two very paltry ones. Do not be afraid to nibble on the pit once you are done cutting; there will be some great, refreshing peppery fruit clinging to it that only a master carver could get to with a knife. Keep some floss handy, too—the fibrous meat of a mango can be worse than corn between your teeth. But it's worth it.

Dicing an onion is more involved than chopping a mango or bell pepper, but the visual payoff is much bigger with an onion. First, because onions are basically round, make a bottom cut to create a flat base. Next, very carefully, make a horizontal cut halfway up from the cutting board almost all the way through the onion, as if you were fashioning a hamburger bun. Do not cut the onion in half; stop short of cutting all the way through. Next, turn the onion so that if the new cut were a mouth, the onion would be facing you to talk to you. Now make four or five vertical cuts from the top of the onion down to the cutting board, spaced equally from left to right. The distance between them depends on what size pieces you ultimately want. Last, turn the onion so that you can make vertical slices perpendicular to the first vertical slices. Here is the payoff: with each slice you will see little squares of onion falling effortlessly to your cutting board. The sheer beauty of this technique might just bring a tear to your eye.

Even if you have never cut up an avocado, if you follow this technique you will look as though you have been doing it for twenty years. There is a smooth, round pit in the center of an avocado. Cut into the skin as if you are going to chop the avocado in half lengthwise. When you reach the pit with the blade, spin the avocado slowly and cut all the way around it (you will not even need to take your blade out of the avocado because the pit will guide it around). Once the cut is continuous, remove the knife and separate the two halves. Take the side without the pit and cradle it in your palm, avocado skin resting against your skin. Using a dull knife—a standard butter knife works well—slice down into the avocado meat either length-wise or widthwise, and when you feel that you have reached the inner skin, scoop out the avocado meat with the knife. The meat will stick to the knife, and you will be able to place it wherever you like. Repeat this move-ment, and you will be able to stack three or four crescent-moon-shaped pieces next to one another. To extract the pit from the other half, gently tap it with the sharp edge of a second knife. Do not use your other hand at any time in this process. Set the avocado pit side up on the counter, and gently chop at it until the knife grips it. You will feel the pit dislodge once the knife has sunk in. Lift this (second) knife, which now holds the pit, and gently tap at the pit with the butter knife; the pit will fall out after a few taps. You can also scoop the pit out with a spoon, but you will almost cer-tainly lose the smooth green surface and then you can kiss your perfect crescent moons good-bye.

Once and for all, here is how you wrap a burrito. First, heat the tortilla for five seconds in the microwave, or on the stove in a skillet for thirty to sixty seconds. Next, lay the tortilla flat and put the ingredients in the mid-dle. Fold the two sides in equally, then fold the edge closest to you over the top of them. With your hands on the tortilla, cinch the food back toward you, as if your hands are on a rolling pin and you are rolling it forward. Once you have created a nice, symmetrical log shape, roll the whole thing forward over the remaining flap and you are done. A fresh, warmed tortilla should stick to itself, which is a big part of the equation.

A wire whisk introduces air into what you are mixing and thus creates volume. A fork cannot do this, and two forks stuck together is just lame. Invest in a nice whisk—they're simple but valuable.

Folding one ingredient into the next is a delicate process. In terms of delivering information to someone, "folding" could be thought of as "breaking the news gently," while mixing would be closer to "blurting it out." You fold lighter ingredients into denser ones, digging deeply into the dense element and delicately lifting it over the lighter one with a rubber spatula. Folding should be done in increments—two or three, at least—and the mixing bowl (make that: folding bowl!) should be rotated often. A little folding goes a long way. Don't overdo it; when the ingredients are combined, you're done.

Mincing requires more patience than skill. Once you've chopped your ingredients into the smallest pieces possible, all you have to do is rock your blade over the pile until it looks as if it could have come out of a blender or food processor. You could even lift your blade and slam it down on the cutting board in rapid succession if rocking is not your thing. Exaggerated chopping like that won't hurt your knife, and you might even get more done in less time. Every so often, use the top side of your blade, the dull side, to scrape the ingredients back into a pile (using the sharp edge to do this will make it dull).

Mushrooms have a tendency, more than most vegetables, to carry dirt and grit on them. Wash them thoroughly under the faucet or soak them in water. They can handle it.

Nonreactive bowls are, quite simply, nonporous bowls. Their material will not react to an ingredient, particularly an acidic one, thus changing its color or flavor. Bowls made of stainless steel, glass, plastic, glazed ceramic, or enamel are nonreactive.

To remove sausage from its casing, run the tip of a knife down the length of the link and the casing should open up like a sleeping bag being unzipped. You should then be able to peel it like a banana and extract the meat.

Literally translated, *al dente* means "to the tooth." It is the Italian philosophy of boiling pasta enough to be cooked but not so much as to be overcooked. Al dente pasta gives a little resistance when you bite down on it.

To hull a strawberry is to pluck the leafy greens off the top and dig out the little white stem beneath them.

Some notes on food and seasonings: When it comes down to it, cooking is about ingredients. Educate yourself.

1. *Cream of tartar* is a powder sometimes used in baking powder. It gives frostings and soufflés body. You can find it in the spice section of a supermarket.

2. *"Pancake syrup" does not come from a tree. "Maple syrup" does.* Pay attention to the wording on labels.

3. *A medium yellow onion* is a little bigger than a baseball.

4. *The heat of peppers is measured in Scoville units.* A green pepper has zero, but an Anaheim has 500 to 1,000; a jalapeño has 2,500 to 7,500; a serrano has 7,500 to 20,000; and a habañero has 100,000 to 300,000. Step. Back. Slowly.

5. *There is never, ever a good reason to leave a bay leaf in a dish you are serving.* Once the cooking is complete, the leaf's mission has been fulfilled. Fish it out and throw it away.

6. *Herbes de Provence is a preordained mix of herbs—it's sort of like saying "taco seasoning"—that usually consists of rosemary, basil, thyme, sage, savory, marjoram, and some other herbs,* depending upon who is doing the mixing. You can find it in a supermarket's spice section or order it online.

7. *Vidalia onions are named for a town in Georgia.* The onions are often more squatty than, say, a round yellow onion. Vidalias are so pleasantly sweet that there are people who will pick one up and bite into it as if it were a Georgia peach. Just to be safe, never do this before going on a date.

8. *Meyer lemons are a cross between a common lemon and a mandarin orange.* Their skin is deeper yellow in color and smoother than a traditional lemon's skin. A Meyer lemon's juice is also less acidic than a regular lemon's, with hints of lime, lemon, and mandarin orange. Meyer lemons are now commonly grown in California, but they originated in China.

9. *Five-spice powder is the Chinese equivalent of Herbes de Provence (see above) or taco seasoning.* Five-spice is a preordained mixture usually containing cloves, fennel, star anise, cinnamon, and Szechuan pepper. You can find it in a supermarket's spice section.

10. *A large onion is bigger than a navel orange, smaller than a grapefruit.*

11. *Small brussels sprouts are more tender than big ones.*

12. *Tandoori spice* is a blend of black peppercorns, cumin seeds, coriander seeds, cloves, turmeric, paprika, cayenne, cinnamon, nutmeg, and salt. Buy it at a specialty store or online, or mix your own.

13. *Garam masala* is a blend of warm Indian spices such as cinnamon, cumin, cardamom, nutmeg, and cloves. It is best ground with a mortar and pestle or in a spice grinder just prior to use. Some commercial brands are made of garlic, ginger, mustard seeds, turmeric, coriander, fennel, cumin, dried chili peppers, and bay leaves.

14. *A fragrant sauce from Spain, sofrito* is made by sautéing annatto seeds in pork fat with chopped onions, green peppers, garlic, and pork. The Italian version includes chopped celery, onions, green peppers, garlic, and herbs sautéed in olive oil. Both are used to add flavor to sauces, soups, and stocks.

DIFFERENT NAME, SAME THING

Often in cooking, two words, such as "stovetop" and "range," refer to the same thing. Why do we need both words? Of course we don't need them, but as long as we have them you should be aware of them.

DIFFERENT NAME, SAME PROTEIN
tofu, bean curd
It is made from curdled soy milk, which is the extracted liquid of cooked soybeans.

DIFFERENT NAME, SAME HERB
cilantro, coriander
Its pungent flavor stands up well to spice, which is why you see it often in Latin and Asian dishes. Cilantro is the leaves of the plant, while coriander is the seeds (although some people also refer to the leafy part as coriander).

DIFFERENT NAME, SAME CONDIMENT
chutney, salsa, relish
Any of them can include chopped-up fruits, vegetables, spices, or all three.

DIFFERENT NAME, SAME LEGUME: PART I
edamame, soybean
Beans, peas, soybeans, and even peanuts are legumes because they grow inside pods
Party trivia: A peanut is a not a nut.

DIFFERENT NAME, SAME LEGUME: PART II
chickpea, garbanzo bean
Party riddle: When is a bean a pea? When it is a chickpea.

DIFFERENT NAME, SAME LEGUME: PART III
lima bean, butter bean
One name honors the capital of Peru (and you've been mispronouncing it all these years); the other is a southern colloquialism. Party trivia: Where do Lima (LAI-muh) beans come from? Lima! (LEE-muh).

DIFFERENT NAME, SAME TUBER
sunchoke, Jerusalem artichoke
Despite the name, this sunflower-family, potato-like tuber neither hails from Jerusalem nor is an artichoke. This is why people started calling them sunchokes.

DIFFERENT NAME, SAME GREEN: PART I
arugula, rocket
The flavor is bitter and peppery, and the leaves are flat and soft.

DIFFERENT NAME, SAME GREEN: PART II
Chinese cabbage, Napa cabbage
It has thinner leaves and a much milder taste than the plain old cabbage we are used to.

DIFFERENT NAME, SAME TECHNIQUE
bake, roast
Usually cakes and breads are "baked" and meats and vegetables are "roasted," but they are all cooked inside a hot, dry oven. This is why someone found it acceptable at some point to cross over and name a dish "baked chicken." As yet, no one has had the audacity to introduce "roasted cookies" to the world.

DIFFERENT NAME, SAME ROOT
ginger, gingerroot
We associate ginger with sushi and Chinese cooking, but the majority of it grows in Jamaica.

DIFFERENT NAME, SAME COOKWARE
frying pan, omelet pan, skillet
The pan has shallow, sloping sides, as opposed to the deeper, straight sides of a sauté pan.

DIFFERENT NAME, SAME SPREAD

jam, preserves

Technically, jam is more pureed and preserves are chunkier, but they both consist of fruit cooked with sugar and pectin.

DIFFERENT NAME, SAME LEAF

bay, laurel

This aromatic leaf comes from the laurel tree and is used in savory cooking. A little goes a long way. Snap a leaf in half if you are cooking only a small portion of food.

DIFFERENT COLOR, SAME CAPSICUM

bell pepper

Green, red, orange, or yellow (or purple or brown), if it's a pepper and it looks like an elongated apple—or bell—it's a bell pepper. In fact, a red pepper is a green pepper that was picked later. In Britain a pepper is known as a capsicum because it belongs to the genus *Capsicum.* So formal, they are over there.

DIFFERENT COLOR, SAME FOOD

white egg, brown egg

A white or brown eggshell will tell you what breed of hen laid the egg, but the egg inside will be essentially the same regardless of the color of the shell. There are different qualities of eggs, but shell color alone will not help anyone distinguish them.

DIFFERENT DIRECTION, SAME FLAME

grilling, broiling

When you grill, you cook *over* an open flame. When you broil, you cook *under* an open flame.

DIFFERENT NAME, SAME TOOL

chef's knife, French knife

Call it whatever you like, but it is the big chopping knife you will use most.

DIFFERENT NAME, SAME WINE

Champagne, sparkling wine

By law only the bubbly produced in the Champagne region of France can be labeled Champagne. French sparkling wine produced outside Champagne is called *crémant.* In Spain, sparkling wine is called *cava.* In Italy, it is *spumante* or *prosecco.* In Germany it is *Sekt,* and in the United States and Australia it is simply sparkling wine.

DIFFERENT NAME, SAME WINE GRAPE
shiraz, syrah
Australians and South Africans call it shiraz, the French call it syrah, and Americans call it both.

SAME NAME, DIFFERENT TOOL *(the exception to the rule)*
spatula
A rubber spatula helps you scrape the last bit of fat-free mayonnaise from a jar; the other kind of spatula, also called a "turner," helps you flip a pancake or an omelet.

WHAT'S THE DIFFERENCE?

These cooking techniques are similar but not the same.

WHAT'S THE DIFFERENCE?
Sweating softens an ingredient and releases its juices ("sweats" it) in butter, oil, or cooking spray over low heat.
Sautéing browns and caramelizes an ingredient in butter, oil, or cooking spray over high heat.
Toasting "sautés" an ingredient without using butter, oil, or cooking spray. All three techniques require either a sauté pan (with straight sides) or a standard frying pan (with flared sides).

WHAT'S THE DIFFERENCE?
To **boil** something is to cook it in hot, bubbling water.
To **poach** something is to cook it in water that is just shy of boiling.
To **blanch** something is to plunge it into boiling water, then plunge it into cold water.

WHAT'S THE DIFFERENCE?
Braising is a way to cook meat or vegetables in shallow liquid at a low temperature for a long time. "Low and slow" is the operative phrase.
Stewing uses the same technique but with more liquid, which usually thickens and is served as part of the dish.

SHOPPING AND THE HOME PANTRY

The pantry is the key to your home-cooking kingdom. Keeping a well-organized, well-stocked pantry is not a new idea; it's been done for centuries, especially at times when the availability of certain necessary foods was not always guaranteed. You will find that maintaining a well-managed home pantry will help you considerably in bringing meals to the table more quickly and easily.

This book is all about eating smarter, and that begins with shopping smarter. How is that done? One way is to know exactly what you want before you leave home for the market. Unfortunately, many shoppers go to the supermarket without a shopping list, which, in my opinion, is like driving a car without a license. First, you must know what you want, and that often starts with a recipe. We have created a collection of healthy recipes and options for you and your family that allows you to begin to shop smarter for foods. For example, shop for fresh food every two to three days rather than every day. When shopping for dry goods, shop two to three weeks in advance or even monthly.

To make the use of this book more practical and enjoyable, I recommend creating an organized list before shopping using columns to separate dairy products, dry products, seafood, etc. You become a more efficient shopper, which means less time at the supermarket and more time for you and your family. Over time, once you incorporate more of these recipes into your kitchen repertoire, your list and shopping experience will become simpler and more efficient.

Today's family seeks out foods that are less refined, healthier, and often in their freshest state—especially when attention is being paid to weight management. For some of us, growing an herb and/or vegetable garden is possible, while many of us in urban areas must rely on green markets and grocery/produce stores. Although most families I know eat fresh vegetables raw or slightly cooked, there are also good-quality canned products, such as Del Monte organic tomatoes and corn. Frozen vegetables are also a convenient and healthy alternative when a fresh produce market is unavailable.

What I find most important is to really know your markets and the people who work in them. For example, when shopping for fresh seafood, it's very important to buy from someone you trust. I encourage you to become familiar with what "fresh" smells and tastes like.

I cook and shop for food all over the world, and I've learned how very important it is to have great resources for fresh food available when you need them. We've selected a group of contacts that we know will help you shop for your family and facilitate better health.

HEALTHFUL INGREDIENTS TO STOCK YOUR KITCHEN WITH

Having a well-stocked pantry will continue to guide and encourage you to live a healthy life. Most of us call out for a food delivery when we have nothing in the house to make dinner with. I am not saying you have to swear off your favorite pizza or Chinese restaurant; I am suggesting that you indulge only every now and then. In the meantime, stock your pantry with healthy snacks and groceries. I have listed some of the items that I always have on hand in my kitchen. Once your pantry is stocked, make a trip to a farmers' market or the produce section of your favorite grocery store and purchase some fruits and vegetables in the height of their season. It is best to purchase perishable fruits and vegetables a few times a week to ensure their freshness.

Whole Grains and Flours

Almond flour
Amaranth flour
Brown rice
Buckwheat noodles
Bulghur wheat
Flaxseed, ground
Quinoa
Rolled oats
Rye flour
Spelt flour
Spelt or rice pasta
Steel-cut oats
Whole-wheat couscous

Nuts and Seeds

Almonds
Cashews
Flaxseed
Pine nuts
Pumpkin seeds
Sunflower seeds

Dried Herbs and Spices

Asian rub
Bay leaf
Cinnamon
Coriander
Cumin
Curry powder
Dill
Garam masala
Ground garlic
Herbes de Provence
Nutmeg
Onion powder
Paprika
Peppercorns
Red chili flakes
Sesame seeds

Oils and Vinegars

Balsamic vinegar
Canola oil
Extra-virgin olive oil
Olive oil cooking spray
Red wine vinegar
Rice wine vinegar
Sherry vinegar
White wine vinegar

Canned Goods

Canned artichoke hearts (in water)
Canned Italian tomatoes
Canned legumes:
- Black beans
- Cannellini beans
- Garbanzo beans (chickpeas)
- Kidney beans

Canned tuna (in water)
Lentils: red and black
Low-sodium vegetable broth

Refrigerator Staples

Basil: fresh and pesto
Capers
Chili paste
Cilantro
Dill
Italian parsley
Kefir
Low-sodium soy sauce
Miso
Olives
Rosemary
Shiritake (soy noodles)
Thyme
Tofu
Whole-grain mustard

Freezer Staples

Organic berries
Organic corn kernels
Organic peas, fava beans, and edamame
Soy burgers
Veggie sausages

PRODUCE SEASONALITY GUIDE

■■■■■■■■

Today, with the luxury of FedEx, we can obtain a perfectly ripe peach from Australia in December. Many fruits and vegetables are available year-round because of the efficiency of air freight. But many of us still live by and crave local foods in the height of their season. That is how I like to eat, and I believe in supporting my local farmers' market. In Chicago, where I live, we are blessed with many farmers' markets every day in different neighborhoods. The Chicago Green City Market is my favorite market. It believes in supporting farmers who support the land. It supports small family farms that sustainably raise produce and other food products. Its mission is to improve the availability and diversity of high-quality foods; see www.chicagogreencitymarket.org. There are many farmers' markets all over the country that have the same core belief system as Chicago Green City Market, and I hope you will make an effort to visit one in your area. You will be delighted at what you discover at the farmers' market!

When Produce Is in Season

Item	Jan	Feb	Mar	Apr	May	Jun	Jul	Aug	Sep	Oct	Nov	Dec
Apples				■	■	■	■	■	■			
Apricots				■	■	■	■	■				
Artichokes			■	■	■				■	■	■	
Arugula		■	■	■	■	■	■	■	■	■		■
Asian greens	■	■	■	■	■	■	■	■	■	■	■	■
Asparagus			■	■	■	■						
Avocados		■	■	■	■	■	■	■	■			
Basil					■	■	■	■	■	■		
Beans, fava				■	■	■						
Beans, green						■	■	■	■	■		
Beans, shelling							■	■	■	■		
Beans, wax						■	■	■	■	■		
Beets	■	■	■	■	■	■	■	■	■	■	■	■
Blackberries						■	■	■	■			
Blueberries						■	■	■				
Broccoli	■	■	■	■	■				■	■	■	■
Brussels sprouts	■	■	■	■					■	■	■	■
Buddha's hand	■	■										■
Burdock root	■	■	■	■			■	■	■	■	■	■
Cabbage	■	■	■	■	■	■	■	■	■	■	■	■
Cactus	■					■	■	■	■	■		■
Cardoon stalk	■	■	■	■	■	■	■	■	■	■		■
Carrots	■	■	■	■	■	■	■	■	■	■	■	■
Cauliflower	■	■	■	■	■							
Celery	■				■	■	■	■	■	■	■	■
Celery root	■	■	■	■	■				■	■	■	■
Chard	■	■	■	■	■	■	■	■	■	■	■	■
Cherries	■	■	■	■				■	■	■	■	■
Collard greens	■	■	■	■	■	■	■	■	■	■	■	■
Corn										■		

Shaded cells (●) indicate that the item is in season.

Item	Jan	Feb	Mar	Apr	May	Jun	Jul	Aug	Sep	Oct	Nov	Dec
Cress	●	●	●			●	●	●	●	●	●	●
Cucumbers					●	●	●	●	●	●	●	
Dates								●	●	●	●	●
Eggplants							●	●	●	●		
Endive	●	●	●	●	●	●	●	●	●	●	●	●
Fennel	●	●	●	●	●	●	●	●	●	●	●	●
Figs							●	●	●	●		
Garlic	●	●	●	●	●	●	●	●	●	●	●	●
Grapes							●	●	●	●		●
Grapefruit	●	●	●	●	●						●	●
Green garlic		●	●	●	●	●						
Horseradish	●	●	●	●	●	●	●	●	●	●	●	●
Kale	●	●	●	●	●	●	●	●	●	●	●	●
Kiwis	●	●	●	●							●	●
Kohlrabi	●	●	●	●	●	●	●	●	●	●	●	●
Kumquats	●	●	●	●							●	●
Leeks	●	●	●	●	●	●	●	●	●	●	●	●
Lemons	●	●	●	●	●	●	●	●	●	●	●	●
Lemons, Meyer	●	●	●	●							●	●
Lettuces	●	●	●	●	●	●	●	●	●	●	●	●
Limes	●	●	●	●					●	●	●	●
Limes, Key						●	●	●	●			
Melons						●	●	●	●			
Mushrooms, wild	●	●	●	●	●						●	●
Nectarines						●	●	●	●			
Okra						●	●	●	●	●		
Olives									●	●	●	●
Onions	●	●	●	●	●	●	●	●	●	●	●	●
Onions, green	●	●	●			●	●	●	●	●	●	●
Onions, small bulb						●	●	●	●			
Onions, sweet						●	●	●	●			

Item	Jan	Feb	Mar	Apr	May	Jun	Jul	Aug	Sep	Oct	Nov	Dec
Oranges	■	■	■	■						■	■	■
Oranges, mandarins/tangerines	■	■	■	■								
Parsnips	■	■	■	■								
Peaches	■				■	■	■	■		■	■	
Pears	■						■	■	■	■	■	■
Pears, Asian								■	■	■	■	
Peas, green				■	■	■		■	■			
Peas, snow				■	■	■						
Peas, sugar snap				■	■	■						
Peppers, sweet							■	■	■	■		
Peppers, hot							■	■	■	■		
Persimmons									■	■	■	
Plums							■	■	■	■		
Pomegranates									■	■	■	
Pomelos	■	■	■	■	■							■
Potatoes	■	■	■	■	■	■	■	■	■	■	■	■
Potatoes, sweet			■	■	■	■	■	■	■	■		
Radishes			■	■	■	■	■	■	■	■		
Ramps/wild leeks				■	■	■			■	■	■	■
Rapini/broccoli rabe	■	■	■	■	■	■		■	■	■	■	■
Raspberries					■	■	■	■	■	■		
Rhubarb				■	■	■						
Rutabagas	■	■	■	■	■					■	■	■
Salsify							■	■	■	■	■	■
Shallots					■	■	■	■	■	■		
Spinach				■	■	■	■	■	■	■		
Squash blossoms					■	■	■	■	■			
Squash, summer						■	■	■	■			
Squash, winter	■	■	■	■						■	■	■
Strawberries				■	■	■	■	■				
Sunchokes/Jerusalem artichokes	■	■								■	■	■
Tomatillos						■	■	■	■	■	■	
Tomatoes						■	■	■	■	■		
Turnips	■	■	■	■	■					■	■	■

ART'S PANTRY AND KITCHEN EQUIPMENT SOURCES

FOODS

Adagio Teas
www.adagio.com

Camellia Beans
Harahan, LA
www.camelliabrand.com
(504) 733-8155

Del Monte Foods
San Francisco, CA
www.delmonte.com

Fiji Water
Los Angeles, CA
www.fijiwater.com
(888) 426-3454

Global Palate
East Hampton, NY
www.globalpalate.com

Organic coffee: Beantrees
Sacramento, CA
www.beantrees.com
(916) 451-3744

Organic Trade Association
Greenfield, MA
www.usorganicproducts.com
(413) 774-7511

Pete's Fresh Produce
Chicago, IL
(773) 523-4600

Quaker Oats
www.quakeroats.com

Safeway Foods
www.safeway.com

Select Fish of Whole Foods Market
Seattle, WA
(206) 767-2642

Superior Tofu
Vancouver, BC, Canada
www.superiortofu.com
(604) 251-1806

Whole Foods Market
Austin, TX
www.wholefoods.com
(512) 477-4455

KITCHEN EQUIPMENT

Bridge Kitchenware
New York, NY
www.bridgekitchenware.com
(800) 274-3435

Sur La Table
Seattle, WA
www.surlatable.com
(800) 243-0852

Viking
Greenwood, MS
www.vikingrange.com
(888) VIKING1

EPILOGUE

Thank you for this opportunity to be of service. I hope this book has been useful to you. It represents the best and most useful of what my colleagues and I have learned in more than thirty years of conducting research and working with people from around the world on improving their health and well-being.

This book is based on science, and science is continually evolving. As I described in chapter 4, because this field is so rapidly progressing, my colleagues and I are developing a website (www.OrnishSpectrum.com) that will offer additional support and resources in personalizing a way of living and eating beyond what this or any other book can provide.

Also, genetic testing may progress in the near future to a point that could be very useful.

Wishing you a lifetime filled with health, joy, and, love.

Dean Ornish, M.D.

ACKNOWLEDGMENTS

Gratitude bestows reverence, allowing us to encounter everyday epiphanies, those transcendent moments of awe that change forever how we experience life and the world.

—John Milton (1608-1674)

No one is as capable of gratitude as one who has emerged from the kingdom of night.

—Elie Wiesel

■ ■ ■ ■ ■ ■ ■ ■ ■ ■

Gratitude is a powerful portal to happiness. Lately, I tend to walk around in a more-or-less constant state of appreciation, so I feel happier than ever. In large part, this is due to being with my wife, Anne, and son, Lucas. Being with Anne, my True Love, best friend, lover, closest colleague, and confidante, has completely transformed my life in ways that I couldn't even imagine before. Words are so inadequate to convey the depths of love and appreciation I feel for her. As the Taoist philosopher Wei Wu Wei once wrote, "Truth cannot be communicated. It can only be laid bare." And as Lucas once asked me, "Will you come inside my dreams with me?"

I love writing this section. It provides an opportunity for me to meditate on the many people who have made such a meaningful difference in my life. The attitude of gratitude.

Let me begin by extending my heartfelt thanks to Chef Art Smith, who created the recipes and cooking section for *The Spectrum*. Art is a chef's chef, one of the best in the world. What impresses me even more, though, is his commitment to service.

Art founded Common Threads, a nonprofit organization whose mission is to educate children on the importance of nutrition and physical well-being and to instill an appreciation of our world's diversity through the food and art of different cultures (www.commonthreads.org). Common

Threads provides after-school programming to children eight to twelve years old who are on the free- or assisted-lunch program. It promotes physical fitness and culture and provides a day camp for six weeks during the summer where children learn to plant, harvest, and cook fresh vegetables from the Common Threads World Garden. In recognition of his extraordinary work, Art won the 2007 James Beard Foundation Humanitarian of the Year Award.

Special appreciation to Al Gore for raising awareness of the need to address global warming.

I have worked with Esther Newberg at ICM and Michael Rudell at Franklin, Weinrib, Rudell, and Vassallo on my books for almost thirty years. My professional esteem and personal affection for them only continues to grow over time. Thanks also to Don Walker at the Harry Walker Agency. Deepest appreciation to Skip Brittenham for his friendship and always-brilliant advice and support, and to Kathy Hallberg, who works with him.

Heartfelt thanks to everyone at the Random House/Ballantine Books Publishing Group who made this book possible, especially Executive Editor Caroline Sutton, as well as Gina Centrello, Libby McGuire, Kim Hovey, Brian McLendon, Tom Perry, Christina Duffy, Gene Mydlowski, Christine Cabello, Stacey Witcraft, Rachel Bernstein, Jack Perry, Kelle Ruden, Patricia Nicolescu, and Carol Schneider.

I am indebted to Sandee Lamotte, Elaine Widner, Nan Forté, and Wayne Gattinella at WebMD and to Joey Tucker, Nancy Bielenberg, and David Turner at VTA in Atlanta for making the DVD of guided meditations available, especially under such a tight deadline (the irony was not lost on any of us . . .). Very special thanks to Norman Seeff for his extraordinary photography and direction of the DVD and for the deep friendship that he and his wife, Sue, provide.

All of my books are based on research conducted with my colleagues at the nonprofit Preventive Medicine Research Institute (PMRI), which I founded in 1984. None of my books—especially this one—would have been possible without their expert advice and support.

These include Executive Vice President Jennifer McCrea and Vice Presidents Colleen Kemp, Terri Merritt-Worden, Anne Ornish, and Dr. Gerdi Weidner. I am grateful to Alice Pierce for keeping my life organized. Others at PMRI include Ellen Beller, Donna Platt, Steven Frenda, Annie Schmidt, Dr. Rebecca Campo, Claudia Pischke, Dr. Joanne Frattaroli, and Loren Yglecias, as well as consultants Bryce Williams, Glenn Perelson, Dr. Bob Avenson, Dr. Ruth Marlin, Caren Raisin, Lila Crutchfield, Antonella Dewell, Stacey Dunn-Emke, Sarah Govil, Dr. Damien McKnight, Dr. Jordan Fein, Marcia and Jim Billings, Melanie Eller, Billy Gao, Patty McCormac, Heather Amador, Dennis Malone, Christine Chi, Erin Hansen, Michael Sumner, Deanna McCrary, Jean-Marc Fullsack, Joel Goldman, Bob Lieber, and Dr. Lee Lipsenthal.

I remain deeply grateful to the PMRI board of directors for supporting our vision and making it real. These include Jenard and Gail Gross, Henry Groppe, Brock Leach, Ken Hubbard, Bruce Rohde, Fenton Talbott, and Jay Walker. Heartfelt gratitude to Niko Canner and Katzenbach Partners, Pierre and Pam Omidyar, Randy Ching, Greg Simon, Adam Bosworth, Mats Lederhausen, Bill Mayer, Richard Decker, Steve and Mary Swig, Gary Burstein, Vinod and Neeru Khosla, Warren Hellman, Nick Jacobs, John Whyte, and Jeff Walker for their strategic vision, planning, and friendship.

Deep appreciation to Dr. Peter Carroll for the opportunity to collaborate with him on both the Prostate Cancer Lifestyle Trial and the GEMINAL gene array study. Dr. Carroll is, to me, the leading urologist in the world. We both appreciate the privilege of collaborating with Dr. Elizabeth Blackburn on the telomere study in cooperation with Drs. Chris Haqq, Mark Magbanua, Millie Hughes-Fulford, Jue Lin, June Chan, Jennifer Daubenmier, Elissa Epel, and others. Special thanks to the late Dr. William Fair and Dr. Ann Dnestrian of Memorial Sloan-Kettering Cancer Center; Drs. Jim Barnard, Tung Ngo, and Bill Aronson of UCLA; Nick Jacobs from Windber Hospital; Dr. Elaine Pettengill from UCSF; and Dr. Nancy Mendell from SUNY for their important roles in the Prostate Cancer Lifestyle Trial Study.

Our research would not be possible without the generosity, advice, and support of many people, for which I remain deeply grateful. These include the National Institutes of Health (5P50CA089520), the U.S. Department of Defense Uniformed Services University grants, the Henry M. Jackson Foundation (via Reps. Nancy Pelosi and John Murtha and Sen. Arlen Specter), the University of California, San Francisco Prostate Cancer Specialized Center of Excellence, the Bravewell Foundation, the Bucksbaum Family Foundation, the Ellison Foundation, the Fisher Foundation, the Gallin Foundation, the Goldman Foundation, Highmark, Inc., the Hines Foundation, the Kaye Foundation, the Sol and Heather Kerzner Foundation, the Koch Foundation, the Prostate Cancer Foundation (Michael Milken), the Resnick Foundation, the Safeway Foundation, the Wachner Foundation, the Walton Family Foundation, the Wynn Foundation, and many others.

Special appreciation to Dr. Gavin Hougham and his colleagues at the John A. Hartford Foundation and the American Geriatric Society, to

Dr. Mark Smith of the California HealthCare Foundation, to Jackie Millan of the PepsiCo Foundation, and to John Paul and Eloise DeJoria for helping us expand the open-source model of our program to those who most need it. Thanks to Dr. David Agus, Ryan Phelan, and Dr. Raymond Rodriguez for helping me learn more about the state of the art in genomics counseling. Thanks to Chris Anderson and his visionary TED conference for stimulating some of the ideas expressed in this book, and to Donna Karan for her Urban Zen initiative.

Thanks to all of the enormously dedicated people at the San Francisco Food Bank, the Quincy Jones Foundation, and the United Nations High Commission on Refugees for allowing me to serve on your boards of directors.

I appreciate the support of everyone at the Centers for Medicare and Medicaid Services who was helpful in making it possible for Medicare coverage to be extended to eligible beneficiaries going through our program for reversing heart disease and to ones like it, especially to former administrators Dr. Bruce Vladeck, Dr. Mark McClellan, and Dr. Nancy-Ann Min DeParle. I remain grateful to Representatives Charles Rangel and Dan Burton, and Senators Maria Cantwell and Max Baucus for their support, without which this would not have occurred, as well as to Dean Rosen and Max Tribble.

Many thanks to friends who continue to make a very meaningful difference in my life, including (in no particular order) Phillip Moffitt and Pawan Bareja, Rachel Remen, Barry and Lizanne Rosenstein, Kim Polese, Larry and Girija Brilliant, Steve and Laurene Jobs, Quincy Jones (my "brother from another mother"), Jennifer McCrea and Jack Maley, Sandra McLanahan, Lawrence Bender, Eric Greenberg, Jerry Inzerillo and Prudence Solomon, Mehmet and Lisa Oz, Richard Baskin, Steven Horowitz, India Arie Simpson, Jon Kabat-Zinn, Clint and Dina Eastwood, Bill and Sandy Nicholson, David and Jan Crosby, Michael and Sharyle Lerner, Peter and Lynda Guber, Edge and Morleigh Steinberg, Bono, Dennis and Phyllis Washington, Alexander Leaf, Cameron Sinclair and Kate Stohr, Craig Venter, Amy Tan and Lou Dimattei, Bob and Marlene Veloz, Rick Smolan and Jennifer Erwitt, Noelle Nelson, Frank Jordan and Wendy Paskin Jordan, Pamela Morgan, David Fenton, Peter and Mary Max, Jim Gordon, Shep and Renée Gordon, Phil and Ashley Jones, John and Lisa Pritzker, Tony and Sage Robbins, and others whom I may have inadvertently omitted. Very special thanks to Peter Max for printing the Spectrum on the cover of this book.

All love to my parents (Dr. Edwin and Natalie Ornish) and to Steven, Marty, Andre, and Miles Ornish, Kathy Ornish and John Olstad, and Laurel Ornish, my father-in-law (Larry Pearce), my late mother-in-law (Ginger Pearce), Rosie Pearce, and to ·Lars and Sandra Pearce, and Lindsey and Steve Foster.

I remain grateful to Joan Abate United Airlines for making it possible for me to travel as much as I do, to Gustavo and Jessica Hornos for showing Anne and me how to move through life gracefully, to Damon Kerby and his colleagues at St. Mark's, and to Susan Lissberger for expanding Lucas's horizons.

Special thanks to Tina Malia for allowing us to use the transformative music from her amazing album *The Silent Awakening* in the guided meditations DVD included with *The Spectrum*.

I wrote this book myself because of my idiosyncratic style of writing. I am especially appreciative to Michael Castleman for his skill in helping me edit it. Thanks also to Domenica Catelli, Sari Zernich, and Michael Austin for their invaluable help in organizing the recipe and cooking section and to Terri Merritt-Worden for providing much of the background information on the Exercise Spectrum described in chapter 8.

Many thanks to Singita in South Africa, where most of this book was written, and to Swami Satchidananda for his ecumenical, transformative teachings that continue to inspire and guide me.

Dr. Mark Hyman was a very helpful source on functional medicine (www.drhyman.com), and Spencer Smith helped organize his information. Thanks to Claudia Pischke for helping organize the references section.

Many thanks to Jon Meacham, editor-in-chief of *Newsweek*, for the privilege of writing a monthly column, and to his colleagues there, including David Noonan, Mark Miller, Deidre Depke, Jennifer Barrett, Barbara Kantrowitz, Deborah Rosenberg, Anna Kuchment, Kathy Deveny, and Ramin Setoodeh, and Geoff Cowley, who is now associate commissioner at the New York City Department of Health and Mental Hygiene.

Sincere appreciation to Mary Berner, Alyce Alston, Eva Dillon, and Jackie Leo at *Reader's Digest*, for the privilege of writing a monthly column, and to their colleagues there, including Julie Bain, Patricia Curtis, Kim Santos, and Beth Turner.

Thanks to CEO Indra Nooyi and former CEO Steve Reinemund of PepsiCo for the opportunity to chair the PepsiCo Blue Ribbon Advisory Board and to their colleagues Nestor Carbonell, Tod MacKenzie, Antonio Lucio, Mike White, Lynn Markley, Dr. Nancy Green, Dr. Derek Yach, and all of the members of the PepsiCo Blue Ribbon Advisory Board.

I appreciate the opportunity to consult closely with current and former members of the leadership at McDonald's, including Jim Skinner and his predecessors (Jack Greenberg, Charlie Bell, and Jim Cantalupo), Ralph

Alvarez, Mary Dillon, Richard Floersch, Don Thompson, Jack Daly, Tim Peters, and Lori Miller, among many others there.

Many thanks to Steve Burd of Safeway for his leadership and to his colleagues Mike Minasi, Ken Shachmut, and Keith Ferrazzi for their innovative approach to employee wellness and to providing state-of-the-art health education for their customers.

I have enjoyed chairing the Google Health Advisory Council and express my deep appreciation to Eric Schmidt, Larry Page, Sergey Brin, Marissa Mayer, Missy Krasner, and the members of the Google Health Advisory Council, and to Adam Bosworth for his vision in helping make it possible.

If I have omitted anyone who should have been included, please remind me and I will add it to the next edition. As Estelle Ramey once said, "I have loved, and I have been loved, and all the rest is just background music."

REFERENCES

■■■■■■■■■■

Chapter 1

9 *patients became pain free* Ornish, D., A. M. Gotto, R. R. Miller, et al. 1979. Effects of a vegetarian diet and selected yoga techniques in the treatment of coronary heart disease. *Clin Res* 27:720A.

Ornish, D., L. W. Scherwitz, R. S. Doody, D. Kesten, S. M. McLanahan, S. E. Brown, E. DePuey, et al. 1983. Effects of stress management training and dietary changes in treating ischemic heart disease. *JAMA* 249(1):54–59.

Ornish, D., S. E. Brown, L. W. Scherwitz, J. H. Billings, W. T. Armstrong, T. A. Ports, S. M. McLanahan, R. L. Kirkeeide, R. J. Brand, and K. L. Gould. 1990. Can lifestyle changes reverse coronary heart disease? *Lancet* 336(8708):129–33.

Gould, K. L., D. Ornish, R. L. Kirkeeide, S. E. Brown, Y. Stuart, M. Buchi, J. Billings, W. Armstrong, T. Ports, and L. Scherwitz. 1992. Improved stenosis geometry by quantitative coronary arteriography after vigorous risk factor modification. *Am J Cardiol* 69(9):845–53.

Gould, K. L., D. Ornish, L. Scherwitz, S. Brown, R. P. Edens, M. J. Hess, N. Mullani, L. Bolomey, F. Dobbs, W. T. Armstrong, et al. 1995. Changes in myocardial perfusion abnormalities by positron emission tomography after long-term, intense risk factor modification. *JAMA* 274(11):894–901.

Ornish, D., L. W. Scherwitz, J. H. Billings, K. L. Gould, T. A. Merritt, S. Sparler, W. T. Armstrong, et al. 1998. Intensive lifestyle changes for reversal of coronary heart disease. *JAMA* 280(23):2001–7.

Ornish, D. 1998. Avoiding revascularization with lifestyle changes: The Multicenter Lifestyle Demonstration Project. *Am J Cardiol* 82(103):72T–76T.

Koertge, J., G. Weidner, M. Elliott-Eller, L. Scherwitz, T. A. Merritt-Worden, R. Marlin, L. Lipsenthal, et al. 2003. Improvement in medical risk factors and quality of life in women and men with coronary artery disease in the Multicenter Lifestyle Demonstration Project. *Am J Cardiol* 91(11):1316–22.

Pischke, C. R., G. Weidner, M. Elliott-Eller, L. Scherwitz, T. A. Merritt-Worden, R. Marlin, L. Lipsenthal, et al. 2006. Comparison of coronary risk factors and quality of life in coronary artery disease patients with versus with out diabetes mellitus. *Am J Cardiol* 97(9):1267–73.

Pischke, C. R., G. Weidner, M. Elliott-Eller, and D. Ornish. 2007 (in press). Lifestyle changes and clinical profile in coronary heart disease patients with an ejection fraction of ≤40 percent or >40 percent in the Multicenter Lifestyle Demonstration Project. *Eur J Heart Fail* 9(9):928–34.

Daubenmier, J. J., G. Weidner, M. D. Sumner, M. Mendell, T. Merritt-Worden, J. Studley, and D. Ornish. 2007. The contribution of changes in diet, exercise, and stress management to changes in coronary risk in women and men in The Multisite Cardiac Lifestyle Intervention Program. *Ann Behav Med* 33(1): 57–68.

Frattaroli, J., G. Weidner, T. Merritt-Worden, S. Frenda, and D. Ornish. 2008 (in press). Effects of cardiac lifestyle intervention programs on angina pectoris and atherosclerotic risk factors. *Am J Cardiol.*

12 *The Cleveland Clinic* Esselstyn, C. B., Jr., S. G. Ellis, S. V. Medendorp, and T. D. Crowe. 1995. A strategy to arrest and reverse coronary artery disease: A 5-year longitudinal study of a single physician's practice. *J Fam Pract* 41(6):560–68.

12 *coronary heart disease* Esselstyn, C. B., Jr. 1999. Updating a 12-year experience with arrest and reversal therapy for coronary heart disease (an overdue requiem for palliative cardiology). *Am J Cardiol* 84(3):339–41, A8.

14 *American Journal of Cardiology* Ornish, D. 1998. Avoiding revascularization with lifestyle changes: The Multicenter Lifestyle Demonstration Project. *Am J Cardiol* 82:72T–76T.

18 *controlled trials of angioplasty* Katritsis, D. G., and J.P.A. Ioannidis. 2005. Percutaneous coronary intervention versus conservative therapy in nonacute coronary artery disease: A meta-analysis. *Circulation* 111:2906–12.

18 *New England Journal of Medicine* Boden, W. E., R. A. O'Rourke, K. K. Teo, et al. 2007. Optimal medical therapy with or with out PCI for stable coronary disease. *N Engl J Med* 356(15):1503–16.

18 *strokes, and premature deaths* Hambrecht, R., C. Walther, S. Möbius-Winkler, S. Gielen, A. Linke, K. Conradi, S. Erbs, et al. 2004. Percutaneous coronary angioplasty compared with exercise training in patients with stable coronary artery disease: a randomized trial. *Circulation* 109(11):1371–78.

18 *those undergoing angioplasty* Pitt, B., D. Waters, W. V. Brown, A. J. van Boven, L. Schwartz, L. M. Title, D. Eisenberg, L. Shurzinske, and L. S. McCormick. 1999. Aggressive lipid-lowering therapy compared with angioplasty in stable coronary artery disease: Atorvastatin versus Revascularization Treatment Investigators. *N Engl J Med* 341(2):70–76.

20 *entered our program* Pischke, C. R., G. Weidner, E. Elliott-Eller, and D. Ornish. 2007 (in press). Lifestyle changes and clinical profile in coronary heart disease patients with an ejection fraction of ≤40 percent or >40 percent in the Multicenter Lifestyle Demonstration Project. *Eur J Heart Fail* 9(9):928–34.

22 *those who were operated on* Elliot-Eller, M., G. Weidner, C. R. Pischke, R. Marlin, M. Li, N. Mendell, L. Lipsenthal, R. Finkel, and D. Ornish. 2003. Clinical events in heart disease patients with low left ventricular ejection fraction: 3 year follow-up results. Abstract presented at the International Academy of Cardiology, 3rd World Congress on Heart Disease, Washington, DC.

Chapter 2

31 *unhealthy than do happy people* New York Times. 2007. Drilling down. Balms for sadness: Salt, grease, sugar. January 8.

32 *and are often sustainable* Hill, J. O., H. R. Wyatt, G. W. Reed, and J. C. Peters. 2003. Obesity and the environment: Where do we go from here? *Science* 299 (5608):853–55.

Chapter 3

41 *convergence of recommendations* Ornish, D. 2004. The Atkins Ornish South Beach Zone Diet. *Time,* June.

42 *higher on intelligence tests* Birch, E. E., S. Garfield, D. R. Hoffman, R. Uauy, and D. G. Birch. 2000. A randomized controlled trial of early dietary supply of long-chain polyunsaturated fatty acids and mental development in term infants. *Dev Med Child Neurol* 42(3):174–81.

43 *who consumed less seafood* Hibbeln, J. R., J. M. Davis, C. Steer, P. Emmett, I. Rogers, C. Williams, and J. Golding. 2007. Maternal seafood consumption in pregnancy and neurodevelopmental outcomes in childhood (ALSPAC study). *Lancet* 369(9561):578–85.

43 *urged to eat fish* Leaf, A. 2006. Prevention of sudden cardiac death by n-3 polyunsaturated fatty acids. *Fundamen Clin Pharmacol* 20(6):525-38.

45 *canola oil and salmon do not* Vogel, R. A., M. C. Corretti, and G. D. Plotnick. 2000. The postprandial effect of components of the Mediterranean diet on endothelial function. *J Am Coll Cardiol* 36(5):1455–60.

45 *improved blood flow* Cortés, B., I. Núñez, M. Cofán, R. Gilabert, A. Pérez-Heras, E. Casals, R. Deulofeu, and E. Ros. 2006. Acute effects of high-fat meals enriched with walnuts or olive oil on postprandial endothelial function. *J Am Coll Cardiol* 48(8):1666–71 (Epub September).

45 *margarine made from canola oil* Trichopoulou, A., T. Costacou, C. Bamia, and D. Trichopoulos. 2003. Adherence to a Mediterranean diet and survival in a Greek population. *N Engl J Med* 348(26):2599–608.
Hu, F. B. 2003. The Mediterranean diet and mortality—olive oil and beyond. *N Engl J Med* 348(26):2595–96.

50 *can make a big difference* Ebbeling, C. B., M. Leidig, H. Feldman, M. Lovesky, and D. Ludwig. 2007. Effects of a low-glycemic load vs low-fat diet in obese young adults. *JAMA* 297(19):2092.

52 *calories intake is the same* Rudel, L. L., and K. Kavanagh. 2006. Trans fat leads to weight gain even on same total calories. Presented at the 66th Annual Scientific Sessions of the American Diabetes Association, Washington, DC.

54 *on a low-fat diet alone* Ello-Martin, J. A., S. R. Liane, J. H. Ledikwe, A. M. Beach, and B. J. Rolls. 2007. Dietary energy density in the treatment of obesity: A year-long trial comparing 2 weight-loss diets. *Am J Clin Nutr* 85(6):1465–77.

55 *associated with protein intake* Ludwig, D. S., M. A. Pereira, C. H. Kroenke, et al. 1999. Dietary fiber, weight gain, and cardiovascular disease risk factors in young adults. *JAMA* 282(16):1539–46.

55 *sulforaphanes, and others* Dewell, A., G. Weidner, M. D. Sumner, C. S. Chi, and D. Ornish. 2007 (in press). A very low-fat vegan diet increases intake of protective dietary factors and decreases intake of pathogenic dietary factors. *J Am Diet Assoc.*

55 *placebo got a little worse* Sumner, M. D., M. Elliott-Eller, G. Weidner, J. J. Daubenmier, M. H. Chew, R. Marlin, C. J. Raisin, and D. Ornish. 2005. Effects of pomegranate juice consumption on myocardial perfusion in patients with coronary heart disease. *Am J Cardiol* 96:810–14.

56 *men outlive the disease* Pantuck, A. J., J. Leppert, H. Zomorodian, W. Aronson, J. Hong, R. J. Barnard, N. Seeram, H. Liker, et al. 2006. Phase II study of pomegranate juice for men with rising prostate-specific antigen following surgery or radiation for prostate cancer. *Clin Cancer Res* 12(13):4018–26.

67 *cardiovascular and other causes*   Harris, T. B. 1999. Associations of elevated interleukin-6 and C-reactive protein levels with mortality in the elderly. *Am J Med* 106(5):506–12.

67 *cardiovascular and other causes*   Macdonald, T. T., and G. Monteleone. 2005. Immunity, inflammation, and allergy in the gut. *Science* 307(5717):1920–25. Review.

67 *decreased blood markers of inflammation*   Lopez-Garcia, E., M. B. Schulze, T. T. Fung, J. B. Meigs, N. Rifai, J. E. Manson, and F. B. Hu. 2004. Major dietary patterns are related to plasma concentrations of markers of inflammation and endothelial dysfunction. *Am J Clin Nutr* 80(4):1029–35.

Hyman, M. Clinical approaches to environmental inputs. *Textbook of Functional Medicine.* Ed. D. S. Jones. Gig Harbor: Institute for Functional Medicine. 2006.

Lutsey, P. L., D. R. Jacobs, S. Kori, E. Mayer-Davis, S. Shea, L. M. Steffen, M. Szklo, and R. Tracy. 2007. Whole grain intake and its cross-sectional association with obesity, insulin resistance, inflammation, diabetes and subclinical CVD: The MESA Study. *Br J Nutr* 98(2):397–405 (Epub March).

68 *generally being more healthful*   Pollan, M. *The Omnivore's Dilemma.* New York: Penguin Press, 2006.

Chapter 4

70 *pills after twelve years*   Christen, W. G., J. E. Manson, R. J. Glynn, J. M. Gaziano, E. Y. Chew, J. E. Buring, and C. H. Hennekens. 2007. Beta carotene supplementation and age-related maculopathy in a randomized trial of US physicians. *Arch Ophthalmol* 125(3):333–39.

Cole, S. W., L. C. Hawkley, J. M. Aravelo, et al. 2007. Social regulation of gene expression in human leukocytes. *Genome Biol* 8:R189.

70 *after 4.5 years of treatment*   Green, A., G. Williams, R. Neale, V. Hart, D. Leslie, P. Parsons, G. C. Marks, et al. 1999. Daily sunscreen application and betacarotene supplementation in prevention of basal-cell and squamous-cell carcinomas of the skin: A randomised controlled trial. *Lancet* 354(9180):723–29.

70 *smokers who did not*   Malila, N., M. J. Virtanen, J. Virtamo, D. Albanes, and E. Pukkala. 2006. Cancer incidence in a cohort of Finnish male smokers. *Eur J Cancer Prev* 15(2):103–107.

70 *regularly took beta-carotene*   Michaud, D. S., D. Feskanich, E. B. Rimm, G. A. Colditz, F. E. Speizer, W. C. Willett, and E. Giovannucci. 2000. Intake of specific carotenoids and risk of lung cancer in 2 prospective US cohorts. *Am J Clin Nutr* 72(4):990–97.

70 *cancer in both groups*   Lee, I. M., N. R. Cook, J. E. Manson, J. E. Buring, and C. H. Hennekens. 1999. Beta-carotene supplementation and incidence of cancer and cardiovascular disease: The Women's Health Study. *J Natl Cancer Inst* 91(24): 2102–106.

70 *developing lung cancer*   Speizer, F. E., G. A. Colditz, D. J. Hunter, B. Rosner, and C. Hennekens. 1999. Prospective study of smoking, antioxidant intake, and lung cancer in middle-aged women. *Cancer Causes Control* 10(5):475–82.

70 *risk of Alzheimer's disease*   Morris, M. C., D. A. Evans, J. L. Bienias, C. C. Tangney, D. A. Bennett, N. Aggarwal, R. S. Wilson, and P. A. Scherr. 2002. Dietary intake of antioxidant nutrients and the risk of incident Alzheimer disease in a biracial community study. *JAMA* 287(24):3230–37.

71 *than all transportation combined*   United Nations Food and Agriculture Organi-

zations. Livestock's Long Shadow Report. http://www.fao.org/newsroom/en/news/2006/1000448/index.html (accessed April 16, 2007).

72 *as much as 20 percent* Cook, N. R., J. A. Cutler, E. Obarzanek, J. E. Buring, K. M. Rexrode, S. K. Kumanyika, L. J. Appel, and P. K. Whelton. 2007. Long term effects of dietary sodium reduction on cardiovascular disease outcomes: Observational follow-up of the trials of hypertension prevention (TOHP). *BMJ* 334(7599): 885 (Epub April).

Boyles, S. 2007. Cut heart risk by eating less salt. Studies show a lower-salt diet lowers risk of heart disease and stroke. *Web MD Medical News,* April 19. http://www.webmd.com/heart-disease/news/20070419/cut-heart-risk-by-eating-less-salt

73 *of no more than one* Rohack, J. 2006. Reducing the population burden of cardiovascular disease by reducing sodium intake. AMA publication. American Heart Association website. http://www.ama-assn.org/ama/pub/category/16413.html.

73 *one cup per day* Kuriyama, S., T. Shimazu, K. Ohmori, N. Kikuchi, N. Nakaya, Y. Nishino, Y. Tsubono, and I. Tsuji. 2006. Green tea consumption and mortality due to cardiovascular disease, cancer, and all causes in Japan: The Ohsaki Study. *JAMA* 296(10):1255–65.

75 *who drank no tea* Sesso, H., J. M. Gaziano, J. Buring, et al. 1999. Coffee and tea intake and the risk of myocardial infarction. *Am J Epidem* 149(2):162-7.

80 *their genes were identical* Atkinson, R. L., N. V. Dhurandhar, D. B. Allison, R. L. Bowen, B. A. Israel, J. B. Albu, and A. S. Augustus. 2005. Human adenovirus-36 is associated with increased body weight and paradoxical reduction of serum lipids. *Int J Obes* (London) 29(3):281–86.

82 *most benefit from tea* Wu, A. H., C. C. Tseng, D. van Den Berg, and M. C. Yu. 2003. Tea intake, COMT genotype, and breast cancer in Asian-American women. *Cancer Res* 63(21):7526–29.

83 *heart disease at an early age* Helgadottir, A., G. Thorleifsson, A. Manolescu, et al. 2007. A common variant on chromosome 9p21 affects the risk of myocardial infarction. *Science* 316(5830):1491–3. http://www.sciencemag.org/cgi/content/abstract/1142842

83 *those of African descent* McPherson, R., A. Pertsemlidis, H. Kavaslar. et al. 2007. A common allele on chromosome 9 associated with coronary heart disease. *Science* 316(5830):1488–91.

84 *increased risk of obesity* Frayling, T. M., N. Timpson, M. Weedon, et al. 2007. A common variant in the FTO gene is associated with body mass index and predisposes to childhood and adult obesity. *Science* 316(5826):889–94.

84 *some of the same genes* Stunkard, A. J., J. R. Harris, N. L. Pedersen, and G. E. McClearn. 1990. The body-mass index of twins who have been reared apart. *N Engl J Med* 322(21):1483–87.

86 *and after five years* Ornish, D., L. W. Scherwitz, J. H. Billings, K. L. Gould, T. A. Merritt, S. Sparler, W. T. Armstrong, et al. 1998. Intensive lifestyle changes for reversal of coronary heart disease. *JAMA* 280(23):2001–2007.

86 *their prostate tumor growth* Ornish, D., G. Weidner, W. R. Fair, R. Marlin, E. B. Pettengill, C. J. Raisin, S. Dunn-Emke, et al. 2005. Intensive lifestyle changes may affect the progression of prostate cancer. *J Urol* 174(3):1065–69; discussion 1069–70.

87 *related to diet and disease* Kallio, P., M. Kolehmainen, D. Laaksonen, et al. 2007. Dietary carbohydrate modification induces alterations in gene expression in abdominal subcutaneous adipose tissue in persons with the metabolic syndrome: The FUNGENUT Study. *Am J Clin Nutr* 85(5):1417–27.

87 *obesity, diabetes, and heart disease* Salsberg, S. L., and D. S. Ludwig. 2007. Putting your genes on a diet: The molecular effects of carbohydrate. *Am J Clin Nutr* 85(5):1169–70.

Chapter 5

116 *lower their telomerase level* Epel, E. S., E. H. Blackburn, J. Lin, F. S. Dhabhar, N. E. Adler, J. D. Morrow, and R. M. Cawthon. 2004. Accelerated telomere shortening in response to life stress. *Proc Natl Acad Sci* 101(49):17312–15 (Epub December).

118 *antidepressants such as Prozac* Caspi, A., K. Sugden, T. E. Moffitt, A. Taylor, I. W. Craig, H. Harrington, J. McClay, J. Mill, J. Martin, A. Braithwaite, and R. Poulton. 2003. Influence of life stress on depression: Moderation by a polymorphism in the 5-HTT gene. *Science* 301(5631):386–89.

118 *signs of being depressed* Bennett, A. J., K. P. Lesch, A. Heils, J. C. Long, J. G. Lorenz, S. E. Shoaf, M. Champoux, S. J. Suomi, M. V. Linnoila, and J. D. Higley. 2002. Early experience and serotonin transporter gene variation interact to influence primate CNS function. *Mol Psychiatry* 7(1):118–22.

120 *again after five years* Ornish, D., S. E. Brown, L. W. Scherwitz, J. H. Billings, W. T. Armstrong, T. A. Ports, S. M. McLanahan, R. L. Kirkeeide, R. J. Brand, and K. L. Gould. 1990. Can lifestyle changes reverse coronary heart disease? *Lancet* 336(8708):129–33.

Ornish, D., L. W. Scherwitz, J. H. Billings, K. L. Gould, T. A. Merritt, S. Sparler, W. T. Armstrong, et al. 1998. Intensive lifestyle changes for reversal of coronary heart disease. *JAMA* 280(23):2001–2007.

Pischke, C. R., L. Schwerwitz, G. Weidner, and D. Ornish. 2007. Long-term effects of intensive lifestyle changes on psychological well-being, health behaviors, and cardiac parameters among CHD patients in the Lifestyle Heart Trial. Annual Meeting and Scientific Sessions of the Society of Behavioral Medicine (SBM), Washington, DC.

126 *Program for Reversing Heart Disease* Ornish, D. *Dr. Dean Ornish's Program for Reversing Heart Disease*. New York: Random House, 1990. Ballantine Books, 1992.

128 *anger and hostility* Pischke, C. R., L. Schwerwitz, G. Weidner, and D. Ornish. 2007. Long-term effects of intensive lifestyle changes on psychological well-being, health behaviors, and cardiac parameters among CHD patients in the Lifestyle Heart Trial. Annual Meeting and Scientific Sessions of the Society of Behavioral Medicine (SBM), Washington, DC.

128 *anxiety in a recent study* Pischke, C. R., L. Scherwitz, G. Weidner, and D. Ornish. 2008 (in press). Long-term effects of lifestyle changes on well-being and cardiac variables among CHD patients. *Health Psychol.*

Chapter 8

141 *brain actually gets bigger* Pereira, A., D. Huddleston, A. Brickman, et al. 2007. An in vivo correlate of exercise-induced neurogenesis in the adult dentate gyrus. *PNAS* 104(13):5638–43.

Colcombe, S. J., K. Erickson, P. Scalf, et al. 2006. Aerobic exercise training increases brain volume in aging humans. *J Geron: Med Sci* 61A(11) 1166–70.

141 *in weight or diet* Kilpeläinen, T. O., T. A. Lakke, D. E. Lanksonen, et al. 2007. Physical activity modifies the effect of SNPs in the SLC2A2 (GLUT2) and

ABCC8 (SUR1) genes on the risk of developing type 2 diabetes. *Physiol Genomics.* July 17 (Epub ahead of print).

142 *than three hundred genes* Melov, S., M. A. Tarnopolsky, K. Beckman, K. Felkey, and A. Hubbard. 2007. Resistance exercise reverses aging in human skeletal muscle. PLoS ONE 2(5):e465. doi:10.1371/journal.pone.0000465.

142 *run up the stairs* Pischke, C. R., L. Scherwitz, G. Weidner, and D. Ornish. 2008 (in press). Long-term effects of lifestyle changes on well-being and cardiac variables among CHD patients. *Health Psychol.*

143 *damaged or non-functioning* Toni, N., E. M. Teng, E. A. Bushong, J. B. Aimone, C. Zhao, A. Consiglio, H. van Praag, M. E. Martone, M. H. Ellisman, and F. H. Gage. 2007. Synapse formation on neurons born in the adult hippocampus. *Nat Neurosci* 10(6):727–34 (Epub May).

143 *functioning in older adults* Colcombe, S. J., K. Erickson, P. Scalf, et al. 2006. Aerobic exercise training increases brain volume in aging humans. *J Geron: Med Sci* 61A(11):1166–70.

143 *a matter of reversing it* Carmichael, M. 2007. Stronger, faster, smarter. *Newsweek,* March.

143 *at least in rats* Jiang, W., Y. Zhang, L. Xiao, et al. 2005. Cannabinoids promote embryonic and adult hippocampus neurogenesis and produce anxiolytic- and antidepressant-like effects. *J Clin Invest* 115(11):3104–16. (Epub October).

144 *found in obese kids* Miller, J., J. Kranzler, Y. Liu, et al. 2006. Neurocognitive findings in Prader-Willi syndrome and early-onset morbid obesity. *J Pediatr* 149(2):192–98.

145 *suggested by the surgeon general* US Department of Health and Human Services. 1996. Physical Activity and Health: A Report of the Surgeon General. US Dept of Health and Human Services, Centers for Disease Control and Prevention, National Center for Disease Control and Prevention and Health Promotion, Atlanta, GA.

147 *attack and stroke in half* Lee, I. M., K. M. Rexrode, N. R. Cook, J. E. Manson, and J. E. Buring. 2001. Physical activity and coronary heart disease in women: Is "no pain, no gain" passe? *JAMA* 285(11):1447–54.

147 *borderline high blood pressure* Church, E. S., C. P. Earnest, J. S. Skinner, and S. N. Blair. 2007. Effects of different doses of physical activity on cardiorespiratory fitness among sedentary, overweight or obese postmenopausal women with elevated blood pressure. *JAMA* 297(19):2081–91.

153 *you have to walk them* Jennings, L. B. 1997. Potential benefits of pet ownership in health promotion. *J Holist Nurs* 15(4):358–72.

153 *been sedentary for a while* Whaley, M. H., P. H. Brubaker, and M. Otto, eds. 2006. *ACSM's Guidelines for Exercise Testing and Prescription.* 7th ed. Philadelphia: Lippincott Williams & Wilkins.

Chapter 9

161 *that promote inflammation* Sies, H., T. Schewe, C. Heiss, and M. Kelm. 2005. Cocoa polyphenols and inflammatory mediators. *Am J Clin Nutr* 81 (Suppl. 1):S304–12.

161 *only modified their diet* Stefanick, M. L., S. Mackey, M. Sheehan, N. Ellsworth, W. L. Haskell, and P. D. Wood. 1998. Effects of diet and exercise in men and postmenopausal women with low levels of HDL cholesterol and high levels of LDL cholesterol. *New Engl J Med* 339(1):12–20.

162 *those who did not* Mansur, A. P., C. V. Serrano, J. C. Nicolau, L. A. César, and J. A. Ramires. 1999. Effect of cholesterol lowering treatment on positive exercise tests in patients with hypercholesterolaemia and normal coronary angiograms. *Heart* 82(6):689–93.

162 *protective cholesterol lipoproteins* Kraus, W. E., J. A. Houmard, B. D. Duscha, K. J. Knetzger, M. B. Wharton, J. S. McCartney, C. W. Bales, et al. 2002. Effects of the amount and intensity of exercise on plasma lipoproteins. *New Engl J Med* 347(19):1483–92.

163 *in your arteries* Liu, S., M. J. Stampfer, F. B. Hu, E. Giovannucci, E. Rimm, J. E. Manson, C. H. Hennekens, and W. C. Willett. 1999. Whole-grain consumption and risk of coronary heart disease: Results from the Nurses' Health Study. *Am J Clin Nutr* 70(3):412–19.

Chapter 10

169 *will eventually become overweight* Vasan, R. D., M. Pencina, M. Cobain, et al. 2005. Estimated risks for developing obesity in the Framingham Heart Study. *Ann Intern Med* 143(7):473–80.

169 *osteoarthritis, and some cancers* Marantz, H. R. 2006. Fat factors. *The New York Times Magazine*, August.

170 *weight five years later* Ornish, D., S. E. Brown, L. W. Scherwitz, J. H. Billings, W. T. Armstrong, T. A. Ports, S. M. McLanahan, R. L. Kirkeeide, R. J. Brand, and K. L. Gould. 1990. Can lifestyle changes reverse coronary heart disease? *Lancet* 336(8708):129–33.

Ornish, D., L. W. Scherwitz, J. H. Billings, K. L. Gould, T. A. Merritt, S. Sparler, W. T. Armstrong, et al. 1998. Intensive lifestyle changes for reversal of coronary heart disease. *JAMA* 280(23):2001–2007.

171 *not to increase it* Rudel, L. L., and K. Kavanagh. 2006. Trans fat leads to weight gain even on same total calories. Presented at the 66th annual Scientific Sessions of the American Diabetes Association, Washington, DC.

171 *DNA damage and insulin levels* Heilbronn, L. K., L. de Jonge, M. I. Frisard, J. P. DeLany, D. E. Larson-Meyer, J. Rood, T. Nguyen, et al.; Pennington CALERIE Team. 2006. Effect of 6-month calorie restriction on biomarkers of longevity, metabolic adaptation, and oxidative stress in overweight individuals: A randomized controlled trial. *JAMA* 295(13):1539–48.

175 *in two important ways* Ahlberg, A. C., T. Ljung, R. Rosmond, B. McEwen, G. Holm, H. O. Akesson, and P. Björntorp. 2002. Depression and anxiety symptoms in relation to anthropometry and metabolism in men. *Psychiatry Res* 112(2): 101–10.

Kyrou, I., G. P. Chrousos, and C. Tsigos. 2006. Stress, visceral obesity, and metabolic complications. *Ann NY Acad Sci* 1083:77–110.

Brunner, E. J., T. Chandola, and M. G. Marmot. 2007. Prospective effect of job strain on general and central obesity in the Whitehall II Study. *Am J Epidem* 165(7):828–37; doi:10.1093/aje/kwk058.

175 *amount of fat they lost* Daubenmier, J. J., G. Weidner, M. D. Sumner, N. Mendell, T. Merritt-Worden, J. Studley, and D. Ornish. 2007. The contribution of changes in diet, exercise, and stress management to changes in coronary risk in women and men in the multisite cardiac lifestyle intervention program. *Ann Behav Med* 33(1):57–68.

176 *belly fat, a double whammy* Kuo, L. E., J. B. Kitlinska, J. U. Tilan, L. Li, S. B.

Baker, M. D. Johnson, and E. W. Lee. 2007. Neuropeptide Y acts directly in the periphery on fat tissue and mediates stress-induced obesity and metabolic syndrome. *Nature Med* 13(7):803–11 (Epub July).

176 *positive or negative ways*   Legendre, A., and R.B.S Harris. 2006. Exaggerated response to mild stress in rats fed high-fat diet. *Am J Physiol Regul Integr Comp Physiol* 291(5):R1288–94.

176 *fat they accumulated*   Brunner, E. J., T. Chandola T, and M. G. Marmot MG. 2007. Prospective effect of job strain on general and central obesity in the Whitehall II Study. Am J Epidem 165(7):828-37; doi:10.1093/aje/kwk058.

177 *anxious and depressed*   Ahlberg, A. C., T. Ljung, R. Rosmond, B. McEwen, G. Holm, H. O. Akesson, and P. Björntorp. 2002. Depression and anxiety symptoms in relation to anthropometry and metabolism in men. *Psychiatry Res* 112(2):101-10.

Chapter 11

180 *United States has hypertension*   Burt, V. L., P. Whelton, E. J. Roccella, C. Brown, J. A. Cutler, M. Higgins, M. J. Horan, and D. Labarthe. 1995. Prevalence of hypertension in the US adult population. Results from the 3rd National Health and Nutrition Examination Survey, 1988–1991. *Hypertension* 25(3):305–13.

181 *was their blood pressure*   Ascherio, A., C. Hennekens, W. C. Willett, F. Sacks, B. Rosner, J. Manson, J. Witteman, and M. J. Stampfer. 1996. Prospective study of nutritional factors, blood pressure, and hypertension among U.S. women. *Hypertension* 27(5):1065–72.

Ascherio, A., E. B. Rimm, E. L. Giovannucci, G. A. Colditz, B. Rosner, W. C. Willett, F. Sacks, M. J. Stampfer. 1992. A prospective study of nutritional factors, and hypertension among U.S. men. *Circulation* 86(5):1475–84.

181 *American Medical Association*   Sacks, F. M., D. Ornish, B. Rosner, S. McLanahan, W. P. Castelli, and E. H. Kass. 1985. Dietary predictors of blood pressure and plasma lipoproteins in lactovegetarians. *JAMA* 254(10):1337–41.

181 *have shown smaller findings*   Rouse, I. L., B. K. Armstrong, and L. J. Beilin. 1983. The relationship of blood pressure to diet and lifestyle in two religious populations. *J Hypertens* 1(1):65–71.

181 *meat and refined carbohydrates*   Appel, L. J., T. J. Moore, E. Obarzanek, W. M. Vollmer, L. P. Svetkey, F. M. Sacks, G. A. Bray; DASH Collaborative Research Group. 1997. A clinical trial of the effects of dietary patterns on blood pressure. *New Engl J Med* 336(16):1117–24.

181 *a low-fat diet, too*   Sacks, F. M., L. P. Svetkey, W. M. Vollmer, L. J. Appel, G. A. Bray, D. Harsha, E. Obarzanek, et al.; DASH-Sodium Collaborative Research Group. 2001. Effects on blood pressure of reduced dietary sodium and the Dietary Approaches to Stop Hypertension (DASH) diet. *New Engl J Med* 344(1): 3–10.

182 *develop high blood pressure*   Blair, S. N., N. N. Goodyear, L. W. Gibbons, and K. H. Cooper. 1984. Physical fitness and incidence of hypertension in healthy normotensive men and women. *JAMA* 252(4):487–90.

Carnethon, M. R., S. S. Gidding, R. Nehgme, S. Sidney, D. R. Jacobs, and K. Liu. 2003. Cardiorespiratory fitness in young adulthood and the development of cardiovascular disease risk factors. *JAMA* 290(23):3092–100.

Paffenbarger, R. S., A. L. Wing, R. T. Hyde, and D. L. Jung. 1983. Physical activity and incidence of hypertension in college alumni. *Am J Epidem* 117(3):245–57.

182 *largely independent of weight loss*   Arroll, B., and R. Beaglehole. 1992. Does physical activity lower blood pressure: A critical review of the clinical trials. *J Clin Epidem* 45(5):439–47.

Whelton, S. P., A. Chin, X. Xin, and J. He. 2002. Effect of aerobic exercise on blood pressure: A meta-analysis of randomized, controlled trials. *Ann Intern Med* 136(7):493–503.

Kelley, G. A., K. S. Kelley, and Z. V. Tran. 2001. Aerobic exercise and resting blood pressure: A meta-analysis review of randomized, controlled trials. *Prev Cardiol* 4(2):73–80.

Kelley, G. A., and K. S. Kelley. 2000. Progressive resistance exercise and resting blood pressure: A meta-analysis of randomized controlled trials. *Hypertension* 35(3):838–43.

Ishikawa, K., T. Ohta, J. Zhang, S. Hashimoto, and H. Tanaka. 1999. Influence of age and gender on exercise training-induced blood pressure reduction in systemic hypertension. *Am J Cardiol* 84(2):192–96.

Seals, D. R., H. G. Silverman, M. J. Reiling, and K. P. Davy. 1997. Effect of regular aerobic exercise on elevated blood pressure in postmenopausal women. *Am J Cardiol* 80(1):49–55.

182 *pressure in hypertensive patients*   Tanaka, H., M. J. Reiling, and R. J. Seals. 1998. Regular walking increases peak limb vasodilatory capacity in older hypertensive humans: Implications for arterial structure. *J Hypertens* 16(4):423–28.

Higashi, Y., S. Sasaki, S. Kurisu, A. Yoshimizu, N. Sasaki, H. Matsuura, G. Kajiyama, and T. Oshima. 1999. Regular aerobic exercise augments endothelium-dependent vascular relaxation in normotensive as well as hypertensive subjects: Role of endothelium-derived nitric oxide. *Circulation* 100:1194–202.

182 *changing their diet and exercise*   Barnard, R. J., E. J. Ugianskis, and D. A. Martin. 1992. The effects of an intensive diet and exercise program on patients with NIDDM and hypertension. *J Cardiopulm Rehabil* 12:194–201.

182 *reductions in blood pressure*   Miller III, E. R., P. Erlinger, D. R. Young, M. Jehn, J. Charleston, D. Rhodes, S. K. Wasan, and L. J. Appels. 2002. Results of the Diet, Exercise, and Weight Loss Intervention Trial (DEW-IT). *Hypertension* 40(5):612–18.

Writing Group of the PCRG. 2003. Effects of comprehensive lifestyle modification on blood pressure control: Main results of the PREMIER clinical trial. *JAMA* 289(16):2083–93.

183 *said the study's lead investigator*   Georgiades, A., A. Sherwood, E. C. Gullette, M. A. Babyak, A. Hinderliter, R. Waugh, D. Tweedy, L. Craighead, R. Bloomer, and J. A. Blumenthal. 2000. Effects of exercise and weight loss on mental stress-induced cardiovascular responses in individuals with high blood pressure. *Hypertension* 36(2):171–76.

184 *effect on your blood pressure*   Everson, S. A., G. A. Kaplan, D. E. Goldberg, and J. T. Salonen. 2000. Hypertension incidence is predicted by high levels of hopelessness in Finnish men. *Hypertension* 35(2):561–67.

184 *negative effects of stress*   Bairey Merz, C. N., W. Kop, D. S. Krantz, K. F. Helmers, D. S. Berman, and A. Rozanski. 1998. Cardiovascular stress response and coronary artery disease: Evidence of an adverse postmenopausal effect in women. *Am Heart J* 135(5 Pt 1):881–87.

184 *another predictor of bad outcomes*   Jennings, J. R., T. W. Kamarck, S. A. Everson-Rose, G. A. Kaplan, S. B. Manuck, and J. T. Salonen. 2004. Exaggerated blood

pressure responses during mental stress are prospectively related to enhanced carotid atherosclerosis in middle-aged Finnish men. *Circulation* 110(15):2198–203 (Epub September).

184 *attendant stressors are high*   Shepard, J. D., M. al'Absi, T. L. Whitsett, R. B. Passey, and W. R. Lovallo. 2000. Additive pressor effects of caffeine and stress in male medical students at risk for hypertension. *Am J Hypertens* 13(5 Pt 1): 475–81.

184 *use of antihypertensive medications*   Schneider, R. H., C. N. Alexander, F. Staggers, D. W. Orme-Johnson, M. Rainforth, J. W. Salerno, W. Sheppard, A. Castillo-Richmond, V. A. Barnes, and S. I. Nidich. 2005. A randomized controlled trial of stress reduction in African Americans treated for hypertension for over one year. *Am J Hypertens* 18(1):88–98.

185 *premature mortality from cancer*   Schneider, R. H., C. N. Alexander, F. Staggers, M. Rainforth, J. W. Salerno, A. Hartz, S. Arndt, V. A. Barnes, and S. I. Nidich. 2005. Long-term effects of stress reduction on mortality in persons > or = 55 years of age with systemic hypertension. *Am J Cardiol* 95(9):1060–64.

185 *In a recent study*   Jakulj, F., K. Zernicke, S. L. Bacon, L. E. van Wielingen, B. L. Key, S. G. West, and T. S. Campbell. 2007. A high-fat meal increases cardiovascular reactivity to psychological stress in healthy young adults. *J Nutr* 137(4):935–39.

185 *oxidative stress showed improvement*   Roberts, C. K., N. D. Vaziri, and R. J. Barnard. 2002. Effect of diet and exercise intervention on blood pressure, insulin, oxidative stress, and nitric oxide availability. *Circulation* 106:2530–32.

185 *to reduce oxidative stress*   Stefano, G. B., and T. Esch. 2005. Integrative medical therapy: Examination of meditation's therapeutic and global medicinal outcomes via nitric oxide. *Int J Mol Med* 16(4):621–30. Review.
Kim, D. H., Y. S. Moon, H. S. Kim, J. S. Jung, H. M. Park, H. W. Suh, Y. H. Kim, and D. K. Song. 2005. Effect of Zen meditation on serum nitric oxide activity and lipid peroxidation. *Prog Neuropsychopharm Biol Psychiatry* 29(2):327–31 (Epub December 2004).

186 *the Spectrum is so beneficial*   Cuevas, A. M., and A. M. Germain. 2004. Diet and endothelial function. *Biol Res* 37(2):225–30.

186 *blood pressure (about 2mm/Hg)*   Taubert, D., R. Roesen, C. Lehmann, N. Jung, and E. Schömig. 2007. Effects of low habitual cocoa intake on blood pressure and bioactive nitric oxide: A randomized controlled trial. *JAMA* 298(1):49–60.

186 *improvement in blood flow*   Heiss, C., A. Dejam, P. Kleinbongard, T. Schewe, H. Sies, and M. Kelm. 2003. Vascular effects of cocoa rich in Flavan-3-ols. *JAMA* 290(8):1030–31.

186 *measured by MRI scans*   Fisher, N. D., F. A. Sorond, and N. K. Hollenberg. 2006. Cocoa flavanols and brain perfusion. *J Cardiovasc Pharmacol* 47(2 Suppl): S210–14.
Francis, S. T., K. Head, P. G. Morris, I. A. Macdonald. 2006. The effect of flavanol-rich cocoa on the fMRI response to a cognitive task in healthy young people. *J Cardiovasc Pharmacol* 47(2 Suppl):S215–20.

Chapter 12

190 *abnormally high blood pressure*   Perez-Pena, R. 2007. One in eight adults in the city has diabetes, a study finds. *New York Times,* January 31.

190 *blindness from diabetes than men*   National Center for Chronic Disease Prevention

and Health Promotion. October 2001. Diabetes and women's health across the life stages: A public health perspective. http://www.cdc.gov/diabetes/pubs/women/ (accessed July 12, 2007).

190 *continued to increase since then* American Diabetes Association. 1996. Diabetes 1996: Vital statistics. American Diabetes Association; Alexandria, VA.

Mokdad, A. H., B. A. Bowman, E. S. Ford, F. Vinicor, J. S. Marks, and J. P. Koplan. 2001. The continuing epidemics of obesity and diabetes in the United States. *JAMA* 286(10):1195–200.

Mokdad, A. H., E. S. Ford, B. A. Bowman, W. H. Dietz, F. Vinicor, V. S. Bales, and J. S. Marks. 2003. Prevalence of obesity, diabetes, and obesity-related health risk factors. *JAMA* 289(1):76–79.

191 *rates are very high* Ravussin, E., M. E. Valencia, J. Esparza, P. H. Bennett, and L. O. Schulz. 1994. Effects of traditional lifestyle on obesity in Pima Indians. *Diabetes Care* 17(9):1067–74.

192 *are not so exposed* National Center for Chronic Disease Prevention and Health Promotion. October 2001. Diabetes and women's health across the life stages: A public health perspective. *http://www.cdc.gov/diabetes/pubs/women/* (accessed July 12, 2007).

192 *intensive lifestyle-change group* Knowler, W. C., E. Barrett-Connor, S. E. Fowler, R. F. Hamman, J. M. Lachin, E. A. Walker, and D. M. Nathan; Diabetes Prevention Research Group. 2002. Reduction in the incidence of type 2 diabetes with lifestyle intervention or metformin. *New Engl J Med* 346(6):393–403.

193 *Diabetes Prevention Program study* Lindström, J., P. Ilanne-Parikka, M. Peltonen, et al. 2006. Sustained reduction in the incidence of type 2 diabetes by lifestyle intervention: Follow-up of the Finnish Diabetes Prevention Study. *Lancet* 368(9548):1673–79.

193 *need for cholesterol-lowering drugs* Pi-Sunyer, X., G. Blackburn, F. L. Brancati, G. A. Bray, R. Bright, J. J. M. Clark, J. M. Curtis, et al.; Look AHEAD Research Group. 2007. Reduction in weight and cardiovascular disease risk factors in individuals with type 2 diabetes: One-year results of the look AHEAD trial. *Diabetes Care* 30(6):1374–83 (Epub March).

193 *reduce their diabetes medications* Pischke, C. R., G. Weidner, M. Elliott-Eller, L. Scherwitz, T. A. Merritt-Worden, R. Marlin, L. Lipsenthal, et al. 2006. Comparison of coronary risk factors and quality of life in coronary artery disease patients with versus with out diabetes mellitus. *Am J Cardiol* 97(9):1267–73 (Epub March).

193 *indicating reduced inflammation* Dewell, A., G. Weidner, M. D. Sumner, R. J. Barnard, R. O. Marlin, J. J. Daubenmier, C. Chi, P. R. Carroll, and D. Ornish. 2007. Relationship of dietary protein and soy isoflavones to serum IGF-1 and IGF binding proteins in the Prostate Cancer Lifestyle Trial. *Nutr Cancer* 58(1):35–42.

194 *increased the risk of diabetes* Van Dam, R. M., E. B. Rimm, W. C. Willett, J. M. Stampfer, and D. B. Hu. 2002. Dietary patterns and risk for type 2 diabetes mellitus in US men. *Ann Intern Med* 136(3):201–209.

194 *reduce the risk of diabetes* Pan, D. A., S. Lillioja, M. R. Milner, A. D. Kriketos, L. A. Baur, C. Bogardus, and L. H. Storlien. Skeletal muscle membrane lipid composition is related to adiposity and insulin action. *J Clin Invest* 96(6):2802–808.

Feskens, E. J., C. H. Bowles, and D. Kromhout. 1991. Inverse association between fish intake and risk of glucose intolerance in normoglycemic elderly men and women. *Diabetes Care* 14(11):935–41.

Feskens, E. J., S. M. Virtanen, L. Rasanen, J. Tuomilehto, J. Stengard, J. Pekkanen, A. Nissinen, and D. Kromhout. 1995. Dietary factors determining diabetes and impaired glucose tolerance. A 20-year follow-up of the Finnish and Dutch cohorts of the Seven Countries Study. *Diabetes Care* 18(8):1104–12.

Salmeron, J., F. B. Hu, J. E. Manson, M. J. Stampfer, G. A. Colditz, E. B. Rimm, and W. C. Willett. 2001. Dietary fat intake and risk of type 2 diabetes in women. *Am J Clin Nutr* 73(6):1019–26.

194 *those on the ADA diet* Barnard, N. D., J. Cohen, D. J. Jenkins, G. Turner-McGrievy, L. Gloede, B. Jaster, K. Seidl, A. A. Green, and S. Talpers. 2006. A low-fat vegan diet improves glycemic control and cardiovascular risk factors in a randomized clinical trial in individuals with type 2 diabetes. *Diabetes Care* 29(8): 1777–83.

194 *such as coronary heart disease* Wellen, K. E., and G. S. Hotamisligil. 2005. Inflammation, stress, and diabetes. *J Clin Investigation* 115(5):1111–19.

194 *shown to reduce inflammation* Liu, S., J. E. Manson, J. E. Buring, M. J. Stampfer, W. C. Willett, and P. M. Ridker. 2002. Relation between a diet with a high glycemic load and plasma concentrations of high-sensitivity C-reactive protein in middle-aged women. *Am J Clin Nutr* 75(3):492–98.

Middleton Jr., E. 1998. Effect of plant flavonoids on immune and inflammatory cell function. *Adv Exp Med Biol* 439:175–82.

194 *to increase insulin sensitivity* Perez-Jimenez, F., J. Lopez-Miranda, M. D. Pinillos, P. Gomez, E. Paz-Rojas, P. Montilla, and C. Marlin. 2001. A Mediterranean and a high-carbohydrate diet improve glucose metabolism in healthy young persons. *Diabetologia* 44(11):2038–43.

195 *reduce their risk significantly* Prediabetes may raise risk for Alzheimer's. *USA Today*. http://www.usatoday.com/news/health/2006-07-16-prediabetes_x.htm (accessed July 16, 2006).

Grady, D., 2006. Link between diabetes and Alzheimer's deepens. *New York Times*. July 17.

195 *was 83 percent higher* Xu, W., C. Qiu, B. Winblad, and L. Fratiglioni. 2007. The effect of borderline diabetes on the risk of dementia and Alzheimer's disease. *Diabetes* 56(1):211–16.

195 *reduce the risk of diabetes* Kilpeläinen, T. O., T. A. Lakka, D. E. Laaksonen, et al. 2007. Physical activity modifies the effect of SNPs in the SLC2A2 (GLUT2) and ABCC8 (SUR1) genes on the risk of developing type 2 diabetes. *Physiol Genomics,* doi:10.1152/physio/genomics.00036.2007 (Epub ahead of print; accessed July 25, 2007).

195 *three hours per week* Lakka, T. A., D. E. Laaksonen, H. M. Lakka, N. Mannikko, L. K. Niskanen, R. Rauramaa, and J. T. Salonen. 2003. Sedentary lifestyle, poor cardiorespiratory fitness, and the metabolic syndrome. *Med Sci Sports Exerc* 35(8):1279–86.

196 *criteria for metabolic syndrome* Katzmarzyk, P. T., A. S. Leon, J. H. Wilmore, J. S. Skinner, D. C. Rao, T. Rankinen, and C. Bouchard. 2003. Targeting the metabolic syndrome with exercise; evidence from the HERITAGE study. *Med Sci Sports Exerc* 35(10):1703–709.

196 *people with metabolic syndrome* Katzmarzyk, P. T., T. S. Church, and S. N. Blair. 2004. Cardiorespiratory fitness attenuates the effects of the metabolic syndrome on all-cause and cardiovascular disease mortality in men. *Arch Internal Med* 164(10):1092–97.

196 *as much as 40 mg/dl* Hübinger, A., A. Franzen, and F. A. Gries. 1987. Hormonal and metabolic response to physical exercise in hyperinsulinemic and non-hyperinsulinemic type 2 diabetics. *Diabetes Res* 4(2):57–61.
Laws, A., and G. M. Reaven. 1991. Physical activity, glucose tolerance, and diabetes in older adults. 1991. *Ann Behav Med* 13:125–31.

196 *by 10 to 20 percent* Sigal, R. J., G. P. Kenny, D. H. Wasserman, C. Castaneda-Sceppa, and R. D. White. 2006. Physical activity/exercise and type 2 diabetes: A consensus statement from the American Diabetes Association. *Diabetes Care* 29(6):1433–38.

196 *after about seventy-two hours* Wallberg-Henriksson, H., J. Rincon, and J. R. Zierath. 1998. Exercise in the management of non-insulin-dependent diabetes mellitus. *Sports Med* 25(1):25–35.

197 *(as measured by hemoglobin A1C)* Daubenmier, J. J., G. Weidner, M. D. Sumner, N. Mendell, T. Merritt-Worden, J. Studley, and D. Ornish. 2007. The contribution of changes in diet, exercise, and stress management to changes in coronary risk in women and men in the multisite cardiac lifestyle intervention program. *Ann Behav Med* 33(1):57–68.

197 *some diabetes-control drugs* Surwit, R. S., M. A. van Tilburg, N. Zucker, C. C. McCaskill, P. Parekh, M. N. Feinglos, C. L. Edwards, P. Williams, and J. D. Lane. 2002. Stress management improves long-term glycemic control in type 2 diabetes. *Diabetes Care* 25(1):30–34.

197 *saturated fat and calories* Fisher, L., M. M. Skaff, J. T. Mullan, P. Arean, D. Mohr, U. Masharani, R. Glasgow, and G. Laurencin. 2007. Clinical depression versus distress among patients with type 2 diabetes: Not just a question of semantics. *Diabetes Care* 30(3):542–48.

197 *more than double the risk* Räikkönen, K., K. A. Matthews, and L. H. Kuller. 2007. Depressive symptoms and stressful life events predict metabolic syndrome among middle-aged women: A comparison of World Health Organization, Adult Treatment Panel III, and International Diabetes Foundation definitions. *Diabetes Care* 30(4):872–77.

Chapter 13

203 *by at least one-third* Critchley, J., and S. Capewell. 2003. Smoking cessation for the secondary prevention of coronary heart disease. *Cochrane Database of Systematic Reviews* Issue 4. Art. No.: CD003041. doi: 10.1002/14651858.CD003041 .pub2.

203 *practiced stress-management techniques* Schuler, G., R. Hambrecht, G. Schlierf, M. Grunze, S. Methfessel, K. Hauer, and W. Kübler. 1992. Myocardial perfusion and regression of coronary artery disease in patients on a regimen of intensive physical exercise and low fat diet. *J Am Coll Cardiol* 19(1):34–42.

204 *deaths from heart disease* Sdringola, S., K. Nakagawa, Y. Nakagawa, S. W. Yusuf, F. Boccalandro, N. Mullani, M. Haynie, M. J. Hess, and K. L. Gould. 2003. Combined intense lifestyle and pharmacologic lipid treatment further reduce coronary events and myocardial perfusion abnormalities compared with usual-care cholesterol-lowering drugs in coronary artery disease. *J Am Coll Cardiol* 41(2):263–72.

205 *heart disease in others* Stefanick, M. L., S. Mackey, M. Sheehan, N. Ellsworth, W. L. Haskell, and P. D. Wood. 1998. Effects of diet and exercise in men and postmenopausal women with low levels of HDL cholesterol and high levels of LDL cholesterol. *N Engl J Med* 339(1):12–20.

205 *developing coronary heart disease*   McCullough, M. L., D. Feskanich, E. B. Rimm, E. L. Giovannucci, A. Ascherio, J. N. Variyam, D. Spiegelman, M. J. Stampfer, and W. C. Willett. 2000. Adherence to the Dietary Guidelines for Americans and risk of major chronic disease in men. *Am J Clin Nutr* 72(5):1223–31.

McCullough, M. L., D. Feskanich, M. J. Stampfer, B. A. Rosner, F. B. Hu, D. J. Hunter, J. N. Variyam, G. A. Colditz, and W. C. Willett. 2000. Adherence to the Dietary Guidelines for Americans and risk of major chronic disease in women. *Am J Clin Nutr* 72(5):1214–22.

Meyerhardt, J. A., D. Niedzwiecki, D. Hollis, et al. 2007. Association of dietary patterns with cancer recurrence and survival in patients with stage III colon cancer. *JAMA* 298(7):754–64.

206 *amount of fruits and vegetables*   Howard, B. V., L. Van Horn, J. Hsia, J. E. Manson, M. L. Stefanick, S. Wassertheil-Smoller, L. H. Kuller, A. Z. LaCroix, et al. 2006. Low-fat dietary pattern and risk of cardiovascular disease: The Women's Health Initiative Randomized Controlled Dietary Modification Trial. *JAMA* 295(6):655–66.

207 *It isn't*   Ornish, D. 2004. Was Dr. Atkins right? *J Am Diet Assoc* 104(4):537–42.

209 *plaque with in only five weeks*   Forrester, J. S., and P. K. Shah. 2006. Emerging strategies for increasing HDL. *Am J Cardiol* 98(11):1542–49.

209 *measured by intravascular ultrasound*   Nissen, S. E., T. Tsunoda, E. Murat Tuzcu, et al. 2003. Effect of recombinant ApoA-I Milano on coronary atherosclerosis in patients with acute coronary syndromes: A randomized controlled trial. *JAMA* 290(17):2292–300.

210 *United States than in China*   Roberts, C. K., and J. R. Barnard. 2005. Effects of exercise and diet on chronic disease. *J App Physiol* 98(1):3–30.

210 *risk of cardiovascular disease*   Jacobs Jr., D. R., K. A. Meyer, L. H. Kushi, and A. R. Folsom. 1998. Whole-grain intake may reduce the risk of ischemic heart disease death in postmenopausal women: The Iowa Women's Health Study. *Am J Clin Nutr* 68(2):248–57.

Liu, S., M. J. Stampfer, F. B. Hu, E. Giovannucci, E. Rimm, J. E. Manson, C. H. Hennekens, and W. C. Willett. 1999. Whole-grain consumption and risk of coronary heart disease: Results from the Nurses' Health Study. *Am J Clin Nutr* 70(3):412–19.

Liu, S., W. C. Willett, M. J. Stampfer, F. B. Hu, M. Franz, L. Sampson, C. H. Hennekens, and J. E. Manson. 2000. A prospective study of dietary glycemic load, carbohydrate intake, and risk of coronary heart disease in US women. *Am J Clin Nutr* 71(6):1455–61.

210 *dense LDL particles*   Dreon, D. M., H. A. Fernstrom, P. T. Williams, and R. M. Krauss. 1999. A very low-fat diet is not associated with improved lipoprotein profiles in men with a predominance of large, low-density lipoproteins. *Am J Clin Nutr* 69(3):411–18.

210 *dense LDL particles*   Beard, C. M., R. J. Barnard, D. C. Robbins, J. M. Ordovas, and E. J. Schaefer. 1996. Effects of diet and exercise on qualitative and quantitative measures of LDL and its susceptibility to oxidation. *Arterioscler Thromb Vasc Bio* 16(2):201–207.

210 *LDL particles, decreased significantly*   Ornish, D., L. W. Scherwitz, J. H. Billings, K. L. Gould, T. A. Merritt, S. Sparler, W. T. Armstrong, et al. 1998. Intensive lifestyle changes for reversal of coronary heart disease. *JAMA* 80(23):2001–2007.

211 *risk of heart disease*   Liu, S., M. Stumpfer, F. Hu, et al. 1999. Whole-grain consumption and risk of coronary heart disease: Results from the Nurses' Health Study. *Am J Clin Nutr* 70(3):412–9.

211 *risk of heart disease* Oomen, C. M., M. C. Ocke, E. J. Feskens, M. A. van Erp-Baart, F. J. Kok, and D. Kromhout. 2001. Association between trans fatty acid intake and 10-year risk of coronary heart disease in the Zutphen Elderly Study: A prospective population-based study. *Lancet* 357(9258):746–51.

211 *eliminated from our diet* American Diabetes Association. 2007. Diabetes, Obesity, CVD News. www.diabetes.org/docnews.

211 *disease and their children* Patsch, J. R., G. Miesenbock, T. Hopferwieser, et al. 1992. Relation of triglyceride metabolism and coronary artery disease: Studies in the postprandial state. *Arterioscler Thromb* 12(11):1336–45.

Uiterwaal, C. S., D. E. Grobbee, J. C. Witteman, et al. 1994. Postprandial triglyceride response in young adult men and familial risk for coronary atherosclerosis. *Ann Intern Med* 121(8):576–83.

Karpe, F., G. Steiner, K. Uffelman, T. Olivecrona, and A. Hamsten. 1994. Postprandial lipoproteins and progression of coronary atherosclerosis. *Atherosclerosis* 106(1):83–97.

212 *help promote inflammation* Middleton Jr., E. 1998. Effect of plant flavonoids on immune and inflammatory cell function. *Adv Exp Med Biol* 439:175–82.

212 *also increase inflammation* Liu, S., J. E. Manson, J. E. Buring, M. J. Stampfer, W. C. Willett, and P. M. Ridker. 2002. Relation between a diet with a high glycemic load and plasma concentrations of high-sensitivity C-reactive protein in middle-aged women. *Am J Clin Nutr* 75(3):492–98.

212 *risk than LDL cholesterol* Ridker, P. M. 2003. Clinical application of C-reactive protein for cardiovascular disease detection and prevention. *Circulation* 107: 363–9.

Ridker, P. M., J. E. Buring, N. R. Cook, and N. Rifai. 2003. C-reactive protein, the metabolic syndrome, and risk of incident cardiovascular events: An 8-year follow-up of 14,719 initially healthy American women. *Circulation* 107:391–97.

Ridker, P. M., J. E. Buring, J. Shih, M. Matias, and C. H. Hennekens. 1998. Prospective study of C-reactive protein and the risk of future cardiovascular events among apparently healthy women. *Circulation* 98:731–33.

212 *heart disease in women* Ridker, P. M., J. E. Buring, N. Rifai, and N. R. Cook. 2007. Development and validation of improved algorithms for the assessment of global cardiovascular risk in women: The Reynolds Risk Score. *JAMA* 297(6): 611–19.

212 *a heart attack occuring* Heilbronn, L. K., and P. M. Clifton. 2002. C-reactive protein and coronary artery disease: Influence of obesity, caloric restriction and weight loss. *J Nutr Biochem* 13(6):316–21.

213 *after only two weeks* Wegge, J. K., C. K. Roberts, T. H. Ngo, and R. J. Barnard. 2004. Effect of diet and exercise intervention on inflammatory and adhesion molecules in post-menopausal women on hormone replacement therapy and at risk for coronary artery disease. *Metabolism* 53(3):377–81.

213 *C-reactive protein levels* Heilbronn, L. K., M. Noakes, and P. M. Clifton. 2001. Energy restriction and weight loss on very-low-fat diets reduce C-reactive protein concentrations in obese, healthy women. *Arterioscler Thromb Vasc Biol* 21(6): 968–70.

213 *by about one third* Jenkins, D. J., C. W. Kendall, A. Marchie, D. A. Faulkner, J. M. Wong, R. de Souza, A. Emam, et al. 2003. Effects of a dietary portfolio of cholesterol-lowering foods vs lovastatin on serum lipids and C-reactive protein. *JAMA* 290(4):502–10.

214 *more than eight years* Blair, S. N., H. W. Kohl, R. S. Paffenbarger, D. G. Clark,

K. H. Cooper, and L. W. Gibbons. 1989. Physical fitness and all-cause mortality: A prospective study of healthy men and women. *JAMA* 262(17):2395–401.

214 *costs, risks, and trauma* Hambrecht, R., C. Walther, S. Möbius-Winkler, S. Gielen, A. Linke, K. Conradi, S. Erbs, et al. 2004. Percutaneous coronary angioplasty compared with exercise training in patients with stable coronary artery disease: A randomized trial. *Circulation* 109(11):1371–78.

214 *also reduces inflammation* Ford, E. S. 2002. Does exercise reduce inflammation? Physical activity and C-reactive protein among US adults. *Epidemiology* 13(5):561–68.

215 *physical or emotional stress* Burke, A. P., A. Farb, G. T. Malcom, Y. Liang, J. E. Smialek, and R. Virmani. 1999. Plaque rupture and sudden death related to exertion in men with coronary artery disease. *JAMA* 281(10):921–26.

216 *monkeys were on the same diet* Kaplan, J. R., S. B. Manuck, T. B. Clarkson, F. M. Lusso, and D. M. Taub. 1982. Social status, environment, and atherosclerosis in cynomolgus monkeys. *Arteriosclerosis* 2(5):359–68.

216 *on a low-cholesteral diet* Williams, J. K., J. A. Vita, S. B. Manuck, A. P. Selwyn, and J. R. Kaplan. 1991. Psychosocial factors impair vascular responses of coronary arteries. *Circulation* 84(5):2146–53.

216 *and lack of exercise* Rosengren, A., S. Hawkin, S. Ounpuu, et al. 2004. Association of psychosocial risk factors with risk of acute myocardial infarction in 11,119 cases and 13,648 controls from 52 countries (the INTERHEART study): Case-control study. *Lancet* 364(9438):953–62.

216 *the majority of patients* Rozanski, A., C. N. Bairey, D. S. Krantz, J. Friedman, K. J. Resser, M. Morell, S. Hilton-Chalfen, L. Hestrin, J. Bietendorf, and D. S. Berman. 1988. Mental stress and the induction of silent myocardial ischemia in patients with coronary artery disease. *N Engl J Med* 318(16):1005–12.

216 *heart to pump blood* Bairey, C. N., D. S. Krantz, and A. Rozanski. 1990. Mental stress as an acute trigger of ischemic left ventricular dysfunction and blood pressure elevation in coronary artery disease. *Am J Cardiol* 66(16):28G–31G.

216 *people with out mental stress* Sheps, D. S., R. P. McMahon, L. Becker, R. M. Carney, K. E. Freedland, J. D. Cohen, D. Sheffield, et al. 2002. Mental stress-induced ischemia and all-cause mortality in patients with coronary artery disease: Results from the Psychophysiological Investigations of Myocardial Ischemia Study. *Circulation* 105(15):1780–84.

216 *buildup in coronary arteries* Matthews, K. A., and B. B. Gump. 2002. Chronic work stress and marital dissolution increase risk of posttrial mortality in men from the Multiple Risk Factor Intervention Trial. *Arch Intern Med* 162(3):309–15.

Orth-Gomer, K., S. P. Wamala, M. Horsten, K. Schenck-Gustafsson, N. Schneiderman, and M. A. Mittleman. 2000. Martial stress worsens prognosis in women with coronary heart disease: The Stockholm Female Coronary Risk Study. *JAMA* 284:3008–14.

Coyne, J. C., M. J. Rohrbaugh, V. Shoham, J. S. Sonnegra, J. M. Nicklas, and J. A. Cranford. 2001. Prognostic importance of marital quality for survival of congestive heart failure. *Am J Cardiol* 88:526–9.

Gallo, L. C., W. M. Troxel, L. H. Kuller, et al. 2003. Marital status, marital quality, and atherosclerotic burden in postmenopausal women. *Psychosom Med* 65(6): 952–62.

217 *having a heart attack* Rozanski, A., J. A. Blumenthal, and J. Kaplan. 1999. Impact of psychological factors on the pathogenesis of cardiovascular disease and implications for therapy. *Circulation* 99(16):2192–217.

Lesperance, F., N. Frasure-Smith, M. Talajic, and M. G. Bourassa. 2002. Five-year risk of cardiac mortality in relation to initial severity and one-year changes in depression symptoms after myocardial infarction. *Circulation* 105(3):1049–53.

217 *other inflammatory proteins*   Anisman, H., and Z. Merali. 2002. Cytokines, stress, and depressive illness. *Brain Behav Immun* 16(6):513–24.

217 *other illnesses as well*   Steptoe, A., N. Owen, S. Kunz-Ebrecht, and V. Mohamed-Ali. 2002. Inflammatory cytokines, socioeconomic status, and acute stress responsivity. *Brain Behav Immun* 16(6):774–84.

217 *reporting low stress levels*   Iso, H., C. Date, A. Yamamoto, H. Toyoshima, N. Tanabe, S. Kikuchi, T. Kondo, et al. 2002. Perceived mental stress and mortality from cardiovascular disease among Japanese men and women: The Japan Collaborative Cohort Study for evaluation of cancer risk sponsored by Monbusho (JACC Study). *Circulation* 106(10):1229–36.

217 *risk of fatal stroke*   Truelsen, T., N. Nielsen, G. Boysen, and M. Grønbaek; Copenhagen City Heart Study. 2003. Self-reported stress and risk of stroke: The Copenhagen City Heart Study. *Stroke* 34(4):856–62 (Epub March).

217 *this can be fatal*   Grady, D. 2005. Something to consider before you all shout, "Surprise, Grandma!" *New York Times.* June 5.

217 *reported more emotional distress*   Hedges, C. 2002. Separating spiritual and political, he pays a price. *New York Times.* June 13.

217 *members of the control group*   Blumenthal, J. A., M. Babyak, J. Wei, C. O'Connor, R. Waugh, E. Eisenstein, D. Mark, A. Sherwood, P. S. Woodley, R. J. Irwin, and G. Reed. 2002. Usefulness of psychosocial treatment of mental stress-induced myocardial ischemia in men. *Am J Cardiol* 89(2):164–68.

Chapter 14

221 *from prostate cancer*   Roemeling, S., M. J. Roobol, R. Postma, C. Gosselaar, T. H. van der Kwast, C. H. Bangma, and F. M. Schröder. 2006. Management and survival of screen-detected prostate cancer patients who might have been suitable for active surveillance. *Eur Urol* 50(3):475–82 (Epub May).
Cooperberg, M. R., J. W. Moul, and P. R. Carroll. 2005. The changing face of prostate cancer. *J Clin Oncol* 23(32):8146–51.

221 *evidence that this is true*   Meng, M. V., E. P. Elkin, S. R. Harlan, S. S. Mehta, D. P. Lubeck, and P. R. Carroll. 2003. Predictors of treatment after initial surveillance in men with prostate cancer: Results from CaPSURE. *J Urol* 170(6 Pt 1):2279–83.

222 *peer-reviewed urology journal*   Ornish, D., G. Weidner, W. R. Fair, R. Marlin, E. B. Pettengill, C. J. Raisin, S. Dunn-Emke, et al. 2005. Intensive lifestyle changes may affect the progression of prostate cancer. *J Urol* 174(3):1065–9; discussion 1069–70.

224 *feelings of vulnerability*   Daubenmier, J. J., G. Weidner, R. Marlin, L. Crutchfield, S. Dunn-Emke, C. Chi, B. Gao, P. Carroll, and D. Ornish. 2006. Lifestyle and health-related quality of life of men with prostate cancer managed with active surveillance. *Urology* 67(1):125–30.
Kronenwetter, C., G. Weidner, E. Pettengill, et al. 2005. A qualitative analysis of interviews of men with early stage prostate cancer: The Prostate Cancer Lifestyle Trial. *Cancer Nurs* 28(2):99–107.

225 *35 percent or more*   Freedland, S. J., E. B. Humphreys, L. A. Mangold, M. Eisenberger, F. J. Dorey, P. C. Walsh, and A. W. Partin. 2005. Risk of prostate

cancer-specific mortality following biochemical recurrence after radical prostate-ctomy. *JAMA* 294(4):433–39.

225 *with recurrent prostate cancer* Saxe, G. A., J. M. Major, J. Y. Nguyen, K. M. Freeman, T. M. Downs, and C. E. Salem. 2006. Potential attenuation of disease progression in recurrent prostate cancer with plant-based diet and stress reduction. *Integr Cancer Ther* 5(3):206–13.

225 *between the two diseases* Coffey, D. S. 2001. Similarities of prostate and breast cancer: Evolution, diet, and estrogens. *Urology* 57(Suppl 4A):31–8.

226 *healthier end of the Spectrum* Ibid.
Kolonel, L. N. 2001. Fat, meat, and prostate cancer. *Epidemiologic Rev* 23(1): 72–81.

226 *are especially carcinogenic* Strickland, P. T., Z. Qian, M. D. Friesen, N. Rothman, and R. Sinha. 2002. Metabolites of 2-amino-1-methyl-6-phenylimidazo(4,5-b)pyridine (PhIP) in human urine after consumption of charbroiled or fried beef. *Mutat Res* 506–507:163–73.
Weisburger, J. H. 1998. Worldwide prevention of cancer and other chronic diseases based on knowledge of mechanisms. *Mutat Res* 402:331–37.

226 *ever getting prostate cancer* Stroup, S. P., J. Cullen, B. K. Auge, J. O. L'esperance, and S. K. Kang. 2007. Effect of obesity on prostate-specific antigen recurrence after radiation therapy for localized prostate cancer as measured by the 2006 Radiation Therapy Oncology Group-American Society for Therapeutic Radiation and Oncology (RTOG-ASTRO) Phoenix consensus definition. *Cancer* 110(5):1003–1009.

227 *prostate and breast cancer* Coffey, D. S. 2001. Similarities of prostate and breast cancer: Evolution, diet, and estrogens. *Urology* 57(Suppl 4A):31-38.

228 *average follow-up period* Prentice, R. L., B. Caan, R. T. Chlebowski, R. Patterson, L. H. Kuller, J. K. Ockene, K. L. Margolis, et al. 2006. Low-fat dietary pattern and risk of invasive breast cancer: The Women's Health Initiative Randomized Controlled Dietary Modification Trial. *JAMA* 295(6):629–42.

228 *the diet has no effect* Kolata, G. 2006. Low-fat diet does not cut health risks, study finds. *New York Times.* February 8.

229 *a few more caveats* Gillette, F. 2006. A heaping serving of baked Kolata, hold the caveats. *The Columbia Journalism Review.* February 9.

229 *food frequency questionnaire* Freedman, L. S., A. Schatzkin, A. C. M. Thiebaut, M. Potischman, A. F. Subar, and F. E. Thompson. 2007. Abandon neither the Food Frequency Questionnaire nor the Dietary Fat-Breast Cancer Hypothesis. *Cancer Epidemiol Biomarkers Prev* 16(6):1321–22.

230 *risk of breast cancer* Thiébaut, A. C., V. Kipnis, S. C. Chang, A. F. Subar, F. E. Thompson, P. S. Rosenberg, A. R. Hollenbeck, M. Leitzmann, and A. Schatzkin. 2007. Dietary fat and postmenopausal invasive breast cancer in the National Institutes of Health-AARP Diet and Health Study cohort. *J Natl Cancer Inst* 99(6):451–62.

230 *estrogen-negative breast cancer* Chlebowski, R. T., G. L. Blackburn, C. A. Thomson, D. W. Nixon, A. Shapiro, M. L. Hoy, M. T. Goodman, et al. 2006. Dietary fat reduction and breast cancer outcome: Interim efficacy results from the Women's Intervention Nutrition Study. *J Natl Cancer Inst* 98(24):1767–76.

230 *invasive breast cancer* Thiébaut, A. C., V. Kipnis, S. C. Chang, A. F. Subar, F. E. Thompson, P. S. Rosenberg, A. R. Hollenbeck, M. Leitzmann, et al. 2007. Dietary fat and postmenopausal invasive breast cancer in the National Institutes of Health-AARP Diet and Health Study cohort. *J Natl Cancer Inst* 99(6):451-62.

230 *and polyunsaturated fat* Wirfält, E., I. Mattisson, B. Gullberg, U. Johansson, H. Olsson, and G. Berglund. 2002. Post-menopausal breast cancer is associated with high intakes of 6 fatty-acids (Sweden). *Cancer Causes Control* 13(10):883–93.

230 *risk of breast cancer* Smith-Warner, S. A., and M. J. Stampfer. 2007. Fat intake and breast cancer revisited. *J Natl Cancer Inst* 99(6):418–19.

231 *estrogen in your body* Wu, A. H., M. C. Pike, and D. O. Stram. 1999. Meta-analysis: Dietary fat intake, serum estrogen levels, and the risk of breast cancer. *J Natl Cancer Inst* 91(6):529–34.

Prentice, R., D. Thompson, C. Clifford, S. Gorbach, B. Goldin, and D. Byar. 1990. Dietary fat reduction and plasma estradiol concentration in healthy post-menopausal women. The Women's Health Trial Study Group. *J Natl Cancer Inst* 82(2):129–34.

231 *regulates gene expression* Jump, D. B., and S. D. Clarke. 1999. Regulation of gene expression by dietary fat. *Annu Rev Nutr* 19:63–90.

231 *modulates immune function* Hwang, D. 2000. Fatty acids and immune responses—a new perspective in searching for clues to mechanisms. *Annu Rev Nutr* 20:431–56.

231 *intake, and breast cancer* Holmes, M. D., S. Liu, S. E. Hankinson, G. A. Colditz, D. J. Hunter, and W. C. Willett. 2004. Dietary carbohydrates, fiber, and breast cancer risk. *Am J Epidemiol* 159(8):732–39.

231 *have shown some relationship* Silvera, S. A., M. Jain, G. R. Howe, A. B. Miller, and T. E. Rohan. 2005. Dietary carbohydrates and breast cancer risk: A prospective study of the roles of overall glycemic index and glycemic load. *Int J Cancer* 114(4):653–58.

Lajous, M., W. Willett, E. Lazcano-Ponce, L. M. Sanchez-Zamorano, M. Hernandez-Avila, and I. Romieu. 2005. Glycemic load, glycemic index, and the risk of breast cancer among Mexican women. *Cancer Causes Control* 16(10): 1165–69.

Potischman, N., R. J. Coates, C. A. Swanson, R. J. Carroll, J. R. Daling, D. R. Brogan, M. D. Gammon, D. Midthune, J. Curtin, and L. A. Brinton. 2002. Increased risk of early-stage breast cancer related to consumption of sweet foods among women less than age 45 in the United States. *Cancer Causes Control* 13(10): 937–46.

231 *and prostate cancer* McEligot, A. J., J. Largent, A. Ziogas, D. Peel, and H. Anton-Culver. 2006. Dietary fat, fiber, vegetable, and micronutrients are associated with overall survival in post-menopausal women diagnosed with breast cancer. *Nutr Cancer* 55(2):132–40.

Roberts, C. K., and J. R. Barnard. 2005. Effects of exercise and diet on chronic disease. *J Appl Physiology* 98:3–30.

231 *reduce oxidative stress* Ames, B. N. 1983. Dietary carcinogens and anticarcinogens. Oxygen radicals and degenerative diseases. *Science* 221(4617):1256–64.

231 *and breast cancer* Li, H., M. J. Stampfer, J. B. Hollis, L. A. Mucci, J. M. Gaziano, D. Hunter, E. L. Giovannucci, and J. Ma. 2007. A prospective study of plasma vitamin D metabolites, vitamin D receptor polymorphisms, and prostate cancer. *PLoS Med* 4(3):e103 (Epub ahead of print).

Robien, K., G. J. Cutler, and D. Lazovich. 2007. Vitamin D intake and breast cancer risk in postmenopausal women: The Iowa Women's Health Study. *Cancer Causes Control* 18(7):775–82 (Epub June).

231 *obese and nonobese women* Pierce, J. P., M. L. Stefanick, S. W. Flatt, L. Natarajan, B. Sternfeld, L. Madlensky, W. K. Al-Delaimy, et al. 2007. Greater survival

after breast cancer in physically active women with high vegetable-fruit intake regardless of obesity. *J Clin Oncol* 25(17):2345–51.

232 *7.3-year follow-up period* Pierce, J. P., L. Natarajan, B. J. Caan, et al. 2007. Influence of a diet very high in vegetables, fruit, and fiber and low in fat on prognosis following treatment for breast cancer: The Women's Healthy Eating and Living (WHEL) Randomized Trial. *JAMA* 298(3):289–98.

233 *self-reported dietary data* Gapster, S. M. 2007. Fat, fruits, vegetables, and breast cancer survivorship. *JAMA* 298(3):335.

233 *by promoting weight loss* Thune, I., and A. S. Furberg. 2001. Physical activity and cancer risk: Dose-response and cancer, all sites and site-specific. *Med Sci Sports Exerc* 33(6 Suppl):S530–S550; discussion S609-S610.

233 *by 20 to 40 percent* Harvard Men's Health Letter. 2006. Exercise and malignancy: Can you walk away from cancer? http://body.aolcom/conditions/exercise-and-malignancy-can-you-walk-away-from-cancer.

233 *or intensity of activity* Holmes, M. D., W. Y. Chen, D. Feskanich, C. H. Kroenke, and G. A. Colditz. 2005. Physical activity and survival after breast cancer diagnosis. *JAMA* 293(20):2479–86.

Bianchini, F., R. Kaaks, and H. Vainio. 2002. Weight control and physical activity in cancer prevention. *Obes Rev* 3(1):5–8.

233 *mortality from breast cancer* Holmes, M. D., W. Y. Chen, D. Feskanich, C. H. Kroenke, and G. A. Colditz. 2005. Physical activity and survival after breast cancer diagnosis. *JAMA* 293(20):2479–86.

234 *of major discrimination* Taylor, T. R., C. D. Williams, K. H. Makambi, C. Mouton, J. P. Harrell, Y. Cozier, J. R. Palmer, L. Rosenberg, and L. L. Adams-Campbell. 2007. Racial discrimination and breast cancer incidence in US black women: The Black Women's Health Study. *Am J Epidemiol* 166(1):46–54 (Epub March).

234 *with high social support* Stone, A. A., E. S. Mezzacappa, B. A. Donatone, and M. Gonder. 1999. Psychosocial stress and social support are associated with prostate-specific antigen levels in men: Results from a community screening program. *Health Psychology* 18(5):482–86.

234 *associated with improved survival* Watson, M., J. S. Haviland, S. Greer, J. Davidson, J. M. Bliss. 1999. Influence of psychological response on survival in breast cancer: A population-based cohort study. *Lancet* 354(9187):1331–36.

234 *disease and prostate cancer* Schulz, V., C. R. Pischlee, G. Weidner, J. J. Daubenmier, M. Elliot-Eller, L. Scherwitz, M. Bullinger, and D. Ornish. 2007 (in press). Social support group attendance is related to blood pressure health behaviors, and quality of life in the Multicenter Lifestyle Demonstration Project. *Psychol, Health and Med.*

234 *known to affect survival* Spiegel, D., J. R. Bloom, H. C. Kraemer, and E. Gottheil. 1989. Effect of psychosocial treatment on survival of patients with metastatic breast cancer. *Lancet* 2(8668):888–91.

234 *confirmed these findings* Goodwin, P. J., M. Leszcz, M. Ennis, J. Koopmans, L. Vincent, H. Guther, E. Drysdale, et al. 2001. The effect of group psychosocial support on survival in metastatic breast cancer. *N Engl J Med* 345(24):1719–26.

234 *been easier to detect* Spiegel, D. 2001. Mind matters. Group therapy and survival in breast cancer. *New Engl J Med* 345(24):1767–68.

235 *improved immune function* Sephton, S. E., C. Koopman, M. Schaal, C. Thoresen, and D. Spiegel. 2001. Spiritual expression and immune status in women with metastatic breast cancer: An exploratory study. *Breast J* 7(5):345–53.

235 *rate of breast cancer*   Nkondjock, A., A. Robidoux, Y. Paredes, S. A. Narod, and P. Ghadirian. 2006. Diet, lifestyle and BRCA-related breast cancer risk among French-Canadians. *Breast Cancer Res Treat* 98(3):285–94 (Epub March).

235 *enhancing DNA repair*   Kotsopoulos, J., and S. A. Narod. 2005. Towards a dietary prevention of hereditary breast cancer. *Cancer Causes Control* 16(2):125–38.

235 *BRCA2 gene change*   WebMD. Breast Cancer Health Center. Breast Cancer (BRCA) gene test. http://www.webmd.com/breast-cancer/Breast-Cancer-BRCA-Gene-Test?page=1 (accessed July 12, 2007).

235 *of the BRCA genes*   National Cancer Institute. US National Institutes of Health. Genetic testing for BRCA1 and BRCA2: It's your choice. http://www.cancer.gov/cancertopics/factsheet/Risk/BRCA (accessed July 12, 2007).

235 *chemotherapy to undergo*   Lin, N. U., and E. P. Winer. 2007. Optimal use of aromatase inhibitors: To lead or to follow? *J Clin Oncol* 25(19):2639–41.

ABOUT THE AUTHORS

Dean Ornish, M.D., is the Founder and President of the nonprofit Preventive Medicine Research Institute in Sausalito, California, where he holds the Safeway chair. He is Clinical Professor of Medicine at the University of California, San Francisco. Dr. Ornish received his medical training in internal medicine from the Baylor College of Medicine, Harvard Medical School, and the Massachusetts General Hospital. He received a B.A. in Humanities summa cum laude from the University of Texas in Austin, where he gave the baccalaureate address.

For the past thirty years, Dr. Ornish has directed clinical research demonstrating, for the first time, that comprehensive lifestyle changes may begin to reverse even severe coronary heart disease, without drugs or surgery. Recently, Medicare agreed to provide coverage for this program, the first time that Medicare has covered a program of comprehensive lifestyle changes. Dr. Ornish has also directed the first randomized controlled trial demonstrating that comprehensive lifestyle changes may stop or reverse the progression of prostate cancer. His current research is showing that comprehensive lifestyle changes may affect gene expression.

He is the author of five bestselling books and writes a monthly column for both *Newsweek* and *Reader's Digest* magazines.

The research that he and his colleagues conducted has been published in the *Journal of the American Medical Association, The Lancet, Circulation, The New England Journal of Medicine,* and *The American Journal of Cardiology,* among many others. A one-hour documentary of their work was broadcast on *NOVA,* and was featured on Bill Moyers's PBS series *Healing and the Mind.* Their work has been featured in all major media, including cover stories in *Newsweek, Time,* and *U.S. News and World Report.*

Dr. Ornish is a member of the boards of directors of the U.S. United Nations High Commission on Refugees, the Quincy Jones Foundation, and the San Francisco Food Bank. He was appointed to the White House Commission on Complementary and Alternative Medicine Policy and elected to the California Academy of Medicine. He is Chair of the Google Health advisory council, the PepsiCo Blue Ribbon advisory board, and the Safeway advisory council on health and nutrition, and he consults with the CEO of McDonald's to make more healthful foods and to provide health education to their customers in this country and worldwide.

He has received several awards, including the 1994 Outstanding Young Alumnus Award from the University of Texas, Austin; the University of California, Berkeley, "National Public Health Hero" award; the Jan J. Kellermann Memorial Award for distinguished contribution in the field of cardiovascular disease prevention from the International Academy of Cardiology; a Presidential Citation from the American Psychological Association; the Beckmann Medal from the German Society for Prevention and Rehabilitation of Cardiovascular Diseases; the "Pioneer in Integrative Medicine" award from California Pacific Medical Center; the "Excellence in Integrative Medicine" award from the Heal Breast Cancer Foundation; the Golden Plate Award from the American Academy of Achievement; a U.S. Army Surgeon General Medal; and the Bravewell Collaborative Pioneer of Integrative Medicine award. Dr. Ornish has been a physician consultant to the White House and to several bipartisan members of the U.S. Congress and has consulted with the chefs at the White House, Camp David, and Air Force One to cook more healthfully. He is listed in *Who's Who in Healthcare and Medicine, Who's Who in America,* and *Who's Who in the World.*

Dr. Ornish was recognized as "one of the most interesting people of 1996" by *People* magazine, featured in the *"Time* 100" issue on integrative medicine, and chosen by *Life* magazine as "one of the 50 most influential members of his generation."

Art Smith is a contributing editor to *O: The Oprah Magazine* and is Oprah Winfrey's personal chef. Smith is the recipient of the 2007 James Beard Foundation Humanitarian of the Year Award, and the *New York Times* bestselling author of *Back to the Family* and *Kitchen Life.* He is the Founder of Common Threads, whose mission is to educate children on the importance of nutrition and physical well-being, and to instill an appreciation of our world's diversity through the food and art of different cultures (www.commonthreads.org).

ABOUT THE TYPE

This book was set in Caledonia, a typeface designed in 1939 by William Addison Dwiggins for the Merganthaler Linotype Company. Its name is the ancient Roman term for Scotland, because the face was intended to have a Scotch-Roman flavor. Caledonia is considered to be a well-proportioned, businesslike face with little contrast between its thick and thin lines.